MW00564021

PUBLIC HEALTH BASICS

INTRODUCTION TO PUBLIC HEALTH MANAGEMENT, ORGANIZATIONS, AND POLICY

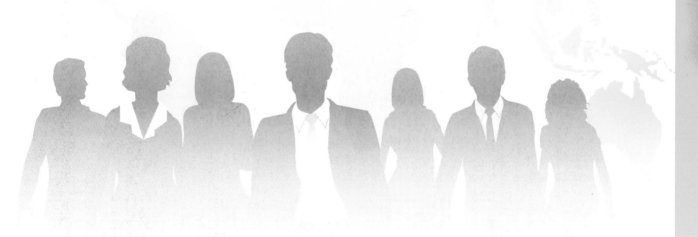

James A. Johnson, Ph.D., M.P.A., M.S.

Series Editor: Carleen H. Stoskopf, Sc.D., M.P.H.

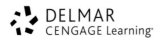

DELMAR
CENGAGE Learning®

Australia • Brazil • Japan • Korea • Mexico • Singapore • Spain • United Kingdom • United States

INTRODUCTION TO PUBLIC HEALTH MANAGEMENT, ORGANIZATIONS, AND POLICY

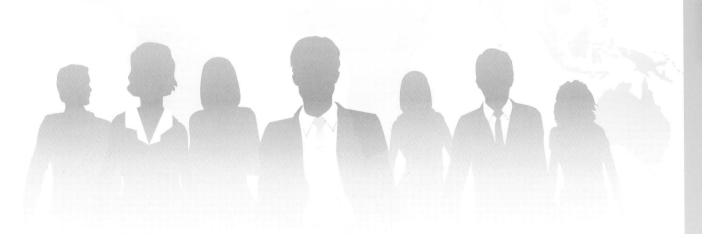

James A. Johnson, Ph.D., M.P.A., M.S.
Series Editor: Carleen H. Stoskopf

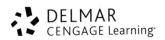

DELMAR
CENGAGE Learning·

Australia · Brazil · Japan · Korea · Mexico · Singapore · Spain · United Kingdom · United States

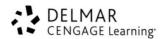

Introduction to Public Health Management, Organizations, and Policy, First Edition
James A. Johnson

Vice President, Careers & Computing: Dave Garza

Senior Acquisitions Editor: Tari Broderick

Director, Development-Careers & Computing: Marah Bellegarde

Associate Product Manager: Meghan E. Orvis

Editorial Assistant: Nicole Manikas

Brand Manager: Wendy Mapstone

Marketing Development Manager: Jonathan Sheehan

Senior Director, Education Production: Wendy A. Troeger

Production Manager: Andrew Crouth

Senior Content Project Manager: Kara A. DiCaterino

Senior Art Director: Jack Pendleton

Media Editor: Bill Overocker

Cover Image: © www.Shutterstock.com

For product information and technology assistance, contact us at
Cengage Learning Customer & Sales Support, 1-800-354-9706

For permission to use material from this text or product,
submit all requests online at **www.cengage.com/permissions.**
Further permissions questions can be e-mailed to
permissionrequest@cengage.com

Library of Congress Control Number: 2012939693

ISBN-13: 978-1-111-54112-5

ISBN-10: 1-111-54112-4

Delmar
5 Maxwell Drive
Clifton Park, NY 12065-2919
USA

Cengage Learning is a leading provider of customized learning solutions with office locations around the globe, including Singapore, the United Kingdom, Australia, Mexico, Brazil, and Japan. Locate your local office at: **international.cengage.com/region**

Cengage Learning products are represented in Canada by Nelson Education, Ltd.

To learn more about Delmar, visit **www.cengage.com/delmar**

Purchase any of our products at your local college store or at our preferred online store **www.cengagebrain.com**

Notice to the Reader

Printed in the United States of America
1 2 3 4 5 6 7 16 15 14 13 12

Contents

PART 1   Fundamentals and Public Health Policy   1

CHAPTER 1   PUBLIC HEALTH MISSION AND CORE FUNCTIONS   2

CHAPTER 2   PUBLIC HEALTH PROFESSIONALISM AND ETHICS   20

PART II Public Health Agencies and Organizations 85

PART III   Public Health Management and Leadership   181

CHAPTER 11 WORKFORCE DEVELOPMENT, DIVERSITY, AND HUMAN RESOURCES 229

CHAPTER 12 COMMUNICATION, INFORMATION SYSTEMS, AND DECISION MAKING 252

CHAPTER 15   PUBLIC HEALTH LEADERSHIP AND THE FUTURE   303

PART V Public Health Management in Practice 327

Foreword

The growing importance of public health is evidenced by its increasing responsibilities. Public health was historically known for its contribution to the reduction and control of infectious diseases through such efforts as environmental sanitation (by securing safe air and water), hygienic practices, the elimination of smallpox and polio (through immunization), and reduction of overcrowding. As chronic diseases replaced infectious diseases as the leading causes of death, public health shifted its focus towards health promotion programs such as lifestyle changes in diet, tobacco, and exercise, along with preventing contemporary health threats including cardiovascular disease, type-2 diabetes, and obesity. In recent years, as a result of a series of natural calamities such as Hurricanes Katrina and Rita and the spread of severe acute respiratory syndrome (SARS) and human created threats such as the 9-11 attack and the possibility of terrorist attacks involving chemical, biological, radiological, or nuclear weapons, public health has again assumed center stage and been called upon to handle these emerging threats. As a result, public health is increasingly challenged by its many demands to have better prepared managers and leaders.

This book, *Introduction to Public Health Management, Organizations, and Policy*, by James Johnson provides one of the essential building blocks needed to address this critical need. Today, students and others who anticipate a career in public health must have at least a basic understanding of public health organizations and management principles. Additionally, some knowledge of health policy and its processes is in increasing demand. This publication—through a combination of substantive text, interviews of public health professionals, and real-world case studies—provides an enriched learning opportunity. It will serve as an excellent foundation for anyone who anticipates working in public health and will be especially useful to those who aspire to be in management or supervisory roles.

Leiyu Shi, Dr.P.H., M.P.A., M.B.A.
Bloomberg School of Public Health
Johns Hopkins University

Preface

James A. Johnson, Ph.D., M.P.A., M.S.

INTRODUCTION

Public health has a long and proud history of accomplishments. From ancient times to present there has been a public health community fighting disease and working to improve lives. Many of the early advances in public health had their roots in management and organization. Ways to more safely manage water resources, disposal of waste, and improvements in food safety came early in human civilization. With the advances in science and medicine that occurred in the nineteenth and subsequent centuries, the role of public health grew in scope and complexity. Today, we have a global public health community working on every imaginable health challenge. Wherever you see a town or city, you will see a public health presence of some kind. Most often, this will be in the form of some type of organization, perhaps a government agency, a volunteer group, or a nongovernmental organization. Each of these entities will be comprised of people committed to promoting the public's well-being by working together in the service of their communities.

WHY I WROTE THIS TEXT

The work of public health could not be done effectively without organizational leaders and managers. These are the individuals who utilize a wide range of processes and tools to enhance the effectiveness of public health organizations and to assure responsiveness and accountability to the communities being served. This book provides the fundamental knowledge base needed for those who might someday become public health managers.

While this text is intended primarily for a student audience, it also could be useful to public health clinicians, technicians, and administrative personnel who are not currently in a management or supervisory role, but want to know more about what managers do or how organizations work. For some, this book might even be a stepping stone to moving from one's current role to a position that has managerial responsibilities.

Regardless of one's path, a better understanding of the public health world, as offered here, will foster greater awareness and enhance one's capabilities to be engaged as change agents for a healthier world.

ORGANIZATION OF THE TEXT

In order to accomplish this goal, the text employs a range of learning devices such as descriptive text, professional interviews, action learning and critical thinking exercises, discussion questions, and case studies. These elements are organized in a way that builds upon a foundational understanding of the mission and functions of public health. Furthermore, the political and social context is described as are the policy processes often used to advance the public health agenda of a healthy nation. From this foundation, the book then proceeds to describe the full range of public health organizations, at all levels: local, state, federal, and global. This helps the student better know the structures, missions, and values of the various agencies they may someday work in. It also underscores the magnitude of the public health presence in our society and around the world. Lastly, the book explores the knowledge, skills, and abilities associated with effective management and leadership. Students will gain valuable insights from practicing public health professionals and will develop competencies in a wide range of management and leadership fundamentals including: decision making, conflict resolution, motivation, communication, team development, planning and evaluation, strategic planning, systems thinking, and so much more.

ANCILLARY PACKAGE

The complete supplement package for *Introduction to Public Health Management, Organizations, and Policy* was developed to achieve two goals:

1. To assist students in learning and applying the information presented in the text.

2. To assist instructors in planning and implementing their courses in the most efficient manner and to provide exceptional resources which will enhance their students' experience.

Instructor Companion Website

ISBN 13: 978-1-111-54113-2

Spend less time planning and more time teaching with Delmar Cengage Learning's Instructor Resources to Accompany *Introduction to Public Health Management, Organizations, and Policy*. The Instructor Companion Website can be accessed by going to www.cengage.com/login to create a unique user log-in. The password-protected Instructor Resources include the following:

Instructor's Manual

An electronic Instructor's Manual provides instructors with invaluable tools in preparing for class lectures and examinations. Following the text chapter-by-chapter, the Instructor's Manual reiterates objectives and provides a synthesized recap of each chapter's main points and goals.

Computerized Test Bank in ExamView™

An electronic test bank makes and generates tests and quizzes in an instant. With a variety of question types, including short answer, multiple choice, true or false, and matching exercises, creating challenging exams will be no barrier in your classroom. This test bank includes a rich bank of 450 questions that test students on retention and application of what they have learned in the course. Answers are provided for all questions so instructors can focus on teaching, not grading.

Instructor PowerPoint Slides

A comprehensive offering of more than 500 Instructor Support Slides created in Microsoft® PowerPoint outlines concepts and objectives to assist instructors with lectures.

CourseMate to Accompany *Introduction to Public Health Management, Organizations, and Policy*

Visit www.cengagebrain.com to access the following resources:

- Printed Access Code ISBN 13: 978-1-111-54119-4
- Instant Access Code ISBN: 978-1-111-54116-3

CourseMate complements your textbook with several robust and noteworthy components:

- An interactive eBook, with highlighting, note taking, and search capabilities.
- Interactive and engaging learning tools including flashcards, quizzes, videos, games, PowerPoint presentations, and much more!
- Engagement Tracker, a first-of-its-kind tool that monitors student participation and retention in the course.

About the Author

James A. Johnson, Ph.D., M.P.A., M.S., is a medical social scientist with a long academic career in public health, policy, and administration. Dr. Johnson is author or co-author of 15 books on a wide range of health organizations topics including *Comparative Health Systems*; *Handbook of Health Administration and Policy*; and *Health Organizations: Theory, Behavior, and Development*. He is also previous editor of the *Journal of Healthcare Management*; *Journal of Management Practice*; and contributing editor for *Journal of Health Services Administration*. Dr. Johnson is author or co-author of over 100 published journal articles and has lectured at Oxford University and Cambridge University in England; University of Beijing in China; University of Dublin in Ireland; University of Colima in Mexico; and St. George's University in Grenada. Additionally, he has worked with the World Health Organization; ProWorld Service Corps; National Diabetes Trust Foundation; Lowcountry AIDS Services; and numerous state and federal health agencies. Dr. Johnson currently holds a faculty position as Professor in the School of Health Sciences at Central Michigan University and is an adjunct professor of Health Administration and Policy at Auburn University-Montgomery. He also serves as a visiting professor at St. George's University in Grenada and is a past Chair of Health Administration and Policy at the Medical University of South Carolina. Dr. Johnson has a Ph.D. in Public Policy and Administration with a specialization in Organizational Behavior and Development from Florida State University.

Acknowledgements

A special thank you for those who contributed to the success of *Introduction to Public Health Management, Organizations, and Policy* with their professional expertise and invaluable knowledge.

Contributors

Chapter 13: Groups, Teams, and Working with the Community

Donald J. Breckon, Ph.D., M.P.A.
President Emeritus of Park University
Parkville, Missouri

Mark J. Minelli, Ph.D., M.P.A.
Professor and Director, Community Health Division
Central Michigan University
Mount Pleasant, Michigan

Chapter 14: Program Planning, Development, and Evaluation

Christine Elnitsky, RN, Ph.D., CHNS
Senior Program Analyst
United States Department of Veterans Affairs Headquarters
Office of the Assistant Secretary for Policy, Planning, and Preparedness
Washington, D.C.

Carolyn K. Lewis, RN, Ph.D., CNAA, BC
Former Assistant Dean and Associate Professor, Nursing Division
Bluegrass Community and Technical College
Lexington, Kentucky

Joanne Martin, Dr.P.H., RN, FAAN
Director of Nurse-Family Partnerships
Goodwill Industries of Central Indiana, Inc.
Indianapolis, Indiana

Chapter 15: Public Health Leadership and the Future

C. William Keck, MD, M.P.H., FACPM
Professor and Chair Emeritus
Community Health Sciences
Northeastern Ohio Universities College of Medicine
Rootstown, Ohio

F. Douglas Scutchfield, MD
Director, National Coordinating Center
Director, Center for Excellence in Public Health Workforce Research and Policy
Director, Center for Public Health Services & Systems Research
University of Kentucky, College of Public Health
Lexington, Kentucky

Chapter 16: Cases in Public Health Management

Scott D. Musch, M.B.A.
Director of Corporate Development
Cambia Health Solutions
Portland, Oregon

Chapter 17: Terms for Public Health Managers

James E. Dotherow IV, M.P.A.
Alabama State University Center for Leadership and Public Policy
Montgomery, Alabama

James Allen Johnson III, M.P.H.
School of Public Health
Georgia Southern University
Statesboro, Georgia

Reviewers

James L. Alexander, Ph.D.
Associate Professor
Coordinator of Practicum Services
School of Rural Public Health
Texas A&M University
College Station, Texas

Minnjuan W. Flournoy, Ph.D., M.P.H, M.B.A
Research Fellow, Health Services Policy and Management
Institute for Partnerships to Eliminate Health Disparities
University of South Carolina
Columbia, South Carolina

Jill Rissi, RN, BSN, M.P.A., Ph.D.
Assistant Professor
Public Health and Public Administration
Portland State University
Portland, Oregon

Susan L. Wilson, Ph.D.
Associate Professor
Department of Health Science
New Mexico State University
Las Cruces, New Mexico

How to Use This Book

A VISUAL WALKTHROUGH

Learning Objectives

Upon completion of this chapter, you should be able to:
1. Define health.
2. Define public health.
3. Be aware of great achievements in public health.
4. Understand the core functions of public health.
5. Grasp the essential services provided in public health.
6. Be familiar with *Healthy People 2010* and *Healthy People 2020* goals.

LEARNING OBJECTIVES: Learning Objectives are presented at the beginning of each chapter and introduce the core concepts you should be able to master after reading and studying each chapter. These can be a great review tool as well.

Key Terms

assessment	*Healthy People 2010*	public health
assurance	*Healthy People 2020*	systems theory
health	policy development	

KEY TERMS: Key Terms introduce important terminology covered in each chapter. Definitions of these terms appear in the margin, closest to where they are first presented in the chapter. This provides a quick and easy way to familiarize you with important terms and concepts.

Chapter Outline

Introduction
Health Defined
Public Health Defined
Systems Approach to Public Health
Public Health Functions
Healthy People 2010 and *Healthy People 2020*
Summary
Public Health Leader Perspective
Discussion and Review Questions
Action Learning and Critical Thinking

CHAPTER OUTLINE: Use the Chapter Outline as an excellent reference guide to direct your learning and ensure that you are competent and knowledgeable about each section of the chapter.

EXHIBITS: Exhibits enhance chapter information with real-life examples and important content that add perspective and understanding to each chapter. From the Universal Declaration of Human Rights to the mission statement of local public health departments, exhibits are invaluable extensions of chapter material.

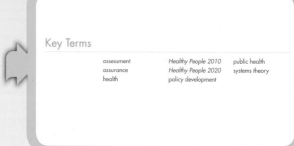

Exhibit 1-1   Essential Public Health Services

- Monitor health status to identify community health problems
- Diagnose and investigate health problems and health hazards in the community
- Inform, educate, and empower people about health issues
- Mobilize community partnerships to identify and solve health problems
- Develop policies and plans that support individual and community health efforts
- Enforce laws and regulations that protect health and ensure safety
- Link people to needed personal health services and assure the provision of health care when otherwise unavailable
- Assure a competent public health care and personal health care workforce
- Evaluate effectiveness, accessibility, and quality of personal and population-based health services
- Research for new insights and innovative solutions to health problems

Source: U.S. Department of Health and Human Services. Retrieved from http://www.hhs.gov

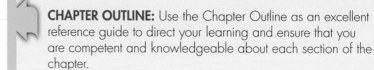

Public Health Professional Perspective

Sandra Schoenfisch, RN, PhD, Consultant to Florida Department of Health, and Retired Public Health Administrator, Tallahassee, Florida

Interview by Dr. James Johnson

(Q): What is your own working definition of an effective manager?

Dr. Schoenfisch: An effective manager is one who can get the job done. One of my favorite books is *Execution: The Discipline of Getting Things Done* by Bossidy and Charan. In a nutshell, it talks about plans and strategies and that they are only good if you can actually execute them. I think an effective manager is the one who understands how things work and has

PUBLIC HEALTH PROFESSIONAL PERSPECTIVE AND PUBLIC HEALTH LEADER PERSPECTIVE: These incredible interviews are assets that you will not find in any other introductory textbook! Two types of interviews are included providing you with a well-rounded perspective of careers in public health administration. The first, Public Health Professional Perspective, consists of interviews with individuals on the ground floor, with a variety of job titles and duties that are making a difference every day. The second, Public Health Leader Perspective, includes interviews with high-profile individuals who have made considerable contributions to the field of public health throughout their careers.

Summary

In the preface to the *Encyclopedia of Public Health*, Lester Breslow describes public health as one of the essential institutions of society existing to promote, protect, preserve, and restore the good health of all people.

As you have seen so far in this introductory chapter, there are many programs, services, organizations, and institutions devoted to public health. With so many entities and varying efforts, it can only be fully understood by embracing a systems perspective. Furthermore, it is important to understand the nature of organizations since that is where most of the work is done. We live in an organizational society and public health is no exception. It is equally important to be aware of the core functions of public health and the goals that keep moving it forward. As Breslow surmises, "Professionals engaged in the field regard it as an organized effort directed at improving the health of populations by assuring the conditions in which people can be healthy." In the next chapter we will be discussing professionalism and ethics with a specific focus on the drive to develop and promote core competencies for public health professionals and managers.

SUMMARY: The chapter Summary is a great place to ensure that you completely understand the information in the chapter and are able to apply it. Look back to the Learning Objectives and make sure that you have met those goals by the end of the Summary.

CASE 1: A FRIEND'S DILEMMA

Situation

Stacy is an administrative assistant at the Los Angeles-Downtown Wellness Center, an HIV testing site funded by the California Department of Public Health (CDPH). In addition to HIV testing, the Wellness Center provides HIV prevention education services, HIV/AIDS medical treatment, and HIV support services such as case management and counseling. Stacy's job primarily involves data entry and processing. Her main responsibility is to assist in filling out the HIV/AIDS case report forms required by the CDPH for confirmed HIV tests.

Although she has worked at the Wellness Center for only eight months, she enjoys the work and recognizes the highly sensitive nature of her job. In the course of her work, she handles patient medical record files and sees the names of patients who have tested positive for HIV. Given the routine of her work, she typically processes the information without much thought to patient names, until this afternoon. In the patient file she is holding, she recognizes the name—Eric—her best friend's boyfriend. He tested positive for HIV and gonorrhea. Linda, her best friend, has been dating Eric exclusively for the last year, and she knows that Linda has not had sexual relations with anyone else during that time.

CASE STUDY CORRELATION: Apply the knowledge you have gained in each chapter and challenge yourself to reading, interpreting, and answering several questions about a case study dealing directly with the chapter content. Look for this box at the end of each chapter, where you will find which case studies in Chapter 16 correspond with the content you have just studied.

Discussion and Review Questions

1. Discuss the definition of health as provided by the World Health Organization. Share your own view or experiences that support or perhaps even expand this definition.

2. Among the great achievements of public health in the last century, which was the most significant and why? In class or online, each student can choose one of the achievements to discuss in more detail.

3. Describe the core functions and services of public health. What area or service might you like to work in sometime in the future?

4. After reading about *Healthy People 2020* and its vision and goals, what do you expect this will accomplish? Are these goals compatible with the core functions and services of public health? If so, how? Give examples.

5. The Director General of the World Health Organization in 2012, Margaret Chan, MD, M.P.H., once stated about goals and objectives, "if you can't measure it, it doesn't exist." Why do you think it is important to have "foundational measures" for *Healthy People 2020*?

DISCUSSION AND REVIEW QUESTIONS: Test your understanding of the information presented in the chapter with discussion questions to help reinforce chapter information. Use this practice to identify areas in the chapter that you may need to go back and reread until you are confident in answering those questions.

Action Learning and Critical Thinking

A. Choose one of the topic foci from *Healthy People 2020* and do a brief online search for current information, issues, and challenges pertaining to this topic. Report your findings back to the class.

B. Interview a local public health professional and ask them what they think about the accomplishments of *Healthy People 2010* and the future of *Healthy People 2020*.

C. Visit the website of the U.S. Office of Disease Prevention and Health Promotion. Review their range of initiatives. Website: http://odphp.osophs.dhhs.gov

D. After reading the interview with Dr. Benjamin, go to the American Public Health Association (APHA) website and learn more about the association. Consider becoming a student member. Go to a national or local conference of APHA. Website: http://www.apha.org/

ACTION LEARNING AND CRITICAL THINKING: Action Learning and Critical Thinking is a unique resource for instructors and students alike. These activities ask for participation, involvement, and go above and beyond the typical review question. Utilize these scenarios and activities to engage yourself and your classroom.

About the Public Heath Basics Series

Led by series editor, Dr. Carleen Stoskopf, PUBLIC HEALTH BASICS is a series that brings to life the interdisciplinary nature of public health and the integration of multiple scientific approaches to public health problem solving through surveillance, critical data analysis, planning and implementation of interventions and programs, evaluation, and management of constrained resources. Through this book series, students will grapple with the major public health issues we are facing locally and globally, while also learning and putting to practice the principles of public health.

PART I

FUNDAMENTALS AND PUBLIC HEALTH POLICY

In these four chapters the fundamentals of public health and the profession is discussed. This includes a description of the core functions of public health and the importance of professionalism and ethics for public health leaders and managers. Additionally, these chapters describe major public health policies and the political structure of policymaking in the United States. This section also discusses policy processes and the role of public health agencies.

Chapter 1

PUBLIC HEALTH MISSION AND CORE FUNCTIONS

Learning Objectives

Upon completion of this chapter, you should be able to:

1. Define health.
2. Define public health.
3. Be aware of great achievements in public health.
4. Understand the core functions of public health.
5. Grasp the essential services provided in public health.
6. Be familiar with *Healthy People 2010* and *Healthy People 2020* goals.

Key Terms

assessment	*Healthy People 2010*	public health
assurance	*Healthy People 2020*	systems theory
health	policy development	

Chapter Outline

INTRODUCTION

This short introductory chapter seeks to help students understand health and public health including functions, core competencies, and long-range national goals. A basic understanding of these functions, services, and goals helps to provide the most fundamental elements of the study of public health and a rudimentary foundation for studying public health organizations and management. While many initiatives, processes, policies, and programs will be discussed in this book, each will in some way come back to the need for an understanding of health and the public nature of this field. After all, public health organizations are created and sustained for the overarching purpose of improving the public's health.

HEALTH DEFINED

A logical starting point in this discussion is the word "health" which can be traced to the Middle English word *hale* which was used to mean hardy and the Old English word *hal* and Old Norse *heill* to mean whole. The word *helthe* emerged from these meanings and started to be used during the twelfth century. These root concepts pertaining to wholeness continue in our understanding of health today in the twenty-first century.

The most widely accepted definition of **health** for the past 60 years is the one published by the World Health Organization (WHO) in its constitution from 1947; the WHO constitution declares, "Health is a state of complete physical, mental, and social well-being and not merely the absence of disease and infirmity." Some scholars have chosen to expand upon this enduring definition in an attempt to be more holistic. One example is describing health in terms of six interacting and dynamic dimensions—physical, emotional, social, intellectual, spiritual, and occupational. From Neighbors and Tannehill-Jones book *Human Diseases*, a graphic image of an expanded definition is presented in Figure 1-1. Graber and Johnson in the *Journal of Healthcare Management* further underscore the importance of spirituality.

health: A state of complete physical, mental, and social well-being and not merely the absence of disease and infirmity.

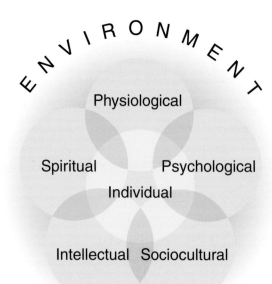

FIGURE 1-1 Holistic View of Health
© Cengage Learning 2013

However, due to the universality of the WHO definition and its impact on the profession of public health, we will use its definition throughout this book with occasional references to or examples from the expanded definitions.

> "It is health that is real wealth and not pieces of gold and silver."
> —*Mahatma Gandhi, Social Justice Lawyer and Activist*

PUBLIC HEALTH DEFINED

public health: The science and art of preventing disease, prolonging life, and promoting physical health and efficiency through organized community efforts for the sanitation of the environment, the control of community infections, the education of the individual in principles of personal hygiene, the organization of medical and nursing services for the early diagnosis and preventive treatment of disease, and the development of the social machinery which will ensure to every individual in the community a standard of living adequate for the maintenance of health.

Many who study the history of public health trace the roots of the WHO definition to American public health leader Charles-Edward A. Winslow. In 1920, Winslow defined **public health** as:

> Public health is the science and art of preventing disease, prolonging life, and promoting physical health and efficiency through organized community efforts for the sanitation of the environment, the control of community infections, the education of the individual in principles of personal hygiene, the organization of medical and nursing services for the early diagnosis and preventive treatment of disease, and the development of the social machinery which will ensure to every individual in the community a standard of living adequate for the maintenance of health.

An interesting, abbreviated history of public health from ancient times to the twentieth century can be read in the *Encyclopedia of Public Health* (2010), or more comprehensive histories can be found in Rosen's *History of Public Health*. As the philosopher

Top 10 Achievements in Public Health in the 20th Century
1. Vaccination
2. Motor-vehicle safety
3. Safer workplaces
4. Control of infectious diseases
5. Decline in deaths from coronary heart disease and stroke
6. Safer and healthier foods
7. Healthier mothers and babies
8. Family planning
9. Fluoridation of drinking water
10. Recognition of tobacco use as a health hazard

FIGURE 1-2 Great Acheivements of Public Health in the 20th Century
Source: Morbidity and Mortality Weekly Report (April 2, 1999). Centers for Disease Control and Prevention: http://www.cdc
.gov/mmwr/preview/mmwrhtml/00056796.htm

George Santayana wrote in 1905, "Those who do not remember the past are condemned to repeat it." Throughout the twentieth century public health had major achievements that improved health in the United States dramatically (see Figure 1-2).

In 1988 the Institute of Medicine (IOM) published *The Future of Public Health*, which defined the mission of public health as "fulfilling society's interest in assuring conditions in which people can be healthy." Furthermore, the report outlined three core functions of public health: 1) **assessment**—the delineation of health problems, their nature, and the means of dealing with them; 2) **policy development**—the formulation and advocacy of what should be done about health problems; and 3) **assurance**—the implementation of policy, either by activities of others or by direct public health activities. Each of these functions are designed to address the needs of communities, families, individuals, and the larger system as shown in Figure 1-3.

> "Public health is concerned with social organization—what René Dubos refers to as ways of life or what Jacques May, a prominent medical ecologist, called the culture that promotes and supports the survival of the group (community, and world)."—*Meredeth Turshen, Urban Studies Professor, Rutgers University*

assessment: The delineation of health problems, their nature, and the means of dealing with them.

policy development: The formulation and advocacy of what should be done.

assurance: The implementation of policy, either by activities of others or by direct public health activities.

Two years later, in their book *Management of Hospitals and Health Services: Strategic Issues and Performance*, Schulz and Johnson described the primary objective of a public health service is to improve the health of the population for which it is responsible, such as a state or local community. Performance is measured by vital statistics, such as incidence and prevalence of disease, mortality and morbidity, and longevity. A second objective is to protect public interests, such as occupational safety, sanitation, safe food, clean water, and air. A third objective of public health services is to implement expectations and policies of elected officials. Traditionally, public health services have included the following:

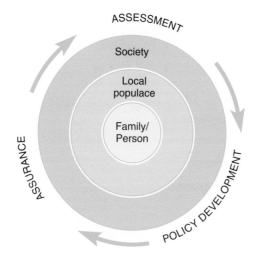

1. ASSESSMENT
- Monitor and surveillance of local health issues
- Protect local population from health hazards and risks

2. POLICY DEVELOPMENT
- Engage and educate community about local health problems
- Develop appropriate health policies and goals

3. ASSURANCE
- Enforcement of health law and regulations
- Evaluation of effectiveness and distribution of health programs

FIGURE 1-3 The Three Core Functions of Public Health
© Cengage Learning 2013

- Communicable (infectious) disease control

- Sanitation

- Maternal and child health

- Public health nursing

- Public health education

- Vital statistics

- Administration of funds by local public health agencies

- Health planning

SYSTEMS APPROACH TO PUBLIC HEALTH

Public health is highly interconnected and interdependent in its relationship to individuals, families, communities, and the larger society, including the global community. To best understand the complex scope of public health, one must take a systems perspective. Using the language of **systems theory**, public health is a complex adaptive system. It is complex in that it is composed of multiple, diverse, interconnected elements, and it is adaptive in that the system is capable of changing and learning from experience and its environment. A model of the public health system as it exists in the United States is provided in Figure 1-4.

A systems approach to public health is more than the inter-organizational relationships that support and facilitate the work of public health. It also includes the mindset of public health professionals and scholars. This is often referred to as "systems thinking" and encompasses the viewpoint that health and health challenges have "determinants" and health behaviors have "outcomes." Table 1-1 identifies many of these determinants including those from the physical environment, social

systems theory: A view of an organization as a complex set of dynamically intertwined and interconnected elements, including all its inputs, processes, outputs, feedback loops, and the environment in which it operates and with which it continuously interacts.

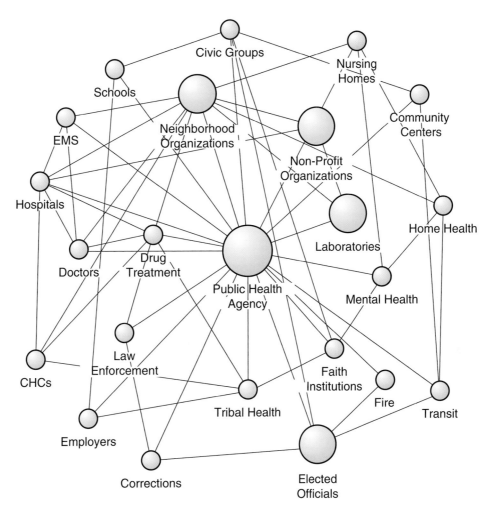

FIGURE 1-4 The Public Health System
© Cengage Learning 2013

environment, policy environment, and the health delivery system, along with both biological and behavioral determinants.

Using the systems perspective, public health addresses many challenges by engaging in health promotion and health improvement. The model adopted for use in *Healthy People 2010* is shown in Figure 1-5. This demonstrates the role of determinants of health in shaping how we look at or engage any public health process, policy, or intervention. In short, this shows how everything is interconnected and interdependent.

Public health utilizes a litany of intervention approaches, processes, and targets to improve the health of populations, including individuals and communities. Each type of intervention or public health initiative may lend itself to a narrow or broad focus as shown in Figure 1-6, sometimes referred to as "The Minnesota Wheel." Here you see in the outer circle a large number of public health tools and processes. More will be discussed about systems theory, systems thinking, and the systems approach to public health throughout this book. It will become clear that we can better understand organizations, communities, and even our own selves through the lens of systems thinking.

TABLE 1-1 Population-Based Health Determinants Assessment Template (Excerpt)

Community Level

Physical Environment

- Housing and geographic location, safety of neighborhoods, community, and school quality

- Environmental quality: air, water, ground, chemical, physical, and biological hazards

- Availability of transportation, communication systems, parks, and recreation facilities

Social Environment

- Community norms, values, and patterns of behavior; political structures within community

- Incidence of crime and violence within the population group and the larger community

- Employment opportunities within community, economic viability of community

Policies and Interventions

- National, state, county, and city health and social policies

- Policies of public, private, and voluntary organizations that provide health and social services

- Policies of health insurance companies, health maintenance organizations, health systems, and health care provider groups

Health Systems Level

Access to Quality Health Care

- Appropriate primary, secondary, and tertiary health services and providers

- Health and social services workforce (numbers, diversity, interdisciplinary mix, deployment, sustainability); educational institutions offering health care provider education and training

- Availability of health and social services resources 24 hours a day, seven days per week

Population Level

Biological

- Demographic data (age, gender, racial/ethnic patterns)

(Continues)

TABLE 1-1 Population-Based Health Determinants Assessment Template (Excerpt) *(Continued)*

- Biological and genetic factors, patterns of health and disease (morbidity and mortality data)

Behavioral

- Education patterns and levels, cultural patterns (lifestyle, languages, religion)

- Socioeconomic status (employment patterns, housing, health and dental insurance)

- Cultural health patterns (health beliefs and self-care practices, nutrition, fitness, previous experiences with health care system, current health providers, family and intergenerational health patterns)

Data Analysis

- Prioritize the health needs of the community and prioritize the vulnerable and at-risk population groups based on need and health status.

- Identify the modifiable and nonmodifiable health risks of the at-risk population.

- Identify the biological, psychosocial, environmental, cultural, political, financial, and iatrogenic causes of the identified health risks.

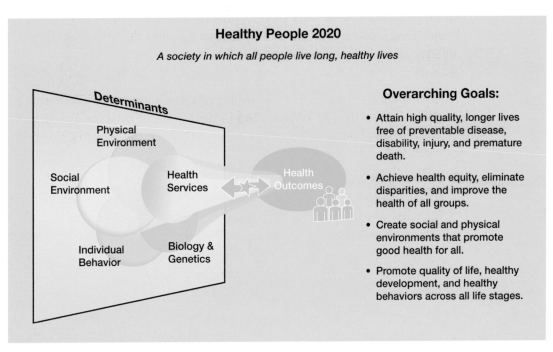

FIGURE 1-5 U.S. Department of Health and Human Services (HHS). Office of Disease Prevention and Health Promotion. (2011) Framework, The Vision, Mission, and Goals of *Healthy People 2020*
(Accessed March 12, 2011, at http://healthypeople.gov/2020/consortium/HP2020Framework.pdf).

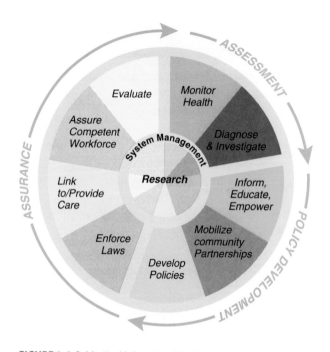

FIGURE 1-6 Public Health Functions Wheel
Source: U.S. Surgeon General, Office of Disease Prevention and Health Promotion; http://www.health.gov/phfunctions/public.htm

PUBLIC HEALTH FUNCTIONS

As you will see, the role, functions, and scope of public health have expanded considerably over the past 20 years. In 1997, a decade after the IOM Report, the World Health Organization took the lead by convening public health leaders from 67 different countries to establish a consensus on what public health is and what its essential functions should be:

1. *Monitoring the health situation.* This includes monitoring morbidity and mortality, the determinants of health (e.g., smoking, sexual behavior, poverty), the effectiveness of public health programs and functions, and assessing population needs and risks.

2. *Protecting the environment.* Environmental protection includes ensuring access to safe water; the control of food safety and quality; provision of adequate drainage, sewerage, solid-waste disposal services, and the control of hazardous substances and wastes; adequate vector control measures; protecting water and soil resources; controlling atmospheric pollution and ionizing radiation are also essential, as is ensuring adequate preventive environmental services and adequate inspection, monitoring, and control of environmental hazards.

3. *Health promotion.* The promotion of community involvement in health; the provision of information and education for health and life-skill enhancement in school, home, work, and community settings; and maintaining linkages with politicians, other sectors, and the community in support of health promotion and public health advocacy are all part of health promotion.

4. *Prevention, surveillance, and control of communicable diseases.* This function includes immunization, disease outbreak control, disease surveillance, and injury prevention.

5. *Public health legislation and regulation.* The review, formulation, and enactment of health legislation, regulations, and administrative procedures are also essential functions of public health. Components include ensuring adequate legislation to protect environmental health; health inspection and licensing; and enforcement of health legislation, regulations, and administrative procedures.

6. *Occupational health.* Setting occupational health and safety regulations, ensuring safety in workplaces, and providing medical and health services for workers are part of this function.

7. *Specific public health services.* These include school health services, emergency disaster services, and public health laboratory services.

8. *Public health management.* Management of public health involves ensuring health policy, planning, and management; the use of scientific evidence in formulating and implementing health policies; public health and health-systems research; and international collaboration and cooperation in health.

9. *Care of vulnerable and high-risk populations.* This involves maternal health care and family planning; infant and child care; and programs to protect the health of refugees, displaced persons, and indigenous peoples.

While this has provided a much needed framework for the nearly 200 countries of the World Health Organization, there is considerable variability in the implementation of the nine essential functions. Some are given higher priority depending on demographics, economics, politics, public health infrastructure, governance, and leadership. From their comparative study of health systems in 20 different countries around the world, in their book *Comparative Health Systems,* Johnson and Stoskopf presented many mitigating factors, especially when considering cost, quality, access, and innovation. Furthermore, due to the wide variability in social determinants of health, the implementation of all of the essential public health functions is much more challenging in some countries than in others.

> "The history of public health must concern itself with two components. One is the development of medical science and technology. Understanding the nature and cause of disease provides a basis for preventive action and control. However, the effective application of such knowledge depends on a variety of nonscientific elements, basically on political, economic, and social factors. This is the other major strand in the fabric of public health."—*George Rosen, Public Health Historian*

In the United States, the most clearly articulated and widely used framework for defining the core functions of public health was also developed in the 1990s. In 1994 the Public Health Functions Steering Committee adopted the public health essential functions and services shown in Exhibits 1-1 and 1-2. The membership of the Steering Committee represented the following organizations:

- American Public Health Association
- Association of Schools of Public Health
- Association of State and Territorial Health Officials
- Environmental Council of the States
- National Association of County and City Health Officials
- National Association of State Alcohol and Drug Abuse Directors
- National Association of State Mental Health Program Directors
- Public Health Foundation
- U.S. Public Health Service
  - Agency for Health Care Policy and Research
  - Centers for Disease Control and Prevention
  - Food and Drug Administration

Exhibit 1-1 Essential Public Health Services

- Monitor health status to identify community health problems
- Diagnose and investigate health problems and health hazards in the community
- Inform, educate, and empower people about health issues
- Mobilize community partnerships to identify and solve health problems
- Develop policies and plans that support individual and community health efforts
- Enforce laws and regulations that protect health and ensure safety
- Link people to needed personal health services and assure the provision of health care when otherwise unavailable
- Assure a competent public health care and personal health care workforce
- Evaluate effectiveness, accessibility, and quality of personal and population-based health services
- Research for new insights and innovative solutions to health problems

Source: U.S. Department of Health and Human Services. Retrieved from http://www.hhs.gov

Exhibit 1-2 Essential Public Health Functions

- Prevents epidemics and the spread of disease
- Protects against environmental hazards
- Prevents injuries
- Promotes and encourages healthy behaviors
- Responds to disasters and assists communities in recovery
- Assures the quality and accessibility of health services

Source: U.S. Department of Health and Human Services. Retrieved from http://www.hhs.gov

---

Exhibit 1-3   U.S. Surgeon General's Public Health Vision and Mission

Vision:

Healthy People in Healthy Communities

Mission:

Promote Physical and Mental Health and Prevent Disease, Injury, and Disability

Source: United States Surgeon General: http:// www. surgeongeneral.gov

---

- Health Resources and Services Administration
- Indian Health Service
- National Institutes of Health
- Office of the Assistant Secretary for Health
- Substance Abuse and Mental Health Services Administration

The Office of Disease Prevention and Health Promotion of the U.S. Department of Health and Human Services (HHS), in its 2004 report *Public Health in America,* lists the ways in which public health serves communities (see Exhibit 1-2).

Exhibit 1-3 is provided by the U.S. Surgeon General to summarize Public Health's Vision and Mission.

HEALTHY PEOPLE 2010 AND HEALTHY PEOPLE 2020

Healthy People 2010: A national initiative setting forth goals of promoting health and preventing disease; an update of Healthy People 2000.

Healthy People 2020: Prepares for the next decade; the initiative aims to unify national dialogue about health, motivate action, and encourage new directions in health promotion, providing a public health roadmap and compass for the country.

To facilitate more strident efforts to serve the nation and its public health needs, HHS has promulgated goals and objectives in a series of 10-year plans. These plans, now in their third edition titled *Healthy People 2010,* have defined the country's health agenda and guided health policy since their inception. Begun in 1979, the Healthy People initiatives are series of health-related goals set out in 10-year increments. The Department of Health and Human Services collects data for baseline statistics and monitors the progress and effectiveness of initiatives designed to reach Healthy People goals. The program sets goals and objectives that are deemed both important and actionable (Exhibit 1-4); that is, the goals are relevant public health concerns, such as the rising rates of obesity in the United States, which we can work toward improving in specific and measurable ways through efforts such as banning vending machines in schools. While still assessing the accomplishments of *Healthy People 2010* and evaluating goals met and unmet, the next set of objectives has been developed for *Healthy People 2020* as shown in Tables 1-2 and 1-3. Howard K. Koh, Assistant Secretary of Health at HHS, states, "As we prepare for the next decade, the initiative aims to unify national dialogue about health, motivate action, and encourage new directions in health promotion, providing a public health roadmap and compass for the country."

Exhibit 1-4 Mission, Vision, and Goals of *Healthy People 2020*

Vision—A society in which all people live long, healthy lives.

Mission—*Healthy People 2020* strives to:
- Identify nationwide health improvement priorities
- Increase public awareness and understanding of the determinants of health, disease, and disability, and the opportunities for progress
- Provide measurable objectives and goals that are applicable at the national, state, and local levels
- Engage multiple sectors to take actions to strengthen policies and improve practices that are driven by the best available evidence and knowledge

- Identify critical research, evaluation, and data collection needs

Overarching Goals
- Attain high quality, longer lives free of preventable disease, disability, injury, and premature death
- Achieve health equity, eliminate disparities, and improve the health of all groups
- Create social and physical environments that promote good health for all
- Promote quality of life, healthy development, and healthy behaviors across all life stages

Source: U.S. Department of Health and Human Services. Retrieved from http://www.healthypeople.gov

TABLE 1-2 *Healthy People 2020* Foundation Measure

Healthy People 2020 includes broad, cross-cutting measures without targets that will be used to assess progress toward achieving the four overarching goals.

Overarching Goals of *Healthy People 2020*	Foundation Measures Category	Measures of Progress
Attain high quality, longer lives free of preventable disease, disability, injury, and premature death	General Health Status	<ul><li>Life expectancy</li><li>Healthy life expectancy</li><li>Physical and mental unhealthy days</li><li>Self-assessed health status</li><li>Limitation of activity</li><li>Chronic disease prevalence international comparisons *(where available)*</li></ul>
Achieve health equity, eliminate disparities, and improve the health of all groups	Disparities and Inequity	Disparities/inequity to be assessed by:<ul><li>Race/ethnicity</li><li>Gender</li><li>Socioeconomic status</li><li>Disability status</li><li>Lesbian, gay, bisexual, and transgender status geography</li></ul>

(Continues)

TABLE 1-2 *Healthy People 2020* Foundation Measure *(Continued)*

Create social and physical environments that promote good health for all	Social Determinants of Health	Determinants can include: • Social and economic factors • Natural and built environments • Policies and programs
Promote quality of life, healthy development, and healthy behaviors across all life stages	Health-Related Quality of Life and Well-Being	• Well-being/satisfaction • Physical, mental, and social health-related quality of life • Participation in common activities

Source: U.S. Department of Health and Human Services. Retrieved from http://www.healthypeople.gov/2020/TopicsObjectives2020/pdfs/HP2020_brochure.pdf (page 3)

TABLE 1-3 Topic Focus of *Healthy People 2020*

The Topic Areas of *Healthy People 2020* identify and group objectives of related content, highlighting specific issues and populations. Each Topic Area is assigned to one or more lead agencies within the federal government that is responsible for developing, tracking, monitoring, and periodically reporting on objectives.

1. Access to Health Services
2. Adolescent Health
3. Arthritis, Osteoporosis, and Chronic Back Conditions
4. Blood Disorders and Blood Safety
5. Cancer
6. Chronic Kidney Disease
7. Dementias, Including Alzheimer's Disease
8. Diabetes
9. Disability and Health
10. Early and Middle Childhood
11. Educational and Community-Based Programs
12. Environmental Health
13. Family Planning
14. Food Safety
15. Genomics
16. Global Health
17. Healthcare-Associated Infections
18. Health Communication and Health Information Technology
19. Health-Related Quality of Life and Well-Being Technology
20. Health-Related Quality of Life and Well-Being
21. Disorders Hearing and Other Sensory or Communication Disorders
22. Heart Disease and Stroke
23. HIV
24. Immunization and Infectious Diseases
25. Injury and Violence Prevention
26. Lesbian, Gay, Bisexual, and Transgender Health
27. Maternal, Infant, and Child Health
28. Medical Product Safety
29. Mental Health and Mental Disorders
30. Nutrition and Weight Status
31. Occupational Safety and Health
32. Older Adults
33. Oral Health
34. Physical Activity
35. Preparedness
36. Public Health Infrastructure
37. Respiratory Diseases
38. Sexually Transmitted Diseases
39. Sleep Health
40. Social Determinants of Health
41. Substance Abuse
42. Tobacco Use
43. Vision

Source: U.S. Department of Health and Human Services. Retrieved from http://www.healthypeople.gov/2020/TopicsObjectives2020/pdfs/HP2020_brochure.pdf (page 4)

Summary

In the preface to the *Encyclopedia of Public Health*, Lester Breslow describes public health as one of the essential institutions of society existing to promote, protect, preserve, and restore the good health of all people.

   As you have seen so far in this introductory chapter, there are many programs, services, organizations, and institutions devoted to public health. With so many entities and varying efforts, it can only be fully understood by embracing a systems perspective. Furthermore, it is important to understand the nature of organizations since that is where most of the work is done. We live in an organizational society and public health is no exception. It is equally important to be aware of the core functions of public health and the goals that keep moving it forward. As Breslow surmises, "Professionals engaged in the field regard it as an organized effort directed at improving the health of populations by assuring the conditions in which people can be healthy." In the next chapter we will be discussing professionalism and ethics with a specific focus on the drive to develop and promote core competencies for public health professionals and managers.

Public Health Leader Perspective

Georges C. Benjamin, MD, Executive Director, American Public Health Association

Dr. Benjamin is well known in the world of public health as a leader, practitioner, and administrator. Benjamin has been the Executive Director of the American Public Health Association (APHA), the nation's oldest and largest organization of public health professionals, since December 2002. He came to that post from his position as Secretary of the Maryland Department of Health and Mental Hygiene. Benjamin became Secretary of Health in Maryland in April 1999, following 4 years as its Deputy Secretary for Public Health Services. As Secretary, Dr. Benjamin oversaw the expansion and improvement in the state's Medicaid program.

   At APHA, Benjamin also serves as the publisher of the nonprofit's monthly publication, *The Nation's Health*, the association's official newspaper, and *The American Journal of Public Health*, the profession's premier scientific publication. He is the author of over 90 scientific articles and book chapters.

   Dr. Benjamin is originally from Gaithersburg, MD, and is a graduate of the Illinois Institute of Technology and the College of Medicine at University of Illinois. He is board-certified in internal medicine and a fellow of the American College of Physicians and also a Fellow Emeritus of the American College of Emergency Physicians.

Interview by Dr. James Johnson

Continues

(Q): What is your own working definition of a leader?

Dr. Benjamin: Leaders are people who have a vision about what should happen and have the capacity to motivate others to achieve it. Sometimes it is overt and sometimes they are part of a group, but everyone in the group knows who they are following.

(Q): What are the biggest challenges you face on a regular basis in your position?

Dr. Benjamin: There are two. The biggest challenge is managing people: Ensuring you are addressing their individual needs and keeping them focused on the larger goals so that they have an understanding of how their individual work fits into the larger picture.

The second biggest challenge is telling people no. You often have to turn down good ideas so you can concentrate on the really great ones. People get very disappointed when they have a good idea but it is off the current game plan for the organization. Sometimes it is cost, sometimes the time is not right, and sometimes we are the wrong group to do it.

(Q): What role does politics or stakeholder relations play in your decision making?

Dr. Benjamin: Politics is an essential component of everything we do. The solution is to understand and stand by your core values and be flexible on everything else. Sometimes that means you retreat before you can advance, and sometimes you take a portion of what you want with the hope of getting the rest later. Also, building collaborations means you can't always have exactly what you want and may have to compromise for the good of the collaboration. The agreed upon goal is the ultimate objective and there are often several ways to achieve it. Often, someone else has to get the credit for it to work, even though you did most of the heavy lifting. You have to get comfortable with you being the only person that knows what your role was.

(Q): What is your favorite project or initiative you are currently working on? Please briefly describe.

Dr. Benjamin: We are in the process of helping build a sustainable public health system to support national health reform. Every health department and public health organization in the country has a role in this transformation and we, at the American Public Health Association (APHA), are working to provide some leadership in this area. We are educating a range of stakeholders about what reform means and why it was necessary; how governmental health departments will need to adapt their programs; and how best to devise new programs to improve the health of individuals and communities.

(Q): Do you consider yourself a "systems thinker"? If so, how or give an example.

Dr. Benjamin: Yes I do. Systems thinkers in management are people that understand how organizations really work. Not what is on the organization chart or what the command structure looks like in boxes, but who really calls the shots. They understand how communication occurs, how decisions are arrived at and who the real decision makers are, how challenges are managed, and most importantly, what the organizational culture is. When one can step back and see the whole picture then you can effect strong management or effect significant change. The goal is to anticipate what will happen when a "lever" gets pulled under normal circumstances and what will happen if a "gear" breaks.

Continues

One example that I frequently face is when people ask me to solve a problem instead of first trying to work with my staff because they believe if they talk to me they will get a command decision that solves their problem faster. Actually, it takes longer. The problem with their approach is I have learned that when my subordinates are not in the loop or are not part of the decision-making process, they get passive. They then refer all decisions on this issue to me and I, in effect, lose the preliminary staff work necessary to either make the best decision and the expert follow-up that has to be done to ensure effective follow-through on the project. So when someone comes to me to get a decision, I usually refer it to the appropriate staff person to keep the system intact. I always have the option of overruling them or adjusting their decision, but this way they are part of the decision-making process. A systems thinker would look at the APHA culture and understand I am in a collaborative management practice with my staff.

(Q): What advice do you have for students who plan a career in public health management or public sector health management?

Dr. Benjamin: Get well educated and have as many experiences as you can. Good management comes from doing and trying to be on the common-sense side of the issue. Anticipate what can go wrong and what can go right and be prepared to act in both situations. Give credit when it is due and tell people early when they are going astray (one of my faults is I sometimes fail to do this quickly enough). Take on challenges whenever possible and have fun doing it. If you are not enjoying what you are doing, change jobs!

End

Discussion and Review Questions

1. Discuss the definition of health as provided by the World Health Organization. Share your own view or experiences that support or perhaps even expand this definition.

2. Among the great achievements of public health in the last century, which was the most significant and why? In class or online, each student can choose one of the achievements to discuss in more detail.

3. Describe the core functions and services of public health. What area or service might you like to work in sometime in the future?

4. After reading about *Healthy People 2020* and its vision and goals, what do you expect this will accomplish? Are these goals compatible with the core functions and services of public health? If so, how? Give examples.

5. The Director General of the World Health Organization in 2012, Margaret Chan, MD, M.P.H., once stated about goals and objectives, "if you can't measure it, it doesn't exist." Why do you think it is important to have "foundational measures" for *Healthy People 2020*?

Action Learning and Critical Thinking

A. Choose one of the topic foci from *Healthy People 2020* and do a brief online search for current information, issues, and challenges pertaining to this topic. Report your findings back to the class.

B. Interview a local public health professional and ask them what they think about the accomplishments of *Healthy People 2010* and the future of *Healthy People 2020*.

C. Visit the website of the U.S. Office of Disease Prevention and Health Promotion. Review their range of initiatives. Website: http://odphp.osophs.dhhs.gov

D. After reading the interview with Dr. Benjamin, go to the American Public Health Association (APHA) website and learn more about the association. Consider becoming a student member. Go to a national or local conference of APHA. Website: http://www.apha.org/

Chapter 2

PUBLIC HEALTH PROFESSIONALISM AND ETHICS

Learning Objectives

Upon completion of this chapter, you should be able to:

1. Describe the concept of professionalism.
2. Be aware of the core competencies for public health.
3. Know how professionalism applies to public health.
4. Relate professionalism and values to leadership.
5. Understand ethics and codes for public health managers.
6. Recognize and understand the purpose of core competencies.
7. Describe the importance of ethics in organizations.

Key Terms

code of ethics   ethical theory   health professionals
Council on Linkages   ethics   servant-leader
ethical issue

Chapter Outline

INTRODUCTION

Public health initiatives and public health organizations are infused with a wide variety of professionals. This includes individuals from the fields of management; education; medicine; nursing; physical sciences such as physics and chemistry; engineering; law; biostatistics; epidemiology; demography; basic medical sciences such as microbiology, physiology, pharmacology, and toxicology; nutrition and dietetics; social and behavioral sciences; and the list goes on. Clearly, public health is multidisciplinary and indeed much of the work done by public **health professionals**, or people working in the field of public health or health care who have some special training and/or education, occurs in groups comprised of individuals from many different educational and experiential backgrounds. A team working on a diabetes program perhaps would include a public health nurse, a nutritionist, an endocrinologist, an epidemiologist, and an education specialist. For more information Chapter 10, "Organizational Behavior, Motivation, and Conflict," will focus on the public health workforce.

In addition to professional diversity in public health organizations, there is a strident emphasis placed on professionalism and ethics. This is central to the ethos of public health which is based on the concepts of serving others, doing no harm, and applying expertise within the confines of law, regulation, and professional ethics.

> "He who has health, has hope. And he who has hope, has everything."
> —*Arabian Proverb*

health professionals: A comprehensive term covering people working in the field of public health or health care who have some special training and/or education. The degree of education, training, and other qualifications varies greatly with the nature of the profession, and with the state regulating its practice.

PROFESSIONALISM

Typically a professional is a person who has obtained specialized knowledge in a field through education. Often this involves advanced education and sometimes certification or licensure by the government, usually the state in which that person practices his or her profession. Classic examples of this include medicine, nursing, and law. However, many professions do not have a requirement for licensure but they do have highly specialized educational requirements. This could include a toxicologist, medical anthropologist, or sociologist. In addition to having certain prescribed educational pathways, most professions have a code of ethics and a professional society or association open to its practitioners and scholars. Within public health organizations, it is not uncommon to have employees who are members of a wide variety of societies, associations, and specialized colleges. A few examples include:

- American Public Health Association
- National Association of County and City Health Officials
- American Nursing Association
- American Medical Association
- American Society for Public Administration
- American College of Healthcare Executives
- American Bar Association
- National Mental Health Association
- American School Health Association
- American Dental Association
- American Dietetic Association
- Society for Public Health Education
- National Environmental Health Association
- American Society for Healthcare Engineering
- American Association of Public Health Physicians
- American Epidemiology Society

These associations and societies typically have state level associations and often also have county chapters. Many have international associations they are affiliated with such as the World Federation of Public Health Associations.

Nearly all professional societies at some time in their history advocated for development and promotion of core competencies that serve to improve the effectiveness, relevance, and stature of their profession. In their book, *The American Medical Association and Organized Medicine*, Johnson and Jones provide a comprehensive study of this phenomenon within the American Medical Association (AMA) from its founding in 1847. Interestingly, the AMA constitution has a significant public health objective. Article II states its mission is "To promote the science and art of medicine and the betterment of public health." The book also describes scores of other associations and societies involved in health and public health, including some from the above list.

The common trend is ever-increasing professionalization as reflected in changes in educational requirements and credentialing, as well as the growth in political clout.

In fact, part of the current landscape for professional societies is advocacy and asserting influence on public policy.

CORE COMPETENCIES FOR PUBLIC HEALTH PROFESSIONALS

Another active area for professions, as mentioned previously, is in the development of competency-based practice. In public health this has had its greatest expression through efforts of the Public Health Foundation and the Council on Linkages between Academia and Public Health Practice which is funded through a cooperative agreement between the U.S. Department of Health and Human Services, Health Resources and Services Administration, and the Association of Schools of Public Health (see Table 2-1). The purpose of the **Council on Linkages** is to help create and maintain links between public health practice and academia. This includes strengthening public health infrastructure and fostering continued education throughout the careers of public health professionals.

The Council on Linkages developed a set of Core Competencies that are designed to cross disciplinary boundaries and unify the diverse areas of public health. Since these Core Competencies are designed to cover multiple areas of public health, they are neither all-encompassing nor complete to any one area of public health practice. The Core Competencies are categorized in the following eight skill sets:

- Analytical

- Policy/Program Development

- Communication

- Cultural Diversity

- Community Operations

- Basic Public Health Sciences

- Financial

- Leadership

Council on Linkages: A public health organization whose mission is to improve public health practices and education by fostering, coordinating, and monitoring links between academia and the public health community.

The eight competencies each apply in different ways to three different levels of employment: front-line staff, senior-level staff, and supervisory and management staff. Front-line staff are the face of public health institutions and include nurses, technicians, educators, and others who carry out day-to-day tasks and possibly some data-collection and organizational tasks. Senior-level staff serve more specialized functions but do not act as managers. They include specialists such as epidemiologists, biostatisticians, and health policy analysts who have increased technical knowledge and may oversee projects or programs. Supervisory and management staff are responsible for the major programs or functions of an organization. This level of skill involves the development, implementation, and evaluation of programs as well as the planning, writing, speaking, recommending, and managing that goes with such tasks.

TABLE 2-1 Members of the Council on Linkages Between Academia and Public Health

American Public Health Association (APHA)

C. William Keck, MD, MPH, Chair of the Council

Northeast Ohio Medical University

American College of Preventive Medicine (ACPM)

Hugh Tilson, MD, DrPH

University of North Carolina

Association for Prevention Teaching and Research (APTR)

Amy F. Lee, MD, MPH, MBA

Consortium of Eastern Ohio Master of Public Health

Association of Accredited Public Health Programs (AAPHP)

Gary Gilmore, MPH, PhD, MCHES

University of Wisconsin

Association of Public Health Laboratories (APHL)

John (Jack) M. DeBoy, MPH, DrPH

Retired Public Health Laboratory Director

Association of Schools of Public Health (ASPH)

Lillian Smith, DrPH, MPH, CHES

University of South Carolina

Association of State and Territorial Health Officials (ASTHO)

Terry Dwelle, MD, MPH

State Health Officer, North Dakota Department of Health

Association of University Programs in Health Administration (AUPHA)

Christopher G. Atchison, MPA

University of Iowa

Centers for Disease Control and Prevention (CDC)

Denise Koo, MD, MPH

CDC Office of Surveillance, Epidemiology, and Laboratory Services

Gregory Holzman, MD, MPH

CDC Office for State, Tribal, Local and Territorial Support

(Continues)

TABLE 2-1 Members of the Council on Linkages Between Academia and Public Health *(Continued)*

Community-Campus Partnerships for Health (CCPH)

Diane Downing, RN, PhD

Georgetown University, School of Nursing & Health Studies

Health Resources and Services Administration (HRSA)

Janet Heinrich, DrPH, RN

HRSA Bureau of Health Professions

National Association of County and City Health Officials (NACCHO)

Larry Jones, MA, MPH

Health Director, City of Independence Health Department

National Association of Local Boards of Health (NALBOH)

John Gwinn, MPH, PhD

University of Akron

National Environmental Health Association (NEHA)

Chuck Higgins, MSEH, REHS

Director of Public Health, US National Park Service

National Library of Medicine (NLM)

Lisa Lang, MPP

Health Services Research Information Division, National Library of Medicine

National Network of Public Health Institutes (NNPHI)

Julia Heany, PhD

Center for Healthcare Excellence, Michigan Public Health Institute

National Public Health Leadership Development Network (NLN)

Louis Rowitz, PhD

University of Illinois at Chicago

Quad Council of Public Health Nursing Organizations (QCPHNO)

Jeanne A. Matthews, MS, PhD

Georgetown University

Society for Public Health Education (SOPHE)

Vincent Francisco, PhD

University of North Carolina at Greensboro

Source: Public Health Foundation. Retrieved from http://www.phf.org/programs/council/Pages/Council_on_Linkages_Members.aspx

Specific Competencies	Front Line Staff	Senior Level Staff	Supervisory and Management Staff
Creates a culture of ethical standards within organizations and communities	Knowledgeable to proficient	Proficient	Proficient
Helps create key values and shared vision and uses these principles to guide action	Aware to knowledgeable	Knowledgeable to proficient	Proficient
Identifies internal and external issues that may impact delivery of essential public health services (i.e. strategic planning)	Aware	Knowledgeable to proficient	Proficient
Facilitates collaboration with internal and external groups to ensure participation of key stakeholders	Aware	Knowledgeable to proficient	Proficient
Promotes team and organizational learning	Knowledgeable	Knowledgeable to proficient	Proficient
Contributes to development, implementation, and monitoring of organizational performance standards	Aware to knowledgeable	Knowledgeable to proficient	Proficient
Uses the legal and political system to effect change	Aware	Knowledgeable	Proficient
Applies the theory of organizational structures to professional practice	Aware	Knowledgeable	Proficient

FIGURE 2-1 Domain 8: Leadership and Systems Thinking Skills

Source: Compiled from Public Health Foundation, Council on Linkages Between Academia and Public Health Practice. Competencies Project.

An example of this for one of the eight domains, "Leadership and Systems Thinking Skills," is presented in Figure 2-1.

A complete list of competencies for each of the eight domains shown in Exhibit 2-1 can be found at the Council on Linkages Between Academia and Public Health Practice website of the Public Health Foundation. They also can be found in the Scutchfield and Keck book, *Principles of Public Health Practice*, where there is a

> **Exhibit 2-1   The Eight Domains of Core Competencies for Public Health Professionals**
>
> 1. Analysis and assessment
> 2. Policy development and program planning
> 3. Communication
> 4. Cultural competency
> 5. Community dimensions of practice
> 6. Basic public health sciences
>
> 7. Financial planning and management
> 8. Leadership and systems thinking
>
> *Source: Council on Linkages Between Academia and Public Health Practice. (2001). Core competencies for public health professionals.*

discussion about how these competencies and skills can be integrated into graduate public health education programs, such as the M.P.H.

In addition to being able to delineate competencies, professions also embrace codes and guidelines for ethical behavior. This is especially important for public health managers who are often the keepers of the public trust. As we see an increase in public–private partnerships and more influence by private enterprise into the domain of public health, the challenge could become even greater. However, with every new challenge there comes opportunity. It is likely the public health profession will continue to evolve and move toward even greater professionalization. This is discussed more in later chapters of this book.

ETHICS FOR PUBLIC HEALTH LEADERS

ethics: The kinds of values, morals, and behaviors an individual, profession, or society finds desirable or appropriate.

ethical theory: A system of rules or principles that serve as guides to making decisions in a particular situation.

ethical issue: An issue either implicitly or explicitly involved in any decision made in the public health arena.

As described by Northouse in *Leadership Theory and Practice*, the development of ethical theory dates back to Plato (427–347 BC) and Aristotle (384–322 BC). The word ethics has its roots in the Greek word *ethos*, which means customs, conduct, or character. **Ethics** is concerned with the kinds of values, morals, and behaviors an individual, profession, or society finds desirable or appropriate. **Ethical theory** provides a system of rules or principles that serve as guides to making decisions in a particular situation. **Ethical issues** are either implicitly or explicitly involved in any decision made in the public health arena. *Principles of Biomedical Ethics* by Beauchamp and Childress provides a foundation for health ethics and others have extended some of the same principles to ethical leadership and management, the origins of which can be traced back to Aristotle's concept of the "ethical citizen." This is reiterated in Johnson's recent book, *Meeting the Ethical Challenges of Leadership: Casting Light or Shadow*. These principles include respect, service, justice, honesty, and community.

In any of the job categories mentioned previously, a public health professional could be in a leadership position. Leaders are not limited to management roles. In public health organizations there are team leaders, project leaders, program leaders, community leaders, task force leaders, committee chairs, and so on. In fact, most professionals will be called upon to be in a leadership position at some time in his or her career. The leader's ethical responsibility to serve others is very similar to the ethical principle in health care of *beneficence*. Beneficence is derived from the Hippocratic tradition, which implies that health professionals should make choices that *benefit* patients. See the ancient Hippocratic Oath in Exhibit 2-2. The modern oath can be found at http://www.pbs.org.

For public health professionals, the Hippocratic principles are instructive; however, since the scope is so large, a broader set of principles applies. As promoted by the Public Health Leadership Society, these are shown in Exhibit 2-3.

One of the models of leadership that is very closely associated with ethics and ethical behavior for those in leadership roles is "servant leadership." This is especially pertinent to public health, which is very service-focused in its core mission.

Exhibit 2-2   Hippocratic Oath: Classical Greek Version

I swear by Apollo the physician, and Asclepius, and Hygieia and Panacea and all the gods and goddesses as my witnesses, that, according to my ability and judgment, I will keep this Oath and this contract:

To hold him who taught me this art equally dear to me as my parents, to be a partner in life with him, and to fulfill his needs when required; to look upon his offspring as equals to my own siblings, and to teach them this art, if they shall wish to learn it, without fee or contract; and that by the set rules, lectures, and every other mode of instruction, I will impart a knowledge of the art to my own sons, and those of my teachers, and to students bound by this contract and having sworn this Oath to the law of medicine, but to no others.

I will use those dietary regimens which will benefit my patients according to my greatest ability and judgment, and I will do no harm or injustice to them.

I will not give a lethal drug to anyone if I am asked, nor will I advise such a plan; and similarly I will not give a woman a pessary to cause an abortion.

In purity and according to divine law will I carry out my life and my art.

I will not use the knife, even upon those suffering from stones, but I will leave this to those who are trained in this craft.

Into whatever homes I go, I will enter them for the benefit of the sick, avoiding any voluntary act of impropriety or corruption, including the seduction of women or men, whether they are free men or slaves.

Whatever I see or hear in the lives of my patients, whether in connection with my professional practice or not, which ought not to be spoken of outside, I will keep secret, as considering all such things to be private.

So long as I maintain this Oath faithfully and without corruption, may it be granted to me to partake of life fully and the practice of my art, gaining the respect of all men for all time. However, should I transgress this Oath and violate it, may the opposite be my fate.

Source: National Library of Medicine. Retrieved from http://www.nlm.nih.gov/hmd/greek/greek_oath.html

Exhibit 2-3   Principles of the Ethical Practice of Public Health

1. Public health should address principally the fundamental causes of disease and requirements for health, aiming to prevent adverse health outcomes.
2. Public health should achieve community health in a way that respects the rights of individuals in the community.
3. Public health policies, programs, and priorities should be developed and evaluated through processes that ensure an opportunity for input from community members.
4. Public health should advocate and work for the empowerment of disenfranchised community members, aiming to ensure that the basic resources and conditions necessary for health are accessible to all.
5. Public health should seek the information needed to implement effective policies and programs that protect and promote health.
6. Public health institutions should provide communities with the information they have that is needed for decisions on policies or programs and should obtain the community's consent for their implementation.
7. Public health institutions should act in a timely manner on the information they have within the resources and the mandate given them by the public.
8. Public health programs and policies should incorporate a variety of approaches that anticipate and respect diverse values, beliefs, and cultures in the community.
9. Public health programs and policies should be implemented in a manner that most enhances the physical and social environment.
10. Public health institutions should protect the confidentiality of information that can bring harm to an individual or community if made public. Exceptions must be justified on the basis of the high likelihood of significant harm to the individual or others.
11. Public health institutions should ensure the professional competence of their employees.
12. Public health institutions and their employees should engage in collaborations and affiliations in ways that build the public's trust and the institution's effectiveness.

Reprinted with permission of Public Health Leadership Society (2002). Principles of ethical practice of public health version 2.2. New Orleans, LA. PHLS.

Servant Leadership

servant-leader: The leadership approach public health managers and professionals should embrace; consists of five foundational principles: 1) a concern for people, 2) stewardship, 3) equity or justice, 4) indebtedness, and 5) self-understanding.

The term "**servant-leader**" probably best describes the leadership approach public health managers and professionals should embrace (see Figure 2-2). Hackman and Johnson, in *Leadership: A Communication Perspective*, elaborate on servant leadership by identifying five foundational principles. The first principle is a *concern for people.* Servant-leaders believe that healthy societies and organizations care for their members. They use terms like civility and community to characterize working relationships. The second principle of servant leadership is *stewardship.* Servant-leaders hold positions and organizations, including their resources, in trust for others. The third principle is *equity or justice*, and the fourth principle of servant leadership is *indebtedness*—a central characteristic of service owing others certain rights such as accountability and commitment. The fifth principle

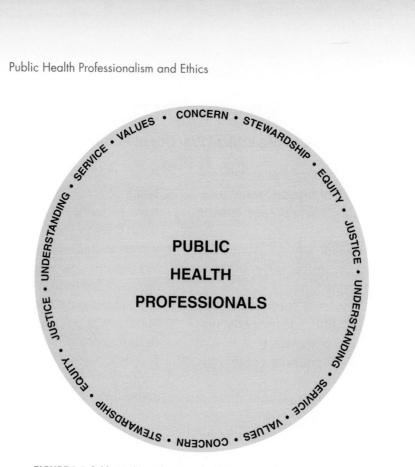

FIGURE 2-2 Public Health Professionals and Managers as Servant-Leaders
© Cengage Learning 2013

for servant-leaders is *self-understanding*. These leaders analyze their motives, seek out opportunities for personal and professional growth, and regularly take time to examine their attitudes and values. They create a positive ethical climate by striving to be trusting, insightful, and open to new ideas.

In addition to embracing a service orientation in leadership and adopting the practices of servant-leaders, the public health manager and professional must also adhere to a range of ethical codes and guidelines. Some of these are broad guiding principles and others are precise rules for a given position. This is especially so, since much of public health is indeed public and involves employment in governmental agencies.

Code of Ethics

There is a Universal Declaration of Human Rights that was adopted by the United Nations in 1948 with fundamental rights shown in Exhibit 2-4.

> "Of all forms of inequality, injustice in health care is the most shocking and inhumane."—*Martin Luther King, Jr., Minister, Social Activist, and Nobel Laureate*

The Public Health Code of Ethics, shown in Exhibit 2-3, has a strong resemblance to these basic human rights principles. Public health ethics call for policies that leave room for community input, respect cultural diversity, work with a variety of agencies and professional disciplines, and enhance the living and working environment (see Exhibit 2-5).

Exhibit 2-4   Universal Declaration of Human Rights

All human beings are born with equal and inalienable rights and fundamental freedoms.

The United Nations is committed to upholding, promoting and protecting the human rights of every individual. This commitment stems from the United Nations Charter, which reaffirms the faith of the peoples of the world in fundamental human rights and in the dignity and worth of the human person.

In the Universal Declaration of Human Rights, the United Nations has stated in clear and simple terms the rights which belong equally to every person.

These rights belong to you.

They are your rights. Familiarize yourself with them. Help to promote and defend them for yourself as well as for your fellow human beings.

Adopted and proclaimed by General Assembly resolution 217 A (III) of 10 December 1948

Preamble

Whereas recognition of the inherent dignity and of the equal and inalienable rights of all members of the human family is the foundation of freedom, justice and peace in the world,

Whereas disregard and contempt for human rights have resulted in barbarous acts which have outraged the conscience of mankind, and the advent of a world in which human beings shall enjoy freedom of speech and belief and freedom from fear and want has been proclaimed as the highest aspiration of the common people,

Whereas it is essential, if man is not to be compelled to have recourse, as a last resort, to rebellion against tyranny and oppression, that human rights should be protected by the rule of law,

Whereas it is essential to promote the development of friendly relations between nations,

Whereas the peoples of the United Nations have in the Charter reaffirmed their faith in fundamental human rights, in the dignity and worth of the human person and in the equal rights of men and women and have determined to promote social progress and better standards of life in larger freedom,

Whereas Member States have pledged themselves to achieve, in cooperation with the United Nations, the promotion of universal respect for and observance of human rights and fundamental freedoms,

Whereas a common understanding of these rights and freedoms is of the greatest importance for the full realization of this pledge,

Now, therefore,

The General Assembly

Proclaims this Universal Declaration of Human Rights as a common standard of achievement for all peoples and all nations, to the end that every individual and every organ of society, keeping this Declaration constantly in mind, shall strive by teaching and education to promote respect for these rights and freedoms and by progressive measures, national and international, to secure their universal and effective recognition and observance, both among the peoples of Member States themselves and among the peoples of territories under their jurisdiction.

Article 1

All human beings are born free and equal in dignity and rights. They are endowed with reason and conscience and should act towards one another in a spirit of brotherhood.

Continues

Article 2

Everyone is entitled to all the rights and freedoms set forth in this Declaration, without distinction of any kind, such as race, colour, sex, language, religion, political or other opinion, national or social origin, property, birth or other status. Furthermore, no distinction shall be made on the basis of the political, jurisdictional or international status of the country or territory to which a person belongs, whether it be independent, trust, non-self-governing or under any other limitation of sovereignty.

Article 3

Everyone has the right to life, liberty and security of person.

Article 4

No one shall be held in slavery or servitude; slavery and the slave trade shall be prohibited in all their forms.

Article 5

No one shall be subjected to torture or to cruel, inhuman or degrading treatment or punishment.

Article 6

Everyone has the right to recognition everywhere as a person before the law.

Article 7

All are equal before the law and are entitled without any discrimination to equal protection of the law. All are entitled to equal protection against any discrimination in violation of this Declaration and against any incitement to such discrimination.

Article 8

Everyone has the right to an effective remedy by the competent national tribunals for acts violating the fundamental rights granted him by the constitution or by law.

Article 9

No one shall be subjected to arbitrary arrest, detention or exile.

Article 10

Everyone is entitled in full equality to a fair and public hearing by an independent and impartial tribunal, in the determination of his rights and obligations and of any criminal charge against him.

Article 11

(1) Everyone charged with a penal offence has the right to be presumed innocent until proved guilty according to law in a public trial at which he has had all the guarantees necessary for his defence.

(2) No one shall be held guilty of any penal offence on account of any act or omission which did not constitute a penal offence, under national or international law, at the time when it was committed. Nor shall a heavier penalty be imposed than the one that was applicable at the time the penal offence was committed.

Article 12

No one shall be subjected to arbitrary interference with his privacy, family, home or correspondence, nor to attacks upon his honour and reputation. Everyone has the right to the protection of the law against such interference or attacks.

Article 13

(1) Everyone has the right to freedom of movement and residence within the borders of each State.

(2) Everyone has the right to leave any country, including his own, and to return to his country.

Continues

Article 14

(1) Everyone has the right to seek and to enjoy in other countries asylum from persecution.

(2) This right may not be invoked in the case of prosecutions genuinely arising from non-political crimes or from acts contrary to the purposes and principles of the United Nations.

Article 15

(1) Everyone has the right to a nationality.

(2) No one shall be arbitrarily deprived of his nationality nor denied the right to change his nationality.

Article 16

(1) Men and women of full age, without any limitation due to race, nationality or religion, have the right to marry and to found a family. They are entitled to equal rights as to marriage, during marriage and at its dissolution.

(2) Marriage shall be entered into only with the free and full consent of the intending spouses.

(3) The family is the natural and fundamental group unit of society and is entitled to protection by society and the State.

Article 17

(1) Everyone has the right to own property alone as well as in association with others.

(2) No one shall be arbitrarily deprived of his property.

Article 18

Everyone has the right to freedom of thought, conscience and religion; this right includes freedom to change his religion or belief, and freedom, either alone or in community with others and in public or private, to manifest his religion or belief in teaching, practice, worship and observance.

Article 19

Everyone has the right to freedom of opinion and expression; this right includes freedom to hold opinions without interference and to seek, receive and impart information and ideas through any media and regardless of frontiers.

Article 20

(1) Everyone has the right to freedom of peaceful assembly and association.

(2) No one may be compelled to belong to an association.

Article 21

(1) Everyone has the right to take part in the government of his country, directly or through freely chosen representatives.

(2) Everyone has the right to equal access to public service in his country.

(3) The will of the people shall be the basis of the authority of government; this will shall be expressed in periodic and genuine elections which shall be by universal and equal suffrage and shall be held by secret vote or by equivalent free voting procedures.

Article 22

Everyone, as a member of society, has the right to social security and is entitled to realization, through national effort and international cooperation and in accordance with the organization and resources of each State, of the economic, social and cultural rights indispensable for his dignity and the free development of his personality.

Article 23

(1) Everyone has the right to work, to free choice of employment, to just and favourable conditions of work and to protection against unemployment.

Continues

(2) Everyone, without any discrimination, has the right to equal pay for equal work.

(3) Everyone who works has the right to just and favourable remuneration ensuring for himself and his family an existence worthy of human dignity, and supplemented, if necessary, by other means of social protection.

(4) Everyone has the right to form and to join trade unions for the protection of his interests.

Article 24

Everyone has the right to rest and leisure, including reasonable limitation of working hours and periodic holidays with pay.

Article 25

(1) Everyone has the right to a standard of living adequate for the health and well-being of himself and of his family, including food, clothing, housing and medical care and necessary social services, and the right to security in the event of unemployment, sickness, disability, widowhood, old age or other lack of livelihood in circumstances beyond his control.

(2) Motherhood and childhood are entitled to special care and assistance. All children, whether born in or out of wedlock, shall enjoy the same social protection.

Article 26

(1) Everyone has the right to education. Education shall be free, at least in the elementary and fundamental stages. Elementary education shall be compulsory. Technical and professional education shall be made generally available and higher education shall be equally accessible to all on the basis of merit.

(2) Education shall be directed to the full development of the human personality and to the strengthening of respect for human rights and fundamental freedoms. It shall promote understanding, tolerance and friendship among all nations, racial or religious groups, and shall further the activities of the United Nations for the maintenance of peace.

(3) Parents have a prior right to choose the kind of education that shall be given to their children.

Article 27

(1) Everyone has the right freely to participate in the cultural life of the community, to enjoy the arts and to share in scientific advancement and its benefits.

(2) Everyone has the right to the protection of the moral and material interests resulting from any scientific, literary or artistic production of which he is the author.

Article 28

Everyone is entitled to a social and international order in which the rights and freedoms set forth in this Declaration can be fully realized.

Article 29

(1) Everyone has duties to the community in which alone the free and full development of his personality is possible.

(2) In the exercise of his rights and freedoms, everyone shall be subject only to such limitations as are determined by law solely for the purpose of securing due recognition and respect for the rights and freedoms of others and of meeting the just requirements of morality, public order and the general welfare in a democratic society.

(3) These rights and freedoms may in no case be exercised contrary to the purposes and principles of the United Nations.

Continues

Article 30

Nothing in this Declaration may be interpreted as implying for any State, group or person any right to engage in any activity or to perform any act aimed at the destruction of any of the rights and freedoms set forth herein.

Source: United Nations, 60th anniversary of the Universal Declaration of Human Rights. Retrieved from http://www.un.org/events/humanrights/udhr60/declaration.shtml

Exhibit 2-5   American Public Health Association Principles on Public Health and Human Rights

1. All human beings are equal in dignity and rights.
2. All human beings are entitled to the enjoyment of all human rights without discrimination.
3. The realization of the highest standard of health requires respect for all human rights, which are indivisible, interdependent, and interrelated.
4. An essential dimension of human rights is the right to health, including conditions that promote and safeguard health and access to culturally acceptable health care.
5. Human rights must not be sacrificed to achieve public health goals, except in extraordinary circumstances, in accordance with the requirements of internationally recognized human rights standards.
6. The active collaboration of public health and human rights workers is a necessary and invaluable means of advancing their common purposes and values.

Source: American Public Health Association (APHA). (2000). Principles on health and human rights. Washington, D.C. Carol Easley Allen.

As promoted in its **code of ethics**, a statement of professional standards of conduct to which the practitioners of a profession subscribe, the American Society of Public Administration advocates ethical behavior for all public service professionals and especially for managers and administrators. These roles and responsibilities, which apply to public health managers working at all levels of government, include the following used with permission from the American Society for Public Administration:

I. Serve the Public Interest

Serve the public, beyond serving oneself. ASPA members are committed to:

1. Exercise discretionary authority to promote the public interest.
2. Oppose all forms of discrimination and harassment, and promote affirmative action.
3. Recognize and support the public's right to know the public's business.
4. Involve citizens in policy decision-making.

code of ethics: A statement of professional standards of conduct to which the practitioners of a profession say they subscribe. Codes of ethics are usually not legally binding, so they may not be taken too seriously as constraints to behavior.

5. Exercise compassion, benevolence, fairness and optimism.

6. Respond to the public in ways that are complete, clear, and easy to understand.

7. Assist citizens in their dealings with government.

8. Be prepared to make decisions that may not be popular.

II. Respect the Constitution and the Law

Respect, support, and study government constitutions and laws that define responsibilities of public agencies, employees, and all citizens. ASPA members are committed to:

1. Understand and apply legislation and regulations relevant to their professional role.

2. Work to improve and change laws and policies that are counterproductive or obsolete.

3. Eliminate unlawful discrimination.

4. Prevent all forms of mismanagement of public funds by establishing and maintaining strong fiscal and management controls, and by supporting audits and investigative activities.

5. Respect and protect privileged information.

6. Encourage and facilitate legitimate dissent activities in government and protect the whistleblowing rights of public employees.

7. Promote constitutional principles of equality, fairness, representativeness, responsiveness and due process in protecting citizens' rights.

III. Demonstrate Personal Integrity

Demonstrate the highest standards in all activities to inspire public confidence and trust in public service. ASPA members are committed to:

1. Maintain truthfulness and honesty and to not compromise them for advancement, honor, or personal gain.

2. Ensure that others receive credit for their work and contributions.

3. Zealously guard against conflict of interest or its appearance: e.g., nepotism, improper outside employment, misuse of public resources or the acceptance of gifts.

4. Respect superiors, subordinates, colleagues and the public.

5. Take responsibility for their own errors.

6. Conduct official acts without partisanship.

IV. Promote Ethical Organizations

Strengthen organizational capabilities to apply ethics, efficiency and effectiveness in serving the public. ASPA members are committed to:

1. Enhance organizational capacity for open communication, creativity, and dedication.

2. Subordinate institutional loyalties to the public good.

3. Establish procedures that promote ethical behavior and hold individuals and organizations accountable for their conduct.

4. Provide organization members with an administrative means for dissent, assurance of due process and safeguards against reprisal.

5. Promote merit principles that protect against arbitrary and capricious actions.

6. Promote organizational accountability through appropriate controls and procedures.

7. Encourage organizations to adopt, distribute, and periodically review a code of ethics as a living document.

V. Strive for Professional Excellence

Strengthen individual capabilities and encourage the professional development of others. ASPA members are committed to:

1. Provide support and encouragement to upgrade competence.

2. Accept as a personal duty the responsibility to keep up to date on emerging issues and potential problems.

3. Encourage others, throughout their careers, to participate in professional activities and associations.

4. Allocate time to meet with students and provide a bridge between classroom studies and the realities of public service.

While Codes of Ethics are adopted by and embraced by professional associations, they often do not carry the weight of law. In fact, there is an overlap, but not direct overlay, of ethics and law, as shown in Figure 2-3. More discussion about law, legislation, regulation, and policy will be provided in the next chapter.

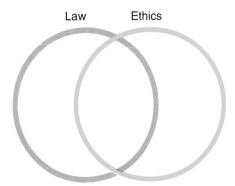

FIGURE 2-3 The Overlap between Law and Ethics
© Cengage Learning 2013

Summary

For anyone who seeks to be a public health manager, leader, or individual with supervisory responsibilities, the duty of abiding by ethical principles and standards is very high. Likewise, management must be approached as a profession with all of the expectations other professions might have. In public health, these expectations can be greater than in other domains due to the importance of health and the nature of the public aspects of public organizations. At the very core of ethics for the public's health is a belief in the universal rights to health and well-being for all people. This is well stated in Article 25 of the Universal Declaration of Human Rights, Exhibit 2-6.

Exhibit 2-6   Article 25 of the Universal Declaration of Human Rights

Everyone has the right to a standard of living adequate for the health and well-being of himself and of his family, including food, clothing, housing and medical care and necessary social services, and the right to security in the event of unemployment, sickness, disability, widowhood, old age or other lack of livelihood in circumstances beyond his control.

Source: United Nations, 60th anniversary of the Universal Declaration of Human Rights: http://www.un.org/events/humanrights/udhr60/declaration.shtml

---

The following case studies in Chapter 16, "Cases in Public Health Management," are directly related to concepts and principles presented in this chapter:

- Case 1: A Friend's Dilemma
- Case 2: Stolen Briefcase
- Case 22: Neglected Tropical Diseases: A Local NGO's Challenges

---

Public Health Leader Perspective

Jan Kirk Carney, MD, MPH, Former Vermont State Health Commissioner

Dr. Carney is known by many as "the People's Doctor," having served for 13 years as the state of Vermont's Commissioner of Health. During this time, Dr. Carney combined the two disciplines of medicine and education in an innovative public health program—*Healthy*

Continues

Vermonters—which significantly reduced levels of lead in baby's brains, made early baby visits almost universal in Vermont, cut the rate of infant child abuse, increased childhood immunizations, and led to improvements in a number of other serious health issues, such as childhood obesity.

Nominating Carney as Vermont's *Local Legend*, United States Congressman Bernie Sanders called her a visionary leader during whose tenure "Vermonters experienced extraordinary gains in their health and well-being."

When she stepped down as Commissioner, the *Burlington Free Press* editorialized, "If Jan K. Carney doesn't return to her old profession as a doctor of medicine, she is well qualified to become a doctor of government!; Carney placed Vermont among the nation's leaders in public health and— Thanks partly to Carney's concerted campaigns against such health threats as breast cancer, AIDS and smoking, and by stressing the importance of early childhood preventative care, health indicators of almost every group of Vermonters have improved!"

Extraordinary accolades for anyone, but for Carney, they signified the fulfillment of a dream of making a difference in people's lives: "I love public health. When I went to public health school, I remember thinking, 'Oh! This is what I intend to do.' I had the great opportunity to be in charge of public health for a whole state, to face all those challenges and see where it didn't work so well and try and do it differently, or where our successes were tremendously gratifying."

Carney earned her undergraduate degree at Middlebury College and received her MD from the University of Cincinnati in 1981. Subsequently, she earned a Master's degree in Public Health (M.P.H.) at the Harvard University, School of Public Health.

Interview by Dr. James Johnson

(Q): What is your own working definition of an effective public health leader?

Dr. Carney: An effective public health leader is credible, knows public health and how to figure out what needs to be done, sets measurable goals, and knows how to accomplish them by working with a wide range of people. I always remember (though I don't know who said it first...) that management is like climbing up a ladder, but leadership means knowing where to put the ladder. In order to achieve your vision, effective communication skills are critical, and you need to work well with people.

(Q): What skills and values are most essential for public health leaders like you?

Dr. Carney: Public health knowledge, from a broad general knowledge of public health, to being able to become a "quick study," on a moment's notice on virtually any subject, is essential. Learning to make important decisions with less-than-complete information is another needed skill. Honesty, integrity, and truly believing in what you are trying to accomplish are at the core of daily values. I always felt that if I did my job in public health well, I could help many, many people, and nothing was more important or rewarding than that.

(Q): What advice do you have for students who plan a career in public health?

Dr. Carney: Expect hard work. It's not easy—there are never enough resources and too many public health needs. But the very things that make it so challenging, also make it incredibly rewarding, and I can't think of a more important career. A small improvement in a public health issue means better health for many, many people.

End

Discussion and Review Questions

1. What is professionalism and why is it important in public health?

2. What is meant by "core competencies" and what are the competency domains we see in public health?

3. Describe the differences in competencies between front line staff, senior staff, and managers. Give examples of each.

4. Why is ethics especially important for health professionals?

5. Within the codes of ethics and declarations discussed in this chapter, are there some common threads or elements? Identify them and discuss.

6. Describe how ethics and law overlaps.

7. What is meant by "servant leadership" and how does this overlap with ethics?

8. Based on the interview in this chapter, would you consider Dr. Carney a "servant-leader"? Explain.

Action Learning and Critical Thinking

A. Look at the competency domains for public health professionals and develop your own personal development plan to help assure you will achieve effectiveness in each of these domains. This might involve college courses, reading books, attending seminars and lectures, doing an internship, participating in a service learning program, engaging in volunteer work, and part-time employment in public health. Your personal development plan should also include a tentative timetable along with the goals and learning activities for each competency domain.

B. Interview a local public health official or public health professional and ask them: 1) to describe their competencies; and 2) how they assure ethical choices and behavior in their role.

C. Write your own professional career plan that includes goals, education required, dream job, and timetable. Describe how professionalism and ethics will be important every step of the way.

Chapter 3

PUBLIC HEALTH POLICY AND POLITICAL STRUCTURE

Learning Objectives

Upon completion of this chapter, you should be able to:

1. Have a broad understanding of the evolution of health policy.
2. Appreciate the role of politics in the policy arena.
3. Discuss major policy initiatives.
4. Be aware of the role of policy at various levels of government.
5. Describe the structure of the United States Government.
6. Understand the role of federalism in policy.
7. Understand multi-sector interdependence in health policy.

Key Terms

endemic

epidemic

federal system

Food and Drug
  Administration
  Amendments Act of
  2007

Food Safety
  Modernization Act of
  2011

laissez faire

policy

Pure Food and Drugs
  Act of 1906

Chapter Outline

INTRODUCTION

policy: A stable, purposeful course of action dealing with a problem or matter of concern. Policy comes in many forms, including: legislative statues, executive orders, court opinions, and agencies (FDA, EPA, FEMA, and so forth). Additionally, policy is the absence of making a decision or taking action. The three main types of policy are distributive, regulatory, and redistributive.

Policy and politics are central to the accomplishment of societal goals; this is especially so when the goal pertains to the public's health. **Policy** is the mechanism whereby resources are allocated or distributed, regulations are refined and enforced, and organizational missions are deployed. In fact, as discussed in Chapter 1, "Public Health Mission and Core Functions," one of the core functions of public health is policy formulation. This chapter provides an overview of public health policy and politics. The fundamentals and foundations provided in this chapter provide a working knowledge that will help with the contextual understanding of many of the remaining topics in this book and any further study of public health.

ORIGINS OF PUBLIC HEALTH POLICY

The intersection of politics, policy, and public health is an ancient one. In fact, whenever humans began to form in communities to meet their food and safety needs for survival, they soon discovered the necessity to establish rules of behavior. These typically were for the purposes of building habitats, keeping order, and sharing resources. As communities grew in size, additional rules developed to assure clean environments, especially as it pertained to waste disposal. As described by George Rosen in the classic book, *A History of Public Health*, evidence of activity connected with community health has been found in the very earliest civilizations. Some 4,000 years ago in northern India, cities were built with broad, paved streets and covered sewers, apparently in accordance with building regulations. Archeologists have found bathrooms and drains were common in many of the buildings. At about the same time in history, cities were built in Egypt by royal command according to a unified plan that dealt effectively with drainage and sewage. Furthermore, securing clean water, a very significant public health need, was effectively done using very ingenious water supply systems in Ancient Crete, the city state of Troy, in modern day Turkey.

In South America, impressive ruins of sewage systems and baths testify to the achievements of the Incas in public health engineering and city planning. As a matter of "public policy," partially related to religious beliefs and a basic understanding of the relationship between the physical environment and health, the Incas celebrated the feast of Citua in September each year, just before the rainy season, which was associated with disease. During this health ceremony, in addition to prayers and offerings, all homes were thoroughly cleaned.

In addition to a basic understanding of the relationship between the physical environment and health that led to fundamental public health rules and regulations (i.e., policy), there was an awareness in some cultures of the transmissibility of disease long before the causes were understood. This came much later in history during the nineteenth century with the research of French chemist Louis Pasteur and the introduction of "germ theory" by the German physician Robert Koch. While not having the precision of these scientists, who benefited from the use of microscopes, the ancient thought-leaders did use philosophical reasoning and observations to realize that health and disease resulted from natural processes. For example, Greek physicians of the fifth-century BC were familiar with malaria, which was thought to be associated with marshes and swamps. In fact, the word malaria comes from *mala aria* meaning bad air, based on the notion that breathing the vapors of these waters caused the disease. Of course, we now know malaria is actually caused by a mosquito-borne parasite and also associated with stagnant water. One of the Greeks writing about the relation between disease and environmental factors was Hippocrates, whose book *Airs, Waters, and Places* established the bedrock for what we now know as population health and informed public health policy. In the book he recognized there were some diseases that were always present in a population, which he called **endemic**, and other diseases that were not always present but did come with some frequency, which he called **epidemic**. Both are terms we still use today. The book also provided his theory of essential factors related to "local endemicity" which he identified as climate, soil, water, mode of life, and nutrition. More than a theoretical treatise, the book was used by Greek leaders to promote health in their communities and to promulgate regulations. It also served to inform colonial expansion as Greek leaders working with physicians established new communities in the Black Sea region and in Italy.

As medical anthropologist Dorothy Porter once stated, "The health of its population is a prerequisite for the survival of all human societies and since ancient times rules and protocols have been devised to promote it."

endemic: Constantly present in a specific population or geographic area. The adjective may be applied, for example, to a disease or an infectious agent.

epidemic: A group of cases of a specific disease or illness clearly in excess of what one would normally expect in a particular geographic area. There is no absolute criteria for using the term epidemic—as standards and expectations change, so might the definition of an epidemic (e.g., an epidemic of violence).

Influences from Europe

Much has happened in the world since the time of the Ancient Incas, Indians, Persians, Egyptians, and Greeks, yet in matters of public health and policy, few events have shaped its course more than epidemics. The bubonic plague that spread in the fourteenth century, commonly known as the "Black Death," caused Renaissance Italian city-states like Venice to create strict civil regulations. Plague epidemics in the sixteenth and seventeenth centuries led English cities to introduce compulsory municipal quarantines. In seeking to address the rapidly spreading social epidemic of smoking, King James I of England and Scotland raised the import tax on tobacco by 4,000 percent and in 1604 wrote a book, *Counterblaste to Tobacco*, stating "Smoking is a custom loathsome to the eye, hateful to the nose, harmful to the brain, dangerous to the lungs." These represent early examples of public health policy, using behavioral economics through taxation and health education. Also at this time, English philosopher and scientist Sir Francis Bacon was developing the scientific method, which is still widely used today in all areas of research, including public health. His work and that of the physicist Sir Isaac Newton contributed to the beginning of what has been called the Age of Reason that contributed to the enlightenment philosophies that influenced the American and French Revolutions in the following century.

In France, the Minister of Finance under Louis XIV established an institutional framework in the late 1600s designed to provide health relief to the poor and to combat epidemics. In 1776 (the year of the American Declaration of Independence) the Royal Society of Medicine was originated to respond to plagues and regulate "remedies" and mineral waters. Following the Revolution of 1789, France embraced an even broader concept of the role of government in public health. Ramsey, in *Public Health in France*, concluded that the revolutionaries agreed that the people enjoyed a right to health. The National Convention working with the Society of Medicine established a committee on health, establishing a law calling for three salaried "health officers" in each district of the country and authorized three new schools to teach medicine and public hygiene. In the early nineteenth century a vigorous public hygiene/public health movement emerged in France led by a committed group of activists within the medical elite. This led to the launching of the first journal of public health in any language, the *Annales d'hygiene publique et de medicine legale* in 1829.

In England, the public hygiene movement was also well engaged to address many of the problems brought about by the Industrial Revolution and rapid urbanization. The 1842 *Report on the Sanitary Condition of the Labouring Population* by social reformer Sir Edwin Chadwick led to the pioneering Public Health Act of 1848. During this time there were cholera outbreaks throughout Britain, Europe, and America, leading to governmental action to secure the public's health.

Public Health Policy in Colonial America

During the colonial period of America's development, public health policy was primarily a local activity focused on preventing the spread of epidemic diseases and the enactment of sanitary laws and regulations. Towns and cities appointed inspectors and had the authority to levy fines against property owners who didn't follow these rules. In the early 1600s, the colony of Virginia required by law the recording of vital statistics (births, deaths, illnesses, marriages) in log books. When the bubonic plague hit London in 1665, port cities in the colonies held British ships offshore in quarantine. Unfortunately, newcomers still brought many infectious diseases, the deadliest being smallpox, which was devastating to the native Indian population. During this era, all the major towns along the eastern seaboard (Boston, Philadelphia, Baltimore, and Charleston) passed quarantine laws. In 1743 a yellow-fever epidemic spread in the colonial cities, claiming an estimated 5 percent of New York City's population. An immigrant physician from Scotland, Cadwallader Colden, recognized a connection between the location of certain homes in the poorest areas with lots of dirty standing water and a higher incidence of disease. He surmised that the cause of yellow fever was poor water supplies, poor diets, and a general condition of filth. His theory translated into a call for clean water and improved sanitation in New York City. This began the sanitarian movement in public health and local government policy that served as the foundational framework for public health policy for the next 150 years as described by Garrett in *The Betrayal of Trust*.

> "If your actions inspire others to dream more, learn more, do more and become more, you are a leader."—*John Quincy Adams, Sixth President of the United States of America*

During 1751 in another port city, Philadelphia, under the leadership of Benjamin Franklin, a scientist and politician, and Thomas Bond, a physician, the first hospital in the colony, Pennsylvania Hospital, was built to care for the "sick-poor and insane who wander the streets of Philadelphia." The founding principles Franklin used in fundraising are still informative today (see Table 3-1) and guided the hospital through many challenging times, including the American Revolution, during which the hospital cared for both Continental and British persons. One of the signers of the Declaration of Independence, Benjamin Rush, a physician, educator, and social reformer, joined the staff.

TABLE 3-1 Five Principles for the Pennsylvania Hospital 1760, Benjamin Franklin

1. Samaritanism—a desire to aid the sick and needy for its own intrinsic value, also called *charity*.

2. Personal health—a desire to improve the health of oneself and one's family to deal more effectively with disease, disability, and death.

3. Public health—a desire for health as a collective or social responsibility to prevent illness and insure a healthy populous while reducing the social burden of disease, disability, and death.

4. Economic value—a desire for the hospital to be a source of income and employment and a desire to benefit the community as a whole.

5. Quality of care—a desire to ensure certain levels of quality and recognizing that poor quality and inefficiency impair the other four principles.

The American Revolution

The Enlightenment philosophy of revolutionary democracy was promulgated in Europe by the ideas of the Geneva philosopher Jean-Jacques Rousseau and the English philosopher and physician John Locke, both of whom had an important ideological influence on eighteenth-century thought about health and the political state. Rousseau's *Discourse on the Origin of Inequality* and *On the Social Contract* are cornerstones in political and social thought and make a strong case for democratic government and social empowerment. Locke's *Essay Concerning Human Understanding*, published in 1690, marked the beginning of the modern Western conception of the self and his *Two Treatises on Government* advocated separation of powers in government and made a case that revolution was not only a right, but in some cases an obligation. He believed in a social contract between governments and citizens, and that everyone had a natural right to defend his "Life, Health, Liberty, or Possessions," which is the basis for the phrase in *The Declaration of Independence* written by Thomas Jefferson as "Life, Liberty, and the Pursuit of Happiness." Jefferson once stated he considered Locke, Bacon, and Newton the greatest men who had ever lived. The influence of these philosophers and scientists is especially evident when Jefferson declared that sick populations were the product of sick political systems, as described by Rosen in *A History of Public Health.* Furthermore, as by Porter in her book, *The History of Public Health and the Modern State*, Jefferson believed despotism produced disease and democracy liberated health. The American Revolution that began in 1776 led to the formation of a new government, independent of England, based on concepts of liberalism as expressed by Thomas Jefferson in the Declaration of 1776 and democracy as written into the Constitution of 1787 by James Madison.

"Democracy is the government of the people, by the people, for the people."—*Abraham Lincoln, 16th President of the United States of America*

STRUCTURE OF THE UNITED STATES GOVERNMENT

The United States Constitution and Bill of Rights, along with the Declaration of Independence, are salient expressions of the unique character of American democracy. Prior to ratification of the Constitution by the States, amendments were added to address fundamental principles of human liberty, which are called the Bill of Rights. These include, among other protections, freedom of speech, a free press, free assembly, free association, and a right to keep and bear arms.

Organization of Government

The organization of government involved the *separation of powers* between three branches: the Executive Branch, comprised of the President and Cabinet; the Legislative Branch, made up of two bodies of Congress (the Senate and House of Representatives) to represent the interests of the people and the states through the process of legislation and oversight; and the Judicial Branch, made up of judges and courts, including the United States Supreme Court. Figure 3-1 illustrates the United States Federal Government's organizational structure.

Furthermore, the Constitution established two levels of government, the federal and the state. This is often called *federalism* and represents a system of government where two or more levels (i.e., national, state, and local) have certain powers and authority (see Figure 3-2). For example, the United States Constitution ensured that there would be shared power between the federal government and the state governments. Typically, each of these levels of government also has a separation of powers between the executive, judicial, and legislative bodies. In a state, the elected executive is the Governor and in a city or town it is the Mayor. The state legislative body is a Legislature or Assembly and the local equivalent would be the City or Town Council, perhaps a County Commission. Likewise, there are federal, state, county, and city judges and courts.

Federalism and Policy

A **federal system** is both a political and philosophical concept that describes how power is given to governments. Federal systems may vary widely in application, but all feature a central government with specific powers over the whole country. In North America the United States, Canada, and Mexico are structured this way, as are many countries around the world. In general, a federal system allows powers that concern the whole nation to be granted to the federal government. For instance, in most countries with a federal system, only the national government can declare war on another country or make international treaties pertaining to trade or foreign policy matters. State power is more focused on issues that directly affect its residents only; Michigan, for example, cannot dictate what laws Indiana enacts. In Canada, the province of Quebec has French language requirements and Ontario does not. Sometimes the state-level governments have to work through problems together. Recently, Georgia, Alabama, and Florida had to work out a water-sharing agreement since rivers and lakes don't always respect state boundary lines and changes in population demographics.

In public health policy there are many examples of intergovernmental programs where all levels of the system—federal, state, and local—are involved, such as the control of air pollution or vaccination programs. Sometimes this also requires the involvement of another federal system, for example the United States working with Mexico and Canada on the H1N1 influenza pandemic in 2009. Intergovernmental initiatives typically also involve the three branches of government since there are issues of law, regulation, funding, authority, and administration. Food and drug regulation is another area that has required the involvement of the executive, judicial, and legislative branches on an ongoing basis, involving government action locally, nationally, and globally to assure the public's health. At the beginning of the twentieth century, the **Pure Food and Drugs Act of 1906** was passed by the United States Congress to provide federal inspection of meat products and prohibit the manufacture, sale, or transportation of adulterated food products and poisonous medicines. As this domain of public health policy grew it was institutionalized in

federal system: A political and philosophical concept that describes how power is given to governments.

Pure Food and Drugs Act of 1906: Passed by the United States Congress to provide federal inspection of meat products and prohibit the manufacture, sale, or transportation of adulterated food products and poisonous medicines.

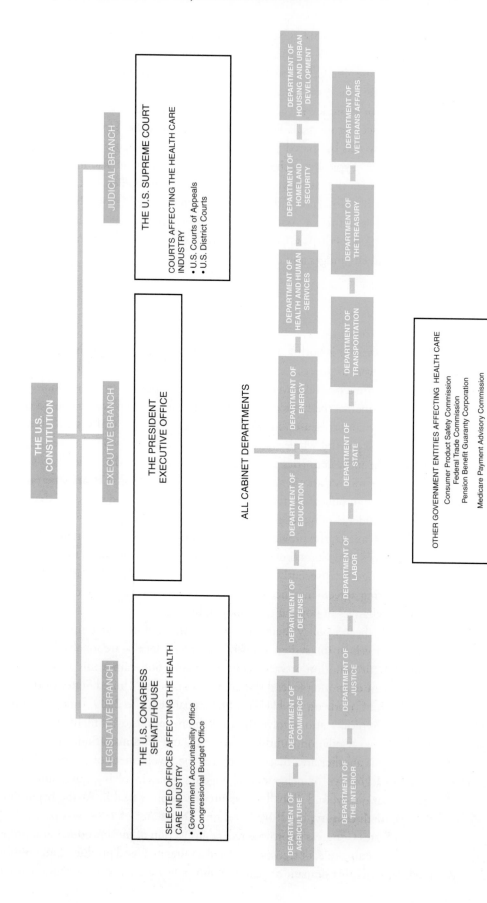

FIGURE 3-1 Organization of the Federal Government
© Cengage Learning 2013

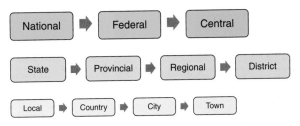

FIGURE 3-2 Levels of Government - National, State, and Local
© Cengage Learning 2013

the Executive Branch, with the establishment of the Food and Drug Administration (FDA) in 1930. Subsequent legislation of more than 200 laws, including the **Food and Drug Administration Amendments Act of 2007** and most recently the **Food Safety Modernization Act of 2011**, broadened the scope of this public health policy area to address ever changing challenges to an increasingly complex and global society. As a result of the interplay between all branches of government, every level of government, private industry, universities, consumer groups, and most importantly, citizens, the United States now has one of the world's most comprehensive and effective networks of public health and consumer protections.

While the original organizational architecture as written in 1787 still exists today, there have been amendments to the Constitution and numerous interpretations by the courts. Numerous public health laws have been enacted by the Congress, state legislatures, and local councils and boards. Furthermore, the number and size of public organizations has grown tremendously into a very complex web of departments, agencies, institutes, offices, centers, and collaboratives. The twenty-first century manifestation of the American experiment with federalist democracy is shown in Part II of this book, which describes the current federal, state, and local organizations responsible for assuring and promoting the public's health. The implications for public health policy are profound now, and have been from the beginning.

Food and Drug Administration Amendments Act of 2007: Legislation reauthorizing and expanding the *Prescription Drug User Fee Act* and the *Medical Device User Fee and Modernization Act*. This amendment allows the FDA to posses the resources needed to conduct the complex and comprehensive review of new drugs and medical devices.

Food Safety Modernization Act of 2011: Sweeping reform to food safety legislation that shifts the focus from reacting to food contamination to preventing it.

HISTORICAL EVOLUTION OF UNITED STATES PUBLIC HEALTH POLICY

Public health policy in the United States borrowed much from developments in Europe where many innovations were being made in cities such as London, Paris, and Venice. After the American Revolution, much of the focus was on sanitation and disease control. Afterwards, over about a 200-year period, public health policy evolved and became central to American culture and society. The innovations continue today in areas such as affordable care, tobacco control, pandemic preparedness, and healthy communities.

Public Health Policy in the Nineteenth Century

In early United States history, public health was primarily a local government activity mostly focusing on sanitation and quarantine. However, there were some challenges, especially epidemics of infectious diseases, where the federal and state governments worked with a local government to formulate public policy and organize public health initiatives. Just prior to the 1800s, several developments were harbingers of the new century (see Exhibit 3-1).

As the United States moved from one century to the next, its industrial activity would increase and its expansion westward would drive much of its development. On the east coast, the port cities grew larger and more crowded, focusing public health efforts on essential urban services. By mid-century, the local governments had an active approach to health problems, while the federal government could be characterized by the French term *laissez faire*, meaning non-interference. Later, public health leaders would become increasingly influenced by the new science of bacteriology that emerged in Europe from the "germ theory" work of Louis Pasteur in France and Robert Koch in Germany.

laissez faire: Non-interference.

Public Health Policy in the Twentieth Century

The late 1800s ended with a new confidence in public health and the ability of governments, at all levels, to be active in mitigating disease. The methods of science, especially bacteriology, were embraced and progress was made in the management of disease. In Massachusetts, William Sedgwick, who had completed his Ph.D. in Bacteriology at Johns Hopkins University in 1881, demonstrated the transmission of typhoid fever by polluted water supplies and had used quantitative methods to measure the presence of bacteria in the air, water, and milk.

Exhibit 3-1   Public Health and Policy in the 1700s

1790: First United States Census was ordered by George Washington. Taken every 10 years thereafter, this would become a cornerstone for population health and community planning.

1793: Yellow Fever epidemic in Philadelphia and other major port cities such as Charleston, Baltimore, New York, and New Orleans, where ships arrived from Central and South America.

1796: Edward Jenner, a general practitioner in England, successfully demonstrated smallpox vaccination. While rudimentary inoculations were being done in the port city of Istanbul in the early 1700s, it was not until Jenner's conclusive research that a vaccine proved to be

successful. The first smallpox vaccinations in the United States began in Boston in 1800.

1796: New York State Legislature passed the nation's first comprehensive public health law (this was in part a response to the economic impact of the smallpox and yellow fever epidemics). A State Commissioner of Health and a New York City Health Office were established.

1798: Congress orders the creation of the Marine Hospital Service to monitor sailors and protect American ports from incoming diseases. This was the forerunner of the U.S. Public Health Service.

Exhibit 3-2   Public Health and Policy in the 1800s

1802: Washington D.C., constructed on swampland, was overrun by yellow fever, smallpox, encephalitis, and malaria which led to the enactment of a series of public health ordinances modeled after those in New York.

1805: New York City created the nation's first Municipal Board of Health. Propelled by the fear of yellow fever and cholera, Boston, Chicago, New Orleans, and many other cities created boards of health based on the New York organizational model.

1855: Louisiana established the first state board of health, primarily focused on the port city of New Orleans.

1861: American Civil War begins and lasts for 4 years, resulting in 620,000 deaths, mostly due to disease, malnutrition, and dehydration. Public health measures were limited, but some sanitation and quarantine measures were used.

1866: New York City passed the Metropolitan Health Bill, the most comprehensive health legislation in the United States at that time.

1869: Massachusetts formed a State Board of Health followed by California (1870), Virginia and Minnesota (1872), Maryland (1874), and Alabama (1875).

1872: American Public Health Association (APHA) began with 10 members and grew rapidly. Today it represents over 50,000 health professionals.

1879: Congress creates a National Board of Health responsible for formulating quarantine regulations between the states. This was a major step toward the growth in federal involvement that would become pervasive in the following century.

1880s: State public health laboratories were established in Rhode Island, Michigan, and Massachusetts.

In describing the impact of the new public health science, he said, "Before 1880 we knew nothing; after 1890 we knew it all; it was a glorious ten years." Going beyond the biological sciences into the social sciences, German economists had begun to calculate the positive financial returns on public health investment. The APHA continued to grow and diversify, with its membership being comprised of scientists, municipal and state officials, physicians, nurses, engineers, and a wide range of social reformers. Exhibit 3-2 showcases public health achievements and advances during the 1800s.

Despite these new insights and advances in public health, the United States entered the twentieth century with life-expectancy at less than 50 years and the old diseases yet to be fully controlled while challenging noninfectious diseases and disabilities were coming to the fore. The limits of a purely bacteriological approach were most evident in the search for the cause of pellagra and rickets, thought to be caused by a bacteria but later found to be the result of vitamin deficiencies. A more comprehensive model of public health and the ability to better inform public policy would be needed in the century ahead. This was best articulated by

Charles-Edward A. Winslow, founder of the Department of Public Health at Yale University in 1915:

> Public health is the science and art of preventing disease, prolonging life, and promoting physical health and efficiency through organized community efforts for the sanitation of the environment, the control of community infections, the education of the individual in principles of personal hygiene, the organization of medical and nursing service for the early diagnosis and preventive treatment of disease, and the development of the social machinery which will ensure every individual in the community a standard of living adequate to the maintenance of health.

These ideals are not far from those of Franklin and Jefferson discussed earlier. If one looks back at the social and economic conditions of the early 1900s, it is easy to see why some of the founding values needed to be reasserted. With rapid urbanization and industrialization, new challenges to the well-being of the nation would arise. There was widespread poverty, growth in chronic illnesses, unsafe working conditions, exploitation of children, high maternal death rates, industrial poisoning, health disparities based on race, and looming threats to health such as polio and major influenza pandemic that killed over 30 million people. Two world wars and the Great Depression were also soon to arrive. Many innovations in public health science, practice, and education would occur along with the expansion of the federal role in health and public policy. (see Exhibit 3-3)

Exhibit 3-3   Public Health and Policy in the 1900s

1902: National Association for the Study and Prevention of Tuberculosis was formed becoming the first national-level volunteer health organization in the United States. Its predecessor was the Pennsylvania Society for the Prevention of Tuberculosis organized in 1892.

1904: William Gorgas led a successful campaign of malaria and yellow fever control in Panama.

1906: Upton Sinclair's book *The Jungle* was published to draw attention to unsafe working conditions in Chicago meat packing plants. That same year Congress passed the Pure Food and Drugs Act.

1906: John D. Rockefeller created a scientific foundation to eradicate hookworm in the American South and later throughout the world. This became one of the many public health accomplishments of what became the Rockefeller Foundation. Ten years later this same foundation donated millions of dollars to create the School of Hygiene and Public Health at Johns Hopkins University in Baltimore.

1910: The first International Congress on Occupational Diseases was held in Chicago. That same year New York passed a Workmen's Compensation Act and over the next 10 years most states had done the same. The Carnegie Foundation commissioned an investigation, led by Abraham Flexner, of medical schools that found severely inadequate training and a lack of science-based approach to medicine.

Continues

In public health, the first degree specific to the field, was awarded at University of Michigan in 1910. Schools and departments of public health would be created somewhat later during this decade at Harvard, Johns Hopkins, Yale, Columbia, Toronto, Michigan, North Carolina, and Minnesota.

1912: The Marine Hospital Service became the U.S. Public Health Service, which was authorized to investigate the causes and spread of diseases, study the problems of sewage, sanitation, and water pollution, and publish health information for the general public.

1913: American Cancer Society was founded.

1916: Polio outbreak in New York spread to cities throughout the United States. The U.S. Surgeon General used what was then a novel approach—warning the public through publicity utilizing newspapers, civic organizations, and schools to teach hygiene as a means of prevention.

1918: Influenza pandemic began in Kansas and circled the globe, killing at least 30 million people.

1923: APHA publishes a national study of municipal health departments finding wide variation in public health practice and organization

1935: Social Security Act was passed to provide a safety net for citizens. This was a central piece of legislation under the leadership of President Franklin Roosevelt to address many of the problems caused by the Great Depression. Under the Venereal Disease Act, the role and authority of the USPHS was expanded. Furthermore, financing was enhanced to allow grants to states for public health education and services. Many state universities responded by establishing new schools and programs in public health to meet a rising demand for public

health professionals. At least a dozen new federal agencies were created between 1933 and 1938 to focus on public health.

1937: National Cancer Institute was established. This was the beginning of what would become a large array of national institutes being developed to address specific illnesses through research. Federal grants to states also continue to grow in size and number.

1939: World War II begins in Europe and the United States enters the war in 1941. Public health was declared a national priority for the armed forces and the civilian population working for the war effort. General James Stevens Simmons, Director of Preventive Medicine for the U.S. Army announced: "A civil population that is not healthy cannot be prosperous and will lag behind in the economic competition between nations." Congress began to see public health as a national security issue and allocated considerably more resources to the U.S. Public Health Service and to communities through the Community Facilities Act. Due to a major problem with malaria in the southern states, the Public Health Service established the Center for Controlling Malaria in Atlanta, Georgia. After the war this organization was transformed into the Communicable Disease Center. Now called the Centers for Disease Control and Prevention (CDC), it is the premier epidemiological center for the United States and the world.

1946: National Hospital Survey and Construction Act. The legislation sponsored by Senator Lister Hill of Alabama and Senator Harold Burton of Ohio is commonly known as the Hill-Burton Act and it sought to answer the national demand for access to medical services by funding construction of hospitals in primarily rural areas.

Continues

1952: Polio vaccine by Jonas Salk at the University of Pittsburgh. This began a nationwide vaccination program and effort to eradicate polio from the United States. Ten years later, based on concerns about the injectable vaccine, Albert Sabin at Cincinnati Children's Hospital and later at the Medical University of South Carolina in Charleston developed an oral version that was both safer and easier to administer.

1955: Indian Health Service (IHS) was established to provide care for American Indians and Alaska Natives.

1956: Health Amendment Act was authorized to provide funding for traineeships for public health professionals from many fields. The APHA had advocated for better and broader training opportunities with its president stating, "Our graduate students needed a better understanding of the social and political swirling about them as they work professionally." He called for graduate public health education to provide a fundamental knowledge of four broad fields: cultural anthropology, human ecology, epidemiology, and biostatistics. The First National Conference on Public Health Training was held in Washington, D.C., in 1958 and the theme of the APHA annual meeting in St. Louis was "The Politics of Public Health." George Rosen, editor of the American Journal of Public Health wrote, "An understanding of political process as it affects the handling of community health problems is as crucial an area of knowledge to health workers as the scientific underpinning of public health practice."

1964: The Civil Rights Act was passed eliminating most legal forms of racial discrimination, including discrimination in the practice of medicine and public health. President Lyndon Johnson also pushed for other major social reforms including a War on Poverty, aid to families and children, and health services for more Americans. Martin Luther King famously declared, "Of all forms of inequality, injustice in health care is the most shocking and inhumane."

1965: Medicare and Medicaid legislation was passed to provide health services to the elderly and the poor, along with Aid to Families with Dependent Children (AFDC)

1970: Clean Air Act was passed and a range of federal agencies had been created in previous decade to address growing concerns about environmental hazards. These included the Environmental Protection Agency (EPA), the Occupational Safety and Health Administration (OSHA), and the National Institute of Occupational Safety and Health (NIOSH).

1976: Health Information and Health Promotion Act was passed and the Office of Disease Prevention and Health Promotion was created. Many public health efforts were designed around the concepts of health promotion with a goal of healthier lifestyles and health behavior. This led the way to the United States Government publication *Healthy People: The Surgeon General's Report on Health Promotion and Disease Prevention* in 1979.

1980: National health goals were published by the Department of Health Education and Welfare (HEW) under the leadership of secretary Joseph Califano in *Promoting Health/Preventing Disease: Objectives for the Nation*. Goals and objectives have been established under the direction of the Department of Health and Human Services (HHS) in every subsequent decade with *Healthy People 2000, Healthy People 2010*, and now *Healthy People 2020*.

1981: AIDS is reported in California and New York. An epidemic had begun and would

Continues

become a global pandemic changing public health organization, practice, and science in profound ways. Unfortunately, as so often in the history of public health, many policy decisions were based more on politics and emotional issues than on science. Nevertheless, a concerted effort to fight the epidemic emerged over the coming decades, bringing together public health professionals from federal agencies such as the CDC, FDA, NIH; state health departments; municipal health agencies; community groups and national associations; universities and private research centers; global organizations like WHO and the United Nations; and foundations large and small.

1988: Institute of Medicine (IOM) released a report, *The Future of Public Health*, based on extensive interviews of public health experts and surveys of health status of every state. It discovered an absence of shared mission among public health agencies and no commonly accepted definition of their duties. The report called for a plan of action for much needed improvements. A summary statement read:

> An impossible responsibility has been placed on America's public health agencies: to serve as stewards of the basic health needs of entire populations, but at

the same time avert impending disasters and provide personal health care to those rejected by the rest of the health system. The wonder is not that American public health has problems, but that so much has been done so well, and with so little.

Many reports pertaining to public health would be provided during the coming decades, including, most recently, the 2010 report titled *For the Public's Health: The Role of Measurement in Action and Accountability* which reviewed current approaches for measuring the health of individuals and communities and created a roadmap for future development.

1996: Health Insurance Portability and Accountability Act (HIPAA) was enacted. Its purpose was to protect health insurance coverage for workers and their families when they change or lose their jobs. It also established national standards for electronic health care transactions and guidelines for health information privacy and security.

1997: State Children's Health Insurance Program (SCHIP) was created as the largest expansion of taxpayer-funded health insurance coverage for children in the United States since Medicaid. Like Medicaid, it was designed as a partnership between the federal and state governments.

The latter half of the twentieth century also had challenges and successes. There were social movements to expand the rights of citizens, including women and minorities. Aggressive legislation and institution-building addressed new threats to public health like chronic diseases, environmental problems, access to care, substance abuse, new infectious disease such as HIV/AIDS and the re-emergence of old ones like tuberculosis. There were also advances in the field of epidemiology and an expanded concept of public health, involving health promotion that informed and shaped public policy. Most fundamental to the new paradigm was the multi-causation disease model, also known as the *epidemiological triangle* (see Figure 3-3). The host represents the organism infected, the agent is the bacteria that causes the disease, and the environment represents external elements that may have caused the disease or allow for easier transmission.

The Epidemiologic Triangle

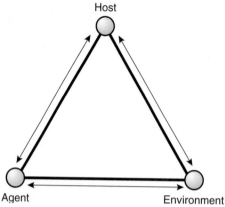

FIGURE 3-3 The Epidemiologic Triangle or Multi-Causation Disease Model
© Cengage Learning 2013

With this perspective, public health policy and practice became more expansive involving agencies at the federal, state, and local levels that were not historically within the domain of public health. Agencies across sectors in housing, environment, transportation, labor, education, social services, and agriculture worked with public health to address large social issues associated with health. Toward the end of the century the United States Government began setting national health goals through the publication of its *Healthy People* reports to guide health policy.

The progress made in the twentieth century to regain the Nation's foundational footing was based on dignity and human rights in a social contract with its government. In 1976, 200 years after the American Revolution, an essay written by Dan Beauchamp, Ph.D., was published in the journal *Inquiry* that equated public health with social justice. In his more recent book, *Social Justice and the Other Great Society*, Beauchamp sees public health as a social and governmental process that is essentially pragmatic in nature, an expression of democracy itself. In words that would surely resonate with Jefferson, Madison, and Franklin, a 1990s leader in the health and human rights movement, Jonathan Mann, argued that promoting the public's health promotes justice and prosperity and is a moral obligation of governments and individuals. In 1999, the last year of the millennium, Mann wrote, "…in the modern world, public health officials have, for the first time, two fundamental responsibilities to the public: to protect and promote public health and to promote human rights."

> "A good leader inspires people to have confidence in the leader, a great leader inspires people to have confidence in themselves."—*Eleanor Roosevelt, Author, Activist, and First Lady of the United States of America*

Public Health Policy in the Twenty-First Century

Public health policy in the twenty-first century is still emerging, but many of the older themes of democracy, federalism, social justice, human rights and dignity continue to provide a link to the Nation's founding principles. The impressive advancements in science during the past 200 years hold even more promise in the years ahead. The Human Genome Project has been completed at the National Institutes of Health, possibly moving biomedical science from the "germ theory era" to the "genome era." Natural and manmade disasters such as the 9/11 attacks on the World Trade Center in New York City; the devastation of New Orleans by Hurricane Katrina; the deadly earthquake in Haiti; and the BP oil spill in the Gulf of Mexico all have resulted in modifications in public health policy. Newly emerging diseases and re-emerging diseases such as H1N1 continue to force the public health community to be constantly vigilant in its goal to protect the public's health. Concerns about the delivery of health care, economics, and changing health demographics will continue and modifications in public health policy will be needed. Likewise, the professionalization of public health through education and training is advancing. Finally, public health policy will increasingly become global health policy as the United States and all countries are further impacted by globalization. The future of public health is discussed in Chapter 15, "Public Health Leadership and the Future." Refer to Exhibit 3-4 for details about public health policy developments of the twenty-first century to date.

Exhibit 3-4   Public Health and Policy in the 2000s

2004: Association of Schools of Public Health in partnership with CDC initiated the Competency and Learning Objectives Development Projects to identify core competencies for public health professionals and advocated their becoming the core framework for public health education at every level, both graduate and undergraduate. The project continues in 2011 and has developed competency guidelines for disaster preparedness, collaborative practice, and global health.

2006: Massachusetts becomes the first state in the United States to establish universal health care with enactment of the Providing Access to Affordable, Quality, Accountable Health Care Act. That same year, San Francisco's Board of Supervisors adopted the Health Care Security Ordinance, the first of its kind in the country, in an attempt to provide universal care for all of its residents.

2010: Patient Protection and Affordable Care Act (hereafter referred to simply as the Affordable Care Act) was enacted in an effort to reform the private health insurance market, provide better coverage for those with pre-existing conditions, college-age citizens, and seniors on Medicare. It included provisions for the establishment of a Center for Medicare and Medicaid Innovation and promoted the use of comparative effectiveness research to inform policy and the management of health systems. As a significant public health measure, it created the Task Force on Preventive Services and Community Preventive Services to develop, update, and disseminate evidenced-based recommendations on the use of clinical and community prevention services. Additionally, it reauthorized and amended the Indian Health Care Improvement Act.

2011: Department of Health and Human Services releases *Healthy People 2020* to establish health goals and objectives for the decade.

Multisector Interdependence

As with everything in the twenty-first century, public health policy is interdependent with other policy domains. It is not unusual for a public health agency to work with the Department of Labor, Department of Agriculture, or Environmental Protection Agency on multi-sector problems. One example that has become quite evident during the "Great Recession" beginning in 2008 is unemployment. Figure 3-4 shows the relationship between the unemployment rate and increases in Medicaid spending by the state and federal government.

In most discussions of health policy today, it is unavoidable that considerations of cost, quality, and access will be discussed. In describing the policy processes, the next chapter takes into consideration and concludes with an evidence-based and systems approach to public health policy.

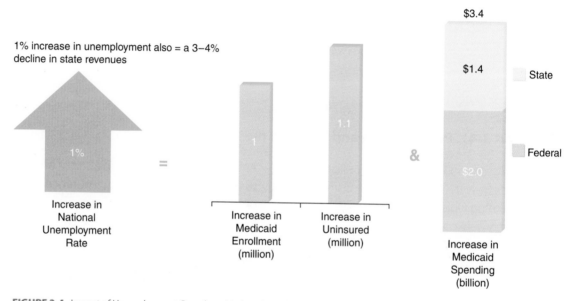

FIGURE 3-4 Impact of Unemployment Growth on Medicaid and the Number of Uninsured
Source: Based on Kaiser Commission on Medicaid and the Uninsured: Rising Unemployment, Medcaid and the Uninsured, January 2009: http://www.kff.org/uninsured/upload/7850.pdf

Summary

Beginning with the early developments of policy in the ancient world and going forward to the complex reality of today, this chapter has demonstrated the significance of policy and politics to the understanding of public health. It is especially important to understand the context of public policy as it is imbedded in a political structure. The United States is a federalist system with different levels of government with shared responsibilities for health. The next chapter discusses how policy is made and evaluated as it continues to evolve in the twenty-first century.

The following case studies in Chapter 16, "Cases in Public Health Management," are directly related to concepts and principles presented in this chapter:

- Case 3: The Anti-Vaccination Paradigm
- Case 8: To Hear This Message in Korean, Press '9'
- Case 11: Budget Cuts in Home Care Program
- Case 12: Don't Ask, But Tell
- Case 14: Collaborative Approach to Diabetes Prevention and Care
- Case 15: Toy Recall Prompts Attention to Lead Poisoning
- Case 17: Top Ten U.S. Public Health Achievements
- Case 22: Neglected Tropical Diseases—A Local NGO's Challenges

---

Public Health Professional Perspective

Sandra Schoenfisch, RN, PhD, Consultant to Florida Department of Health, and Retired Public Health Administrator, Tallahassee, Florida

Interview by Dr. James Johnson

(Q): What is your own working definition of an effective manager?

Dr. Schoenfisch: An effective manager is one who can get the job done. One of my favorite books is *Execution: The Discipline of Getting Things Done* by Bossidy and Charan. In a nutshell, it talks about plans and strategies and that they are only good if you can actually execute them. I think an effective manager is the one who understands how things work and has

Continues

insights into the organization and team members. A good manager is able to recognize team members' skills and strengths and capitalize on the specific capabilities. An effective manager is able to contribute to the organization as well as the team and the growth of individual team members. You get the job done, move forward or accomplish a goal without drawing blood and without the loss of life and limb.

(Q): What are the biggest challenges you face on a daily basis?

Dr. Schoenfisch: The constantly changing environment, competing priorities, and agendas. Trying to keep up with the information overload and being able to separate what is important from the noise.

(Q): What skills are most essential for the work you do?

Dr. Schoenfisch:

- In today's environment effective communication is probably the most important skill needed to succeed. Being able to get your message or information across and being able to interpret the communications you receive can make the difference between success and disaster.
- The ability to accept change and adapt to change quickly is also important. In the current environment it is critical to embrace change and see change as an opportunity. A lot of people say they accept change but if you watch their response and performance, you will see them doing what they have always done or at least striving to do the same thing. Change makes people uncomfortable, they need to know that is okay and natural to experience the discomfort associated with change but they do need to adapt to survive. Usually the end result of change is not as bad as everyone expects and most of the time you can use change to improve things. It is really important to be able to question things.
- There are so many variables and aspects of what you do in a management position. You don't have to have all the answers but you really need to be comfortable with asking questions and making the folks you work with have the same comfort levels.
- Final comment, keep your sense of humor.

(Q): What is your favorite project or initiative you are currently working on?

Dr. Schoenfisch: Right now I have a project that involves looking at the process, impact, and outcomes of a program that has been in place for 10 years. Over the years a number of project managers had moved through the system. A contracting process was used to assist with providing funding to purchase equipment, pay for training, and support exercises to test defined capabilities in hospitals statewide. The good news was that there was a lot of data to review as well as other measures to assess the level of progress. The bad news was that the data was stored in all kinds of formats and files. The information had different "owners" in different offices and teams. None of the information was organized and connected from one year to another. We had no relational databases. Compiling and organizing the data involved staff from four offices. Approximately eight employees, most of whom did not work together on a regular basis, had to start sharing information, complete tasks, and to communicate with each other on a daily basis. A sales pitch on why creating a centralized data base would help all of us received a lukewarm response. One of the "new" team members convinced a key staff person to show us how she collected and stored the data. A copy of the file was made (so that we would not mess up her files) and we proceeded to enter the data from other sources and some additional parameters. The new people were then able to

Continues

generate a descriptive analysis of what had transpired over the 10-year period. It was based on fact and numbers rather than anecdotal information. Many but not all of the findings and observations were positive. We were able to provide documentation of the effectiveness of the contracts and contract managers. However, some weaknesses and challenges also surfaced. Drilling a bit deeper we, as a group, were able to document some items that could be changed and needed to be changed. Almost everyone involved is getting more involved and committed to completing the database and using the findings as a way to improve the process and the program. Right now the data entry is on the fast track, the staff involved have high expectations for the next cycle, and it looks like we will be able to use the analysis to make some evidenced based decisions! On a lighter note, staff members who rarely had contact or spoke to each other are now talking to each other on a regular basis, they meet face-to-face rather than by phone and frequently can be heard laughing, joking, and solving problems to help them get the job done.

(Q): Do you consider yourself a "systems thinker"? If so, how or give an example.

Dr. Schoenfisch: As mentioned earlier, we are all connected and very little of what any of us do, can be done in isolation. We all have to be thoughtful and deliberate in our choices. It is not uncommon for a law or policy that has a good intent to be put in place and result in a negative outcome due to not recognizing the full impact it will have.

The H1N1 campaign was an excellent example of systems. At first glance, it might look like a simple "flu vaccination campaign." Give out the vaccine and have the nurses give people their "shots." Initially there was a shortage of vaccine. The production from the manufacturers could not keep up with the demand. The CDC made recommendations as to who should get the vaccine first, [along with] identification of priority groups.

The campaign was dependent on the vaccine manufacturers, the federal government for allocation and distribution, the states for assuring a network of providers to administer the vaccine, the epidemiologists for advising us on the severity of the outbreak and vulnerable populations. Large chain pharmacies were also engaged as partners and brought with them corporate standards and procedures. In addition to all of the items above, multiple presentations of vaccine were available and that increased the need for effective screening. The message in the beginning of the campaign was "priority" groups, and the "priority" groups were not the same as in previous groups. This meant that after 20 years of telling seniors and persons with chronic health problems that they should get the "flu shot" early and every year that they were not in the top priority group. Rumor control, social media, and anti-vaccine messaging all contributed to the need for a plan that could be operationalized and consistent, accurate messaging from health care providers.

All of the stakeholders had processes and systems in place. Some such as the big box pharmacies were "systems." It became apparent that it was going to take multiple strategies, connections and coordination with all of the key players to make the campaign work and minimize problems. All of our efforts needed to be connected and complementary.

(Q): What advice do you have for students who plan a career in public health management?

Dr. Schoenfisch: Find an area that you really love. Find something you really want to do every day! It is okay to change your mind and go in different directions as long as it is your passion and you pursue it.

I have some other thoughts that I think are important but will probably seem rather basic.

Continues

It is rare that you find a person who comes to work with the idea that they want to fail, create chaos, and antagonize everyone with whom they have contact. However, it is very common that people are hired without having all of the skills and information they need to succeed. An accurate assessment of what they need to be successful is not done. Frequently they are given tasks, assignments, or projects to manage [with] minimal guidance. They are assigned to teams, again [with] little or no support. They are given little or no feedback until they fail or they are micromanaged to the point that they lose their initiative and are fearful of making any decision or completing anything. Almost everyone comes with some skills or knowledge that can be used. Most of the work that I have done for the last 20 years has involved teams or groups of people. The good old days of having an assignment that was "yours" and you could just go about your business and do it are gone. "Teams" were the way work was done due to the scope and diversity of the project. Being able to identify who would be the best person to have lead or complete a certain aspect of the project was critical. You are only as strong as the weakest person on your team.

Silos do not help any of us. Everyone needs information and information in a format they can understand. Good facilitation skills can be more important than degrees, titles, and content.

End

Discussion and Review Questions

1. Identify and discuss three major developments in the ancient world that shaped public health policy at that time. Give examples of this. Do similar policies exist today?

2. Identify and discuss three examples of public health policy initiatives seen in Colonial America or Europe at that time.

3. What is the multi-causation disease model and why is it important when considering public health policy?

4. Review the historical developments in public health and the evolution of public health policy as presented in this chapter and identify other historical events occurring in a given era that might have helped shaped policy.

Action Learning and Critical Thinking

A. Choose any major health policy legislation (Medicaid, Medicare, Affordable Care Act, Clean Water Act, et al.) and using Internet web-searches do the following: 1) describe the political context of the legislation; 2) identify the role of federalism; 3) identify any agencies or interest groups that have advanced the policy and its goals.

B. Watch the movie *And the Band Played On* and discuss your observations about policy in action within the federal, state, and local government sectors represented in the film. Also discuss the role played by nongovernment organizations like the Red Cross, research centers, community activist groups, and private-business interests. The primary focus is on HIV/AIDS policy in its very early phase.

C. Watch the Frontline movie *Sick Around the World* and discuss in class the ways other countries have approached health policy.

D. Watch either or both of the PBS documentaries, *The Great Fever* or *Influenza 1918* and discuss how the United States Public Health System has changed since those times. What role has policy played? How does the "multi-causation model of disease" contribute to our understanding of past health crises like these?

Chapter 4

PUBLIC HEALTH POLICY PROCESSES

Learning Objectives

Upon completion of this chapter, you will be able to:

1. Have a general understanding of public policy in the United States.
2. Better understand the policy-making process.
3. Know more about the legislative and regulatory processes used in public policy.
4. Understand how public health agencies participate in the policy process.
5. Have a basic understanding of policy evaluation.
6. Apply knowledge of policy to the role of public health manager.

Key Terms

advocacy bond

allocate

block grants

categorical grants

outcomes

politics

problem

process measures

public health policy

regulations

stakeholders

Chapter Outline

INTRODUCTION

Public health by its very definition and practice is shaped by public policy. In fact, public health agencies and their funding are established by federal and state policy in the form of legislation. Furthermore, public health organizations are central to the regulatory functions of the government. This is especially evident with the Food and Drug Administration (FDA) and the Department of Health and Human Services (HHS). One of the core functions of public health is policy development, which is often done through the provision of health data and population-based information to policymakers. Furthermore, public health education increasingly requires students to study health policy in order to see the big picture and to understand the constraints and enhancements placed on public health agencies by legislative bodies.

PROCESS OF PUBLIC HEALTH POLICY

public health policy: An attempt by the government at all levels to address a public issue, problem, or concern.

politics: 1) The art or science concerned with guiding or influencing governmental policy. 2) The total complex of relations between people living in a society. 3) Relations or conduct in a particular area of experience, especially as seen or dealt with from a political point of view. 4) In public policymaking, "who gets what, when, and how."

Public health policy is an attempt by the government at all levels to address a public issue, problem, or concern. The government, whether it is city, state, or federal, develops public policy in terms of laws, regulations, codes, decisions, and actions. There are three fundamental parts to public policymaking: problems, stakeholders, and the policy. A fourth dimension, **politics**, is also present and results in a policy process that is dynamic and changeable. Political scientist and scholar Harold Laswell summed up politics as the fight over "who gets what, when, and how."

In public policy, what is referred to as the **problem** is the issue that needs to be addressed, such as clean water. The **stakeholders** are the affected individuals or communities along with those who are influential in forming a plan to address the

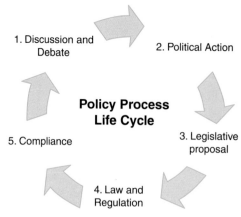

FIGURE 4-1 Public Policy Life Cycles
Source: NIH, National Library of Medicine

problem: An issue that needs to be addressed.

stakeholders: 1) Any individual or group that might be affected by the outcome of something. All decisions have their stakeholders. 2) The affected individuals or communities along with those who are influential in forming a plan to address the problem in question.

problem in question, such as a city. Policy is the finalized course of action decided upon by the government, perhaps in the form of a clean water ordinance. In most cases, policies are widely open to interpretation by nongovernmental players, including those in the private sector. This often leads to the infusion of *politics* before the policy is formulated and after it is implemented. As such, most public policies have a life cycle, as shown in Figure 4-1, and are subject to modification as events and opinions change.

LEGISLATIVE POLICY PROCESS

There are three general categories of public policy in the United States: social, economic, and foreign policy. As can be seen in the examples provided earlier in the section on development of public health policy, it often spans all three domains. This was especially evident in the evolution of policy for food safety with a series of over 200 laws and the establishment of the Food and Drug Administration (FDA) and disease control through municipal ordinances, state and federal laws, and the establishment of the Centers for Disease Control and Prevention (CDC). Both domains, food and disease, cross all three public policy arenas: social, economic, and foreign. Food security is now seen as part of national security, and the economics of food continues to shape health behavior. Likewise disease control, with the emergence of pandemics and the possibility of bioterrorism, spans all three policy arenas with issues such as the economic impact of disease, geopolitics of disease, and the many social justice implications of health disparities associated with disease.

> "The protection and promotion of the health and welfare of its citizens is considered to be one of the most important functions of the modern state."—*George Rosen, Public Health Scholar and Medical Historian*

Given the complexity of public health, it is not surprising that making public policy can be a long and arduous process. Each step requires a significant amount of human resources, expertise, time, and debate, and the five-step process can become a struggle of differing opinions, unforeseen complications, and changes in priorities. The five basic steps, shown in Figure 4-2 are:

1. Identify a problem

2. Draft a policy

3. Enact the policy

4. Execute the policy

5. Assess the policy

The first step of policymaking is to identify a problem. Problems can be identified by individuals and brought to the government's attention, or sometimes lobbyists representing special interests lobby for new policies. Issues can even be identified from executive branches of government, perhaps by the President or a governor, and turned over to Congress or legislature for a resolution. However the issue is identified, policymakers need to consider how many people are or will be affected, whether or not a policy interferes with anyone's civil or human rights, and, increasingly, the economic impact of enacting a given policy.

Once the problem has been identified, a policy must be drafted. Our government is structured so that, ideally, public opinion has a heavy influence on the formulation of policies. Individuals appeal to their members of Congress to vote for or against a policy. The public also influences and is influenced by media campaigns designed to sway public opinion one way or another. Before a policy is complete, relevant experts weigh in and attempt to create a reasonable, actionable policy that takes into account multiple sides of the issue.

Once a policy has been created, the next step is to vote on it. Legislators vote to decide if a policy will become law. Once a policy is enacted, the government must determine the best ways to implement or execute the new policy.

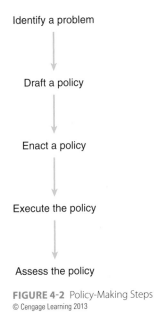

FIGURE 4-2 Policy-Making Steps
© Cengage Learning 2013

After a policy has been enacted for some time, it is assessed for its effectiveness. Data is gathered and research is conducted to evaluate the outcome of the policy's implementation.

Usually the individuals and communities affected by the policy are involved in the process. Community-based participatory research is one tool that is used by the Centers for Disease Control and Prevention (CDC) while comparative effectiveness research is advocated by the Center for Medicaid Administration (CMA).

If the outcomes of enacting and implementing a policy are somewhat different from what was expected, adjustments or amendments can be made, or, if the policy proves to be completely ineffective, it can be done away with altogether. Policymaking is not a perfect process, and laws often need to be fine-tuned and changed over many years. By retracing the history of public health policy discussed earlier, many examples of this change and evolution can be seen.

Another legislative process that needs to be understood is how a proposed bill eventually becomes law. A description of this process and its attributes are provided in Table 4-1, How a Bill Becomes a Law.

TABLE 4-1 How a Bill Becomes Law

Step 1: A Bill Is Born

Anyone may draft a bill; however, only members of Congress can introduce legislation and, by doing so, become the sponsor(s). The president, a member of the cabinet, or the head of a federal agency can also *propose* legislation, but a member of Congress must introduce it.

Step 2: Committee Action

As soon as a bill is introduced, it is referred to a committee. At this point, the bill is examined carefully and its chances for passage are first determined. If the committee does not act on a bill, the bill is effectively "dead."

Step 3: Subcommittee Review

Often, bills are referred to a subcommittee for study and hearings. Hearings provide the opportunity to put on the record the views of the executive branch, other public officials and supporters, experts, and opponents of the legislation.

Step 4: Markup

When the hearings are completed, the subcommittee may meet to "mark up" the bill, that is, make changes and amendments prior to recommending the bill to the full committee. If a subcommittee votes not to report legislation to the full committee, the bill dies. If the committee votes for the bill, it is sent to the floor.

(Continues)

TABLE 4-1 How a Bill Becomes Law *(Continued)*

Step 5: Committee Action to Report a Bill

After receiving a subcommittee's report on a bill, the full committee votes on its recommendation to the House or Senate. This procedure is called "ordering a bill reported."

Step 6: Voting

After the debate and the approval of any amendments, the bill is passed or defeated by the members voting.

Step 7: Referral to Other Chamber

When the House or Senate passes a bill, it is referred to the other chamber, where it usually follows the same route through committee and floor action. This chamber may approve the bill as received, reject it, ignore it, or change it.

Step 8: Conference Committee Action

When the actions of the other chamber significantly alter the bill, a conference committee is formed to reconcile the differences between the House and Senate versions. If the conferees are unable to reach agreement, the legislation dies. If agreement is reached, a conference report is prepared describing the committee members' recommendations for changes. Both the House and Senate must approve the conference report.

Step 9: Final Action

After both the House and Senate have approved a bill in identical form, it is sent to the president. If the president approves of the legislation and signs it, it becomes law. Or, if the president takes no action for 10 days, while Congress is in session, it automatically becomes law. If the president opposes the bill, the president can veto it; or if the president takes no action after the Congress has adjourned its second session, it is a "pocket veto," and the legislation dies.

Step 10: Overriding a Veto

If the president vetoes a bill, Congress may attempt to override the veto. If both the Senate and the House pass the bill by a two-thirds majority, the president's veto is overruled, and the bill becomes a law.

Source: National Human Genome Research Institute. National Institute of Health: http://www.genome.gov/12513982

AGENCY–LEVEL POLICY PROCESS

Not all policy development and implementation follows the legislative model described above. Often, at the agency level, policy is made to meet legislative mandates of agency goals and objectives. In Part II of this book, descriptions of a large array of federal and state public health organizations are provided, along with many of their strategic goals. These goals and the core mission of the agency must be accomplished within the framework of policy. For example, the CDC was created by Congress to control and prevent disease; this is set by law and federal policy, yet the CDC, in seeking to accomplish its mission, might establish a more specific policy that focuses on HIV/AIDS or seasonal influenza. The agency-level policy sets parameters for resources and timetables that are necessary to effectively carry out the policy's intent.

Agency-level policymaking can be described in three general steps: 1) creating an agenda for a policy; 2) considering various options regarding the policy; and 3) implementing the policy. In the first step, agency representatives meet with government officials or other important individuals to identify the problem and decide what they want to achieve with a policy. Then agency policymakers consider multiple ways to carry out the agenda, ultimately deciding what they believe is the best way to achieve the goals set out in the agenda-creating stage. Finally, the policy is implemented.

Ideally, the policy-making process at the agency level would be purely rational and therefore result in the most effective policies that produce the most good. However, personal, business, political, and financial factors often influence policy-making decisions. Regardless, policies enacted by public health agencies are an essential tool for addressing public health concerns. The example mentioned earlier regarding HIV/AIDS policy is one where there have been many policy stakeholders with varying interests and opinions. Throughout the history of HIV/AIDS policy at the agency level (e.g., the CDC and NIH) the personal and professional differences (i.e., community activists vs. scientists vs. physicians) have often shaped policy agendas and influenced program implementation (i.e., prevention vs. cure).

An example of agency-level policy development and policy advocacy is the approach taken by the Texas Department of State Health Services to promote healthy communities. The policy process is graphically shown and described in Exhibit 4-1.

ADMINISTRATIVE POLICY INSTRUMENTS

The Congress, state, and local legislative bodies use two primary instruments to influence public health. One is through the enactment of law and the second is through taxation. Through law, an agency might be created, such as the Environmental Protection Agency (EPA), to carry out legislative mandates to meet the intent of the law, often by enforcing regulations or providing scientific and technical support. A state-level example would be the Commonwealth Health Insurance Authority established by the Massachusetts legislature in its health reform act, to carry out certain goals of the legislation that pertain to the provision of health insurance for those who cannot afford it. A local example would be the high cigarette tax imposed by the City of New York to discourage smoking, one of its most serious public health hazards. As can be seen in both of these examples, and those presented in the history of public health policy earlier, many policy innovations begin at the local and state level.

Exhibit 4-1   Model of Agency-Level Policy Advocacy

*Texas Healthy Communities
Advocacy and Policy Change*

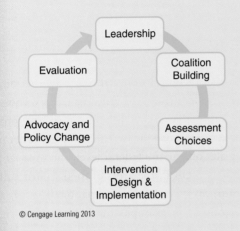

© Cengage Learning 2013

Overview

Policy, environmental, and system change are most challenging:

The potentials for system changes are present and challenging. The lead agency and the partners must remain focused on the importance of their impact on the "map of public health." Each session should incorporate brainstorming, creative activities, concept mapping, one-on-one mentoring, and other forms of organizational development. Using tools that integrate community efforts can result in sustainability and change in policy, environment, and systems.

Communications—Branding and a logo identifies the initiative with credibility:

Internal and external communications are crucial to a healthy community initiative. Creating a marketing guide helps to articulate the coalition's goals and activities to the public as well as bring awareness and notification that system change is in the making. Mapping the coalition's goals and strategies internally provides motivation and purpose to the partners' efforts. Public display of the coalition's progress acknowledges contributions, fosters further commitment, and recruits community involvement. Regular monthly meetings, e-mails, news releases, newsletters, and public media coverage keep the project on the public radar.

Legislative relationships can be very useful in moving system change forward:

Engaging a local legislator with special interests in your issues can become a way to identify a champion for the cause. Learning to write reports, briefs, and correspondence with legislators and their aides helps to put your organization and its issues on their radar. Be well versed in the language of advocacy.

Source: Texas Department of Health Services. Retrieved from http://www.dshs.state.tx.us/layouts/contentpage.aspx?pageid=8589952058&id=8589947295&terms=Texas+Healthy+Communities+Advocacy+and+Policy+Change

"Medicine is a social science, and politics is nothing else but medicine on a large scale."—*Rudolf Virchow, German Physician and Anthropologist*

Public health organizations do not have the same authority to enact law and impose taxes, so they must use a different set of policy instruments to accomplish their goals. Glen Mays, a health policy scholar at the University of Arkansas, School of Public Health, describes four broad categories that a range of administrative policy instruments fall into:

- Regulatory Development and Enforcement
- Health Resource Allocation
- Information Production and Dissemination
- Policy Advocacy and Agenda Setting

Regulation

Public organizations receive their regulatory power either through legislation, as described above, or through executive order (from the President, Governor, or Mayor). Often this authority involves a directive to establish administrative procedures and an infrastructure to enforce **regulations**—a law, rule, or other order prescribed by authority—specified in legislation. At the federal level, the most active areas of public health regulatory activities occur in the areas of food security, drug and medical device development, transportation safety, occupational health and safety, and environmental health protection. For example, the FDA requires rigorous scientific proof of the safety and efficacy of pharmaceutical products before they can be distributed to the general population. The FDA also requires labeling of food products so individuals can be aware of contents that might be harmful or helpful to their health. At the state level, the most active areas of public health regulation have to do with health professions licensure, health services and facilities, public safety, and environmental safety. Local-level regulations by cities and counties vary considerably, as there are over 3,000 local governments in the United States. More about these entities and their roles will be discussed in Chapter 6, "Federal Sector Public Health Agencies."

regulations: A law, rule, or other order prescribed by authority.

Allocation

allocate: To apportion for a specific purpose or to particular persons or things.

categorical grants: A grant that can be used only for specific, narrowly defined activities; grants that are very specific and targeted at selected public health programs and population groups.

block grants: A grant distributed in accordance with a statutory formula for use in a variety of activities within a broad functional area, largely at the recipient's discretion; grants that are allocated more broadly, with activities determined more by the grant recipient.

Most federal public health programs are not carried out through providing public health services directly, but rather through financial and technical support provided to state and local public health organizations. Federal agencies, which receive their funding from Congress, are empowered to **allocate**, or set apart for a particular purpose, funds to public health programs in states, cities, communities, universities, and voluntary health organizations by providing grants. The grants have strict conditions that must be met, and they are monitored by the federal agencies. Some grants are very specific and targeted at selected public health programs and population groups: These are called **categorical grants**. Other grants are allocated more broadly, with activities determined more by the grant recipient: These are called **block grants**. All block grants are given by the agency to the state governments, which are charged with distributing funds appropriately to specific programs, providers, and organizations. The categorical grants give more control over public health funds to federal agencies than do block grants, which allow the states greater discretion. Block grants are often given in such areas as child and maternal health, mental health, substance abuse, and migrant health. An example of a large categorical grant area is the provision of funds to the states for the purchase of health services for low-income families (e.g., Medicaid). There are also grants given to universities, on a competitive basis, for research and health professions training.

Information

All major federal health organizations have some type of research unit. Many are heavily engaged in research, such as the National Institutes of Health (NIH), the CDC, and the Agency for Health Care Research and Quality (AHRQ). Activities of these and other federal agencies include basic and social research, surveillance, and policy studies that produce information for dissemination. Often the agency will partner with universities and the private sector in both research and dissemination. In fact, states depend heavily on federally generated data to inform policy and make decisions about how best to structure public health programs and initiatives. It has often been said that "information is power," and it certainly is a powerful instrument of public health policy. Not only is information used to focus research, promote health, and inform policy, it is also an important tool to draw attention to an emerging or dormant public health issue. One example of this is workshops and conferences sponsored by NIH or CDC to convene important public health stakeholders and researchers around an issue such as tobacco use or obesity.

Advocacy

While federal and state agencies do not have any formal legislative authority, as specified in the Constitution's separation of powers doctrine, they do play an important role in the legislative process. This is primarily in the form of providing information and influence to place public health issues on the legislative agenda. Sometimes agencies are even asked by legislators to design model policies for consideration. They also provide an important counterbalance to information given to legislators by lobbyist and professional associations seeking to shape policy in the directions they prefer. When an agency, a legislative body, and a professional group reach consensus on a public health issue and what needs to be done to address it, a strong **advocacy bond** is formed that typically assures the policy's success. In political science this is called an "Iron Triangle" because it is so formidable, and is detailed in Figure 4-3.

The American Public Health Association (APHA) has developed a set of advocacy recommendations or tips for public health leaders. Public health leaders can help empower constituents to be policy advocates in various ways, such as:

- building trust and credibility with community constituents;

- empowering others to be advocates for public health;

advocacy bond: When an agency, a legislative body, and a professional group reach consensus on a public health issue and what needs to be done to address it.

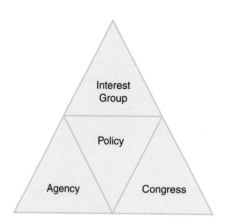

FIGURE 4-3 The "Iron Triangle" that is Vital to Advocacy Goals and Achievement
© Cengage Learning 2013

- providing data and background research on health issues;

- drafting policy statements in the language of legislative bills or municipal ordinances; and

- working with elected officials on legislation and regulations.

AGENDA SETTING FOR PUBLIC HEALTH

A good example of agenda setting by a federal agency is the *Healthy People 2020* report released by the U.S. Department of Health and Human Services, which informs Congress and state legislators, universities, professional associations, foundations, and a wide array of public health organizations and advocates.

The fundamental framework for the Healthy People agenda is to:

- Establish national health objectives.

- Provide data and tools to enable states, cities, communities, and individuals across the country to combine their efforts to achieve them.

Another example of how the policy "iron triangle" can shape policy can be seen in the formation of the Affordable Care Act. President Obama led the effort and promoted it to the public and key interest groups such as the American Medical Association (AMA), American Hospital Association (AHA), American Nurses Association (ANA), Association for the Advancement of Retired People (AARP), and many others. Within Congress there were key committees involved in drafting the legislation and reconciling differences between the two chambers, the Senate and House of Representatives. Furthermore, federal agencies were centrally involved, especially the Department of Health and Human Services (HHS) headed by Secretary Kathleen Sebelius, a former Governor and state Insurance Commissioner for Kansas.

The role of HHS in drafting key elements of the legislation for consideration by the President and Congress is shown in Exhibit 4-2.

Exhibit 4-2   Role of Department of Health and Human Services in 2010 Health Reform Legislation

With the Affordable Care Act, HHS has an opportunity to improve the health of millions of Americans. As the principal federal agency in charge of improving Americans' health and implementing the Affordable Care Act, HHS will seek to drive down costs, put more money in the hands of the American people, and ensure all Americans receive the health care services they need and deserve. These actions will increase transparency, eliminate waste, and put Americans back in charge of their health care.

- *Make Coverage More Secure for Those Who Have Insurance; Extend Affordable Coverage to the Uninsured*
  HHS will enroll eligible children and hard-to-serve populations in health insurance programs; make coverage more stable and secure through insurance market reforms; and establish health insurance exchanges that allow individuals and small businesses to compare plans, buy insurance at affordable prices, and access subsidized health insurance coverage.

- *Reduce Health Care Costs while Promoting High-Value, Effective Care*
  HHS will strengthen program integrity efforts that combat Medicare, Medicaid, and CHIP fraud, waste, and abuse; move Medicare to a system that rewards efficient, effective care and reduces delivery system fragmentation; better align Medicare reimbursement rates with provider costs; and encourage widespread adoption and meaningful use of health information technology while ensuring the privacy and security of electronic health records.

- *Emphasize Primary Care, Prevention, and Wellness*
  HHS will establish Medicare and Medicaid payment and delivery system policies that value primary care and promote prevention and wellness; develop programs that expand the primary care workforce and encourage health care providers to practice in health professional shortage areas; and promote healthy lifestyles, emotional health, and evidence-based disease prevention programs.

- *Improve Health Care Quality and Patient Safety*
  HHS will support patient-centered research; implement payment reforms that reward quality care and reduce health care-associated infections; and institute delivery system reforms that encourage care coordination and improved patient outcomes.

- *Ensure Access to Quality, Culturally Competent Care for Vulnerable Populations*
  HHS will institute policies that encourage care management for patients eligible for both Medicare and Medicaid and patients with chronic illnesses; reduce disparities associated with patients' gender, race, ethnicity, and socioeconomic status; ensure parity for mental and substance use disorders in health insurance; improve early detection and treatment of mental and substance use disorders; and promote coordinated, evidence-based care for individuals with behavioral health issues.

- *Promote Community Living*
  HHS will improve the accessibility and quality of health and support services to enable people with disabilities and seniors with impaired functioning to live in community settings.

Source: U.S. Department of Health and Human Services. Retrieved from http://www.hhs.gov

PUBLIC HEALTH POLICY EVALUATION

Writing for the *American Journal of Public Health*, Kass has provided a framework for the ethical analysis of public health policy and programs. This is designed to advance traditional public health goals while maximizing individual liberties and further social justice. This six-step model was advocated in Ivanov and Blue's *Public Health Nursing Leadership, Policy, and Practice* and is shown in Exhibit 4-3.

Exhibit 4-3   Ethical Framework for Public Health Policy Analysis

1. *What are the public health goals of the proposed program?* Program goals should be expressed in terms of public health improvement (i.e., the reduction of morbidity or mortality). Even though more specific goals may be formulated, for example, that the participants of a health education program will learn a certain amount of information, the ultimate goal of decreased morbidity and mortality must be in view. The program may also be part of a group of interventions that share in reaching the ultimate public health goal.

2. *How effective is the program in achieving its stated goals?* The program must be based on the belief that it will achieve its stated goals. For example, health education programs may be effective in transmitting information, but the recipients show little or no behavioral change. It is important that the outcomes of public health programs are evaluated to ensure that the desired changes have occurred and that these changes have had an effect on the morbidity and mortality of the target group. Again, the proposed program may be part of a group of programs that have the same ultimate goal.

3. *What are the known or potential burdens of the program?* Public health programs may involve a number of burdens or harms, but most cluster into three main categories: risks to privacy and confidentiality, particularly in data collection; risks to liberty and self-determination, especially in public health activities designed to contain the spread of disease; and risks to justice, often seen when public health interventions are targeted only to certain groups with the risk of stigmatization. There may be physical risks as well. For example, mandatory immunization programs may impose health risks to individuals or spraying to prevent mosquito-borne viruses may endanger individuals who are sensitive to the chemicals being sprayed.

4. *Can burdens be minimized? Are there alternative approaches?* Those who propose public health programs are obligated to seek to lessen burdens and harms once they are identified in step 3. Contact tracing in sexually transmitted infections programs is routine; however, this practice may pose a threat to confidentiality and privacy. Yet, contact tracing is voluntary; there are no penalties for

Continues

those who refuse to participate. Therefore, public health professionals have an ethical obligation to inform individuals of their right to refuse to disclose the names of their sexual partners or to contact their partners themselves. In addition, if more than one alternative exists to meet a public health goal, public health professionals are required ethically to choose the alternative that poses the fewest risks to moral concerns such as liberty, privacy, or justice, while not compromising the benefits of the program

5. *Is the program implemented fairly?* This question determines whether or not the demands of distributive justice are satisfied in the fair distribution of the benefits and burdens of the proposed program. This aspect is of vital importance if the program includes restrictive measures. Social harms can result if stereotypes are created or perpetuated such as the notion that certain population groups are more vulnerable to sexually transmitted infections or domestic violence. This problem may be intensified if other population groups use such stereotyping to come to the erroneous belief that they are at little or no risk because they do not fit the risk profile.

Another issue is whether public health professionals have an ethical obligation to right existing social injustices, such as poverty or hunger, that have an adverse effect on the public's health.

6. *How can the benefits and burdens of a program be fairly balanced?* After the first five steps of the framework have been addressed, a decision must be made as to whether the expected benefits of the proposed program will justify the identified burdens. Inevitably, there will be disagreements over the potential burdens and benefits inherent in the details of a particular program. For instance, taxpayers may focus on the financial burdens of a clean water program that may benefit future generations, while public health professionals see only its benefits. Procedural justice requires that a fair process of decision making is used to resolve such disagreements. This process must seek a balance between communal interests and the liberty rights of individuals, realizing that some infringements on individual liberty are unavoidable. Democratic processes and open hearings can help to ensure that minority positions are presented and considered.

"There are those that look at things the way they are, and ask why? I dream of things that never were, and ask why not?"—*Robert Kennedy, United States Senator and Attorney General*

The Centers for Disease Control and Prevention (CDC) employ a multi-stage policy-evaluation process that is also used to evaluate programs that result from implementation of public policy. These programs are designed to carry out the intent of the public policy and must be evaluated to ensure the intent is being met and in a timely, cost effective manner. Figure 4-4 shows the framework for policy evaluation, and Exhibit 4-4 describes how CDC adapts this to the evaluation of its programs by focusing on both outcomes and processes.

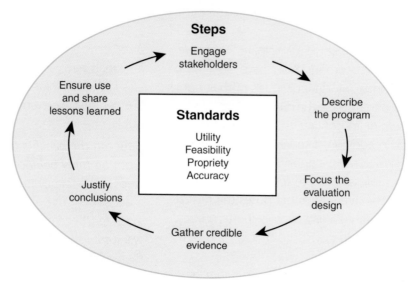

FIGURE 4-4 CDC Evaluation Process
Source: Centers for Disease Control and Prevention (CDC)

Exhibit 4-4   CDC Evaluation Process

Defining the Program and Forming the Evaluation:

In the framework's early steps, it is important to define the program in sufficient detail so that those conducting the evaluation can engage key stakeholders, identify their preferences and needs, and use that information to decide which parts of the program must be evaluated to determine if the activity is worth continuing or improving. A series of questions are part of these tasks:

- What is the "program"? (What are the key activities of the program and what are the key outcomes it aspires to achieve?)
- What is the larger "environment" of the program? (What resources are available to conduct the activities? What elements of the larger context or situation might help or hinder program success?)
- What aspects of the program will be considered by decision makers (i.e., senior leaders) when judging program performance? (e.g., Quality implementation of activities? Achieving outcomes? Which outcomes?)

- What benchmarks (e.g., type or level of performance), if any, must these activities or outcomes reach for the program to be considered successful?
- What kinds of evidence on performance are most credible to key decision makers in making judgments about how the program has performed?
- How will the lessons learned from the inquiry be used? (e.g., To help improve program effectiveness in the next round? To make a decision on program continuation?)

Evaluate Both Outputs and Outcomes over Time:

Clearly, these questions encompass both program implementation and program effectiveness. Either can be the focus of a given evaluation, but usually aspects of both need to be addressed. Ideally, evaluation planning has been integrated with implementation planning, and it is a simple task to identify the main processes (e.g., activities or outputs) employed by the program as well as the intended short-term and long-term

Continues

outcomes (sometimes reflected in the goals and objectives) for the planned programs.

Process Measures:

Process measures examine all the steps and activities taken in implementing a program and the outputs they generate, such as the number and type of educational materials for a stress management class that are developed and given to employees. They are useful for keeping implementation of the program on track and also for determining if program implementation met the quality and other standards to which the program aspired. This is important so that, if a program does not achieve its intended outcomes, it can be determined if the program was the wrong approach or if it was a strong program that simply was not implemented correctly. Process measures also can assess issues such as the costs of operating a program, the numbers of employees reached, the most successful program locations, or comparisons of the program's design and activities to others.

Outcome Measures:

Outcomes are events or conditions that indicate program effectiveness. They generally are displayed as short-, intermediate-, or long-term. Long-term measures, in the context of workplace health promotion, typically relate to things like reductions in disease or injury and the costs associated with them. These are often similar to the goals of

process measures: Examine all the steps and activities taken in implementing a program and the outputs they generate.

outcomes: Events or conditions that indicate program effectiveness.

the program and these long-term outcomes often take years to observe.

Short- and intermediate-term measures, by contrast, relate to the intermediate steps and "drivers" necessary to achieve the long-term outcomes, such as individual employee reductions in healthy lifestyle risks like tobacco use, or process changes such as implementing a new health-related policy or benefit at the organizational level that supports lifestyle changes.

Whatever program components have been included in the evaluation, it is important that they be both measurable and realistic. "Measureable" means that the activity or outcome has been phrased in a way that lends itself to data collection. "Realistic" means that the outcomes are ones which a well-implemented intervention can be reasonably expected to produce. When goals or outcomes are unrealistic it is often because: 1) the program has not been in place long enough to produce the outcome of interest, or 2) the program simply is not broad or intense enough to produce it.

Finally, once the key outcomes have been identified and written as measureable and realistic, identify when each will be measured (e.g., every 6 months, every 12 months, etc.), assign this tracking responsibility to a specific individual, and require regular reports. Some outcomes may be measured only early or late in the program while others may be measured several times for as long as the program is active.

Source: U.S. Department of Health and Human Services, Centers for Disease Control and Prevention (CDC). Retrieved from http://www.cdc.gov

Summary

While much can be done at the organizational and community level to address public health challenges, many issues and problems are so large and difficult that policy instruments such as law and regulation must be used. Policy is one domain of public health that is heavily infused with politics and for the most part takes place in a political context. Thus an understanding of the political process and related influences is critical to know how policy works and how it is changed over time. The public health community is actively engaged in policy formulation and implementation and also plays a major role in advocacy for the benefit of the public at large.

The following case studies in Chapter 16, "Cases in Public Health Management," are directly related to concepts and principles presented in this chapter:

- Case 3: The Anti-Vaccination Paradigm
- Case 14: Collaborative Approach to Diabetes Prevention and Care
- Case 16: Healthy Lifestyles Start at Home
- Case 17: Top Ten U.S. Public Health Achievements
- Case 19: Smoking Cessation Program Implementation
- Case 21: Community Coalitions and the Built Environment

Public Health Leader Perspective

Teresa C. Long, MD, M.P.H., Health Commissioner, Columbus, Ohio

Dr. Teresa C. Long became the first female Health Commissioner for Columbus in 2002. Prior to this appointment, she served as Medical Director and Assistant Health Commissioner for the Columbus Health Department from 1986 until 2002. Before coming to Columbus, Dr. Long served on the front lines of the emerging AIDS epidemic as a physician specialist with the San Francisco Department of Public Health. She conducted her preventive medicine residency with the California Department of Health Services where she developed perinatal AIDS guidelines. Dr. Long is a Clinical Associate Professor at the Ohio State University of College of Medicine and Public Health. She was the first recipient of the Elizabeth Blackwell Award for Pioneering Efforts to Improve Women's and Community Health. She holds a Doctor of Medicine Degree from the University of California, San Francisco and a Master of Public Health from the University of California, Berkeley.

Interview by Scott Musch

Continues

(Q): Tell us about your position as Health Commissioner for Columbus Public Health.

Dr. Long: I have the privilege of serving as Health Commissioner for the residents and visitors of Columbus which may swell to a million plus in any given day. In that job, my role is to work with many professionals to create the support and conditions in which all of our residents and visitors can be healthy, safe, and achieve their optimal health. As you may have recognized, my background is as a medical doctor, so I think of my patient base as being the roughly one million residents and visitors. Columbus is now the sixteenth largest city in the country, so it takes more than just me but many people to orchestrate, coordinate, and oversee the overall public health programming. We try to get as many residents themselves, stakeholders, partners, and all of our health care organizations aligned in a similar direction to promote health, safety, and well-being in everybody's lives.

(Q): What are your main responsibilities?

Dr. Long: Part of my responsibility is being a leader, coordinator, and spokesperson for all kinds of health issues. You may have realized that as soon as anyone thinks they have a really big problem, they call it a public health issue, so it is quite amazing to see the diversity of issues that come our way. My direct responsibilities involve leading and managing a comprehensive set of public health programs and services that make up the Columbus Public Health organization. These include many traditional public health services and then some that are broader than what non-metropolitan health departments would likely consider. For instance, we have traditional services such as a large environmental health division that covers food, air, and water. We have 8,000 licensees that we work within all kinds of areas. When thinking of public health, people typically think of food and water, but they might not think of tattoo parlors, hazardous materials, and working with the fire department to respond to emergencies or evacuations. We are concerned about all types of animal diseases as well, including rabies. We have a very large area that focuses on infectious and communicable diseases. Influenza is a really big issue now. We would like to think that we have been really smart and protected everyone with vaccines, but we have seen many of these communicable diseases come roaring back and become big issues in our community and across the country. Tuberculosis is another good example.

We have a responsibility, as part of our protectionist role, to monitor the 86 reportable diseases in Ohio that must be reported to the local health department. We take those reports and investigate all of them. We then pass them to our state health department who then passes them to the CDC. Through a lens that starts at the community level we get a good picture of what issues are being faced across the country. We also have a large group focused on the health of women and children, and reducing infant mortality. Infant mortality is a leading indicator in the world of the well-being of any country, state, or community, because it is such a broad indicator of social, environmental, and health conditions, so we spend a lot of time and energy trying to understand and address why infants are being born too early or dying before their first birthday here in Columbus. In addition, we have a community health group where a lot of our systems-work is focused. In community health, we have a variety of programs in alcohol and drug treatment, addictions, dental services, and connections with our partners to provide primary care. Our free clinic partner acts as a springboard to many in our community who are having trouble making ends meet, to try to springboard them into the help and health care system. Our final area of responsibility is in planning, which houses much of our systems-coordination work. We work with a lot of different systems and work directly with residents to understand what it is they are facing and how we can address those issues. We focus on how we can direct others as we do not do this work alone, it involves partnerships.

Continues

(Q): It sounds like you have adopted a systems thinking approach.

Dr. Long: Absolutely. Systems thinking has become one of the clearest competencies for public health workers and especially for public health managers and leaders. We have got to think systems-wide as there will never be enough resources in any one organization to take on a problem and handle it alone. The reality is we live in systems. We are very focused on thinking about the environment in which we can create these conditions in which people are healthy. The way we think about it now is that it really matters where we live, where we learn, where we work, and where we play. This is a framework for how we think about many of the current issues we face, whether it be obesity, health disparities, or chronic diseases. We have got to take on this systems work because, for instance, we are not experts in housing, but I can assure you that housing policy is health policy. The same is true of education. Schools really matter. We have got to be both smarter and more strategic in addressing these structural determinants of health.

(Q): How many years have you worked in public health?

Dr. Long: I have been connected to public health for about 30 years. I came to it, believe it or not, from a background of marine biology from my undergraduate and some of my graduate work. This is one of those good examples of how people come to public health from so many different directions. I ended up in medical school to get a Ph.D., but found I liked medicine and continued in medical school and residency in San Francisco.

(Q): Why did you choose to go into the field of public health?

Dr. Long: I did my clinical training in pediatrics. This is where I had one of those "transformation" experiences. My experience was that I spent too much time in intensive care nurseries caring for gravely ill infants and their families, who needed all sorts of care. I kept thinking that there has to be a better way for me to try to keep people out of this situation that was so devastating and resource intensive. I actually went back to school and got a Master's degree in Public Health and my thesis was on this issue—the cost of intensive-care nurseries, looking at both the resource cost and the epidemiology of who ended up in the intensive-care nurseries. It was really the experience of realizing that I wanted to keep people healthy. My real interest was in how we could preserve and promote the good health or at least optimal health that we each have.

(Q): What are the most rewarding aspects about your job in public health?

Dr. Long: It's very exciting, it's constant intellectual stimulation, thinking about how can we, and how can I, think of a better, faster, less resource-intensive way to help people stay healthier, eat healthier, and be safer. It is very different work from illness diagnosis and the "sick-care" system we have in this country. It is equally or more challenging to think about the tools and approaches, which are very broad, that are available at the community level. There is both art and science, not only medical science but also sciences such as psychology and economics. It really requires intellectual rigor to not go down paths that are not likely to be fruitful. It involves promoting and protecting health, as well as communicating. These are some of the areas I would have never thought about originally. I'm now running a large business of 450 to 500 employees. I'm committed to a very clear return on investment and I spend a lot of my time communicating in many different ways, in many different venues. These are essential tools that you were never taught in medical school.

Continues

(Q): What are some of the biggest management challenges you face as a leader in public health and within your organization?

Dr. Long: I have been very fortunate in retaining and recruiting talented staff that are committed and come from a variety of backgrounds. That being said, I think some of the biggest challenges are resources—the right human resources, amount of resources, and financial resources. It is also connected to the resource challenges that our population is facing, because frankly some of the biggest challenges involve a population that isn't well educated, doesn't read at a high level, has trouble paying their bills, has multiple jobs, and has high stress levels. All of these are such huge issues in our community, and across the country, that challenge people's health and well-being every day.

Next, I think that people don't understand public health and so a major challenge is that if you don't understand it, you tend not to resource it appropriately. You won't have a broader understanding of systems work. I think it's very American that we tend to find one problem and try to resolve that, and as a result, we have created five others. It's being able to step back and think about the systems issues and how do we collectively think about how we are going to approach something. These issues about the environment and systems really matter, again, where we live, work, learn, and play. Systems work is hard work. It takes a long time to see results in some cases. We are very concerned right here in Columbus about global climate change and what that is going to mean with infectious diseases, food, and nutrition not only across the globe, but here in Columbus as well. It's a challenge for us to show to our investors, so to speak, the return on investments when so many of us connected to health care are used to touching the elephant on patient care. Having people understand the difference is important.

(Q): What future trends do you see shaping the field of public health as a career opportunity?

Dr. Long: There are more people learning about public health—I'm not sure if they are going to call it public health, but rather prevention. People are going to be involved in prevention work, population-based work, and community work at every level. All of this is public health, so there will be many opportunities connected to prevention. People really need to have a diverse background and a real understanding of systems thinking, as well as have expertise in some content area, whether the health sciences, economics, or social and behavioral sciences, all of which are going to be really important fields for public health in the future. I think the opportunities are going to be increasingly in the private and nonprofit sectors, both locally, nationally, and around the globe. Medical education is still very focused on diagnosis and intervention, and I understand why. But there is so much further we can go. Like in so many other areas, governmental work is not where change will happen first, but rather it will be in the private sector. It is so interesting to watch the population-based health initiatives that are coming out of insurance companies and now coming out of employers. The opportunities are vast.

(Q): What advice would you have for anyone interested in entering the field of public health?

Dr. Long: There really is a place for everyone who has an interest in public health, who have diverse backgrounds and interests. I would encourage people—find out what makes you tick and what your passions are. Sometimes it takes time to do that, but learn all you can while you do it. The course work in public health is broad for a good reason. It is a very broad-level science and art, and there is a theory behind it. It is important to take those practical opportunities in schooling, internships, or even in early jobs to put that theory into practice and learn on the job. Keep open to possibilities. Learn all you can and try to create value in yourself that will be useful to an employer. Be open to the possibility that the area you thought you might start in might not be [where you begin]. It is about connecting your specific interests and talents with the possibilities.

End

Discussion and Review Questions

1. Identify and discuss any policy from the previous chapter and describe how it applies today. How might the policy processes described have been used to develop and implement the policy you are discussing?

2. Discuss the Affordable Care Act and identify its major elements.

3. Describe the public policy life-cycle and discuss why it is important to understand.

4. What is meant by an "iron triangle"? Give an example at the federal level. Give an example at the state level.

5. What are the five basic steps in making policy?

6. Discuss administrative policy instruments and explain why they are useful in public health.

7. Briefly describe how a bill becomes a law. Give a recent example.

8. Describe the steps in the policy evaluation process. What are some ethical considerations?

9. If you were in Dr. Long's position (refer to interview), what elements of the policy process discussed in this chapter might be helpful to you? Explain and discuss.

Action Learning and Critical Thinking

A. Using the Affordable Care Act and Internet web-searches, do the following: 1) describe the political context of the legislation; 2) identify any "iron triangles" that helped support the policy or that served as a barrier to the policy; 3) identify any "administrative instruments" that have been used to advance the policy and its goals.

B. Watch the movie *Contagion* and discuss your observations about policy-in-action within the federal, state, and local government sectors represented in the film.

C. Watch the movie *Money Driven Medicine* and discuss in class the various policy implications and challenges that are evident.

D. Identify a public health policy that has affected you on a personal level and do an online search to better understand the intent and purpose of the policy. Has this made your life better? Safer? Worse? How so? What changes in the policy would you recommend to the Congress or legislature?

PART II

PUBLIC HEALTH AGENCIES AND ORGANIZATIONS

The four chapters in this section provide a descriptive overview of organizations at every level of public health including local, state, national, and global. Many agencies are described, as are their primary functions and missions. Furthermore, the structure and functions of organizations in general are discussed in order to facilitate an understanding of the centrality of organizations in the public health arena. Specifically, public sector and nonprofit organizations are highlighted, as are the responsibilities a manager has in these organizations.

Chapter 5

STRUCTURE AND FUNCTIONS OF ORGANIZATIONS

Learning Objectives

Upon completion of this chapter, you should be able to:

1. Define important terms pertaining to organizations.
2. Identify and describe the functions of organizations.
3. Understand the organization as a complex system.
4. Be knowledgeable about the unique role and challenges of public organizations.
5. Be aware of public-sector values as they apply to organizations.
6. Better understand the organizational environment.

Key Terms

adaptation	maintenance	organizational culture
boundary spanning	management	production
governance	organization	sustainability

Chapter Outline

INTRODUCTION

Public health managers work in and with organizations. The organizational setting is one that must be understood for the public health manager to be effective. This chapter addresses many of the basics needed to understand what organizations are, how they function, what values are important, and what role the manager has in all of this. The complex nature of organizations as changing systems is also explored with the added need to approach organizational management from a sustainability framework.

ORGANIZATIONS DEFINED

organization: A structured social system consisting of groups and individuals working together to meet agreed-upon objectives.

Our understanding of organizations comes through many lenses. While everyone has a mental model drawn from their own experience with organizations, it is important to avoid ambiguity by providing a commonly accepted formal definition. As described by Greenberg and Baron in *Organizational Behavior*, an **organization** is a structured social system consisting of groups and individuals working together to meet agreed-upon objectives. Thus organizations consist of people who strive to attain common goals. Johnson's book *Health Organizations* traces the history of organizations and asserts that as long as there have been human endeavors, there have been people engaged in organizing. This inclination probably grew out of a need for survival in the hostile world of early humankind where food, shelter, and safety required some form of cooperation. In nature itself, we see evidence of organization. Thus it was not unlikely for early organizers in small groups to observe and mimic important lessons from their surrounding environment. Some of the basics might have included forming encampments on high ground for safety from floods, organizing daily life near a water source for sustenance, or banding together in groups to help build shelter and to share the burdens of work.

Theoretical biologist Ludwig von Bertalanffy developed the *general system theory* which helped to explain the phenomenon of organization from a biological and social science perspective. This interdisciplinary approach builds on the idea that organizations, like organisms, are open to their environment and must achieve an appropriate relation with that environment if they are to survive. Not only can organisms and organizations be viewed as open systems, they are also best understood as complex adaptive systems. Begun, Zimmerman, and Dooley, in *Advances in Health Care Organization Theory*, tell us that complex adaptive systems are omnipresent in the natural and social world. Examples include stock markets, human bodies, organs and cells, trees, and health clinics. As they state, *complex* implies diversity—a wide range of elements. *Adaptive* suggests the capacity to alter or change—the ability to learn from experience. A *system* is a set of connected or interdependent "things" (i.e., person, molecule, cell, etc.). Furthermore, complex adaptive systems like organizations are characterized by their dynamic state due to the many feedback loops that inform them. For the health clinic a feedback loop that leads to change and adaptation might come in the form of a client survey, an inspection from an outside agency, or suggestions offered by an advisory board member.

ORGANIZATIONS AS COMPLEX SYSTEMS

Suffice it to say, organizations are very complex social systems that interact with their environment in order to respond to feedback and adapt to change. When we look at health organizations specifically, there is a constant tension between the need for predictability, order, and efficiency competing with the need for openness, adaptability, and innovation according to Shortell and Kaluzny. To help better understand this complexity and its associated dynamics, Kettl and Fesler, in *Politics of the Administrative Process*, provide an interesting range of ways to describe organizations. This is summarized below:

- An organization is both a policy-program-decision making set of processes that also involves execution of those policies, programs, and decisions.

- It is both a way of dividing up work and a way of coordinating work.

- It is a formal, prescribed structure of relations among organizational units and an arena for dynamic conflict and expansion of personal power.

- It both persists over time despite changes in personnel and at any single point in time is a particular group of individuals, each with his or her special set of needs and frustrations.

- It is both a top-down system of authority and compliance and a down-up system for the flow of innovative ideas, problem solutions, and improvement opportunities.

- It sometimes involves a headquarters staff and a distant field service, often with challenges to effective linkages.

- It is an information storage and retrieval system and a communication network including informal grapevines.

- Its decision-making process must embrace the broad choices in which the value preferences and educated guesses of elected and politically appointed officials play a large part. It must provide for other choices for which quantified data and scientific evidence inform decisions.

- It looks both inward and outward, having to maintain internal effectiveness and to adapt to the external environment that brings pressures from other organizations, crises within the society, and needs of stakeholders.

- It can be likened to a physical system such as a machine (an outdated metaphor) or a biological system such as a living organism.

- It can be judged successful if it simply survives, or instead it can be so judged only if it achieves its goals.

> "I believe that we have only just begun the process of discovering and inventing the new organizational forms that will inhabit the twenty-first century. To be responsible inventors and discoverers, though, we need the courage to let go of the old world, to relinquish most of what we have cherished, to abandon our interpretations about what does and doesn't work. We must learn to see the world anew."—*Margaret Wheatley, Management Professor and President of The Berkana Institute*

ORGANIZATION FUNCTIONS

Despite this range of perspectives on organizations and their characteristics, the classic and widely accepted work, *The Social Psychology of Organizations*, by Katz and Kahn is used as a foundation for the study of organization in the fields of public administration, business administration, educational administration, and health administration. All organizations, including those involved in public health, have six primary functions: production, boundary spanning, maintenance, adaptation, management, and governance, as presented in Shortell and Kaluzny's *Essentials of Health Care Management*, and a seventh overarching function, sustainability, added by Johnson in *Health Organizations*.

Production

production: An organization's essential product or service.

An organization's **production** is its essential product or service. It is represented by such items as the inspections of a food inspector, the diagnosis and treatment of patients by the staff in a community health clinic, the vaccinations given by a county health department, or the health-promotion brochures developed and produced in a diabetes campaign. The production function can vary in many aspects, including time, cost, knowledge or skills required, resources needed, and many more, depending on the nature of the product.

Boundary Spanning

boundary spanning: An organization's relationship to its external environment.

Boundary spanning refers to an organization's relationship to its external environment. Changes in community expectations, disease patterns, politics, and countless other determinants affect a public health organization's boundary spanning. Other factors such as the organization's size and function help determine its ability to change and its compatibility with outside forces. Many large organizations staff individuals or designate a department whose function is to take on a boundary-spanning role. In other organizations, managers and others in leadership roles are expected to take on boundary-spanning activities.

Maintenance

maintenance: Deals with the aspects (fiscal, physical, human) that need maintenance in some form or another.

The **maintenance** function in an organization deals with the aspects (fiscal, physical, human) that need maintenance in some form or another. It includes securing and maintaining the budget, maintaining and upgrading the physical facilities, and recruiting and training (or retraining) staff. Demands are placed on the maintenance function in response to changes in the external environment.

Adaptation

adaptation: An organization's capacity to change in response to external or internal factors.

An organization's **adaptation** function, as the name suggests, is its capacity to change in response to external or internal factors. The adaptation function uses information from boundary spanning and knowledge from within the organization in order to alter the organization as necessary. This function is vital for the survival of public health organizations because public health is an area of constant change. Adaptation may include changes in the organization's infrastructure, production, or strategy. A critical aspect of the adaptation function is that it emphasizes the organization's ability to innovate.

Management

management: Permeates all other functions and subsystems of the organization. It involves those in charge of all the other functions.

The **management** function permeates all other functions and subsystems of the organization. It involves those in charge of all the other functions. See Figure 5-1 below for a range of activities and responsibilities ascribed to managers in public health and other organizations.

Governance

governance: Holds those within the organization, especially management, accountable. It also governs the organization's direction and guides its actions.

The **governance** function is important because of the need for public trust and social responsibility. The governance function holds those within the organization, especially management, accountable. It also governs the organization's direction and guides its actions. There are many pressures on organizations involved in public health to demonstrate greater accountability in regard to ethics, financial efficiency, effectiveness, and measurable outcomes.

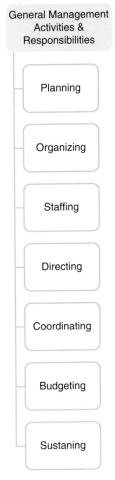

FIGURE 5-1 A General List of Management Activities and Responsibilities That One Might Encounter in a Career in Public Health
© Cengage Learning 2013

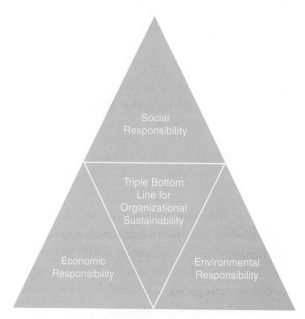

FIGURE 5-2 The "Triple Bottom Line" Is Often Utilized as a Strategy for Sustainability
© Cengage Learning 2013

Sustainability

sustainability: Focuses on the organization's environmental practices in balance with fiscal and social responsibility to assure the long-term success of the organization and its programs.

The **sustainability** function is fairly new for many organizations. It focuses on the organization's environmental practices in balance with fiscal and social responsibility to ensure the long-term success of the organization and its programs. This function helps to ensure that managers and staff make decisions and engage in actions that improve quality of life while also protecting the environment (ecosystem). Within the organization a "triple bottom line" approach is embraced focusing concurrently on financial, social, and environmental responsibility. See Figure 5-2.

DEMANDS ON ORGANIZATIONS

All organizations in the twenty-first century are faced with many competing demands and pressures and must, as social systems, continue to adapt. Kilpatrick and Johnson, in the *Handbook of Health Administration and Policy,* and Johnson, in *Health Organizations,* have discussed various pressures and their associated challenges as they pertain to health organizations. Some of them that are particularly relevant to public health include the following:

- *Increasing complexity and size of organizations.* Health organizations are larger today and often more diversified. The resulting complexity and sometimes over-bureaucratization that emerge serve to isolate employees from both the organization and the environment in which the institution or agency must operate. Managing financial, physical, and human resources efficiently and effectively has become more than just a challenge; it is essential for organizational survival and growth. Rapid growth and demand for public health services result in the need for ongoing improvement and expansion of skills and knowledge for health professionals and managers. There is an increasing amount of specialization required to meet the needs of providing a wide range of services to populations previously underserved.

- *Governments' need to control costs.* At all levels—state, local, and federal—budgets have a direct effect on staff levels and resources needed for program effectiveness. In an era of financial challenges, such as the recent recession, there will be an ever-increasing focus on fiscal responsibility and constraint.

- *Increasing professionalization of the workforce.* Public health occupations require training and education commensurate with their duties. This is especially true for clinicians, scientists, and engineers who must have professional credentials and for technicians and managers who are expected to have education and training.

- *Changing values of the workplace.* The **organizational culture**, the pattern of shared values, beliefs, and norms—along with associated behaviors, symbols, and rituals—that are acquired over time by members of an organization, is expected to support healthy behaviors for its staff and address a greater expectation of rewards, autonomy, and the opportunity to influence the organization. This is especially evident with the current generation of new graduates from colleges and universities.

organizational culture: The pattern of shared values, beliefs, and norms—along with associated behaviors, symbols, and rituals—that are acquired over time by members of an organization.

- *Diversity in the workplace.* There has been a rapid expansion of the multicultural and diverse workforce that reflects the communities being served. Human resource policies and practices must respect differences, many of which, such as age, gender, religion, national origin, ethnicity, sexual orientation, and disability, are protected by law.

ORGANIZATION ENVIRONMENT

The range of conditions and number of external forces are so numerous they cannot all be addressed in any single book. However, in the study of organizations, there are certain general conditions in the organization's environment that can be categorized. Typically these include the following seven conditions:

- Technological
- Legal
- Political
- Economic
- Demographic
- Ecological
- Cultural

Some examples of conditions from each category that potentially could affect public health organizations are included in Table 5-1.

TABLE 5-1 Environmental Conditions of Organizations

- **Technological:** Generally speaking, technological conditions are those that are impacted by knowledge in the fields of science, computers, engineering, and medicine. The technological environment is also impacted by our capacity to communicate, manage, and utilize information in various forms.

- **Legal:** The legal environment is the way in which current laws and regulations affect an organization and its actions.

- **Political:** Political conditions include the form of government, political-party agendas, and policy initiatives of governing officials.

- **Economic:** Wages, taxes, inflation, interest rates, labor costs, and government expenditures make up the economic conditions of an organization.

- **Demographic:** Demographic conditions are the features of a population as they affect an organization. Demographics may refer to race, ethnicity, gender, age, religion, or any number of factors.

- **Ecological:** Ecological conditions include climate, geography, pollution, population density, and other physical features of the environment.

- **Cultural:** A society's values, beliefs, and customs make up the cultural conditions that affect an organization. These cultural conditions help form political and religious systems, family organization, ethics, sexuality, work orientation, and countless other social components.

PUBLIC ORGANIZATIONS

While not all organizations involved in public health are public agencies, most are. In subsequent chapters there are descriptions of public health activities of private nonprofit organizations, associations, universities (many of which are public), and private sector corporations. When considering federal, state, and local government initiatives in public health, it is important to be aware of the distinctive issues that are at the forefront of the public organization.

The distinctions for public organizations are often evident, but not always in an utterly black-and-white, absolute way. For example, many private corporations have to deal with politicians, though they are not subordinate to them in the same way a public organization is. While private businesses have some of the constraints, oversights, and pressures of public organizations, the fact is the influence is not as pervasive on a day-to-day basis. Figure 5-3 provides a fairly common configuration

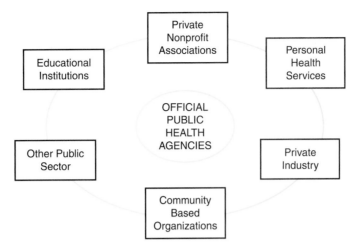

FIGURE 5-3 Public Health Agency Interconnections
© Cengage Learning 2013

of organizations that interconnect on public health issues; at the core of which is typically the public health agency.

According to Christopher Pollitt, author of *The Essential Public Manager*, the public sector organization or agency faces the issues in Table 5-2 more often or with more magnitude than private businesses. However, Hal Rainey, at the University of Georgia, who has done numerous comparative studies of public and private

TABLE 5-2 Issues and Challenges Facing Public Managers

- Managing in a social-political system

- Working with public pressure and potential protest

- An ever-present sense of accountability

- The need to understand public behavior

- The challenge of rationing resources

- Having to manage influence responsibly

- Assessing multi-dimensional performance

- Being open and responsive to the media

- Understanding a wider responsibility to a changing society

© Cengage Learning 2013

sector organizations, finds increasing similarities between the two sectors. This has been especially evident since 2000 in the United States and other countries where we have seen publicly owned industries privatized and some private corporations being "taken over" by the public sector. Furthermore, many public services have been contracted out to the private sector and public-private partnerships have seen dramatic growth.

> "Managers are not confronted with problems that are independent of each other, but with dynamic situations that consist of complex systems of changing problems that interact with each other."—*Russell Ackoff, Past-president of the International Society for Systems Sciences*

VALUES IN THE PUBLIC SECTOR

In addition to the organizational processes and functions, competing demands, environmental conditions, and organizational sector distinctions, there are critical overarching values that must guide public agencies. The Task Force on Public Service Values and Ethics at the Canadian Center for Management Development has identified the following:

- *Democratic values*, such as serving the common good, promoting public accountability, supporting elected representatives, and always observing the law.

- *General ethical values*, such as integrity, honesty, equity, and fairness.

- *Professional values*, such as putting the client's interest first, impartiality, continuous improvement, and effectiveness.

- *People values*, such as reasonableness, civility, respecting differences, and kindness.

Many public-sector professionals, actually all professionals, tend to view problems and challenges through their own professional lenses, as was discussed in Chapter 2, "Public Health Professionalism and Ethics." However, one example observed by the late Massachusetts Institute of Technology (MIT) professor Donald Schon, who extensively studied the "mental models" of professionals, is provided in Owens and Valesky's *Organizational Behavior and Education*:

> A nutritionist, for example, may convert a vague worry about malnourishment among children in developing countries into a problem of selecting an optimal diet. But agronomists may frame the problem in terms of food production; epidemiologists may frame it in terms of diseases that increase the demand for nutrients or prevent their absorption; demographers tend to see it in terms of a rate of population growth that has outstripped agricultural activity; engineers, in terms of inadequate food storage and distribution; economists, in terms of insufficient purchasing power or the inequitable distribution of land or wealth.

Summary

Organizations, both public and private, are complex, multifaceted, adaptive social systems. Those involved in public health have overarching values and an overriding mission to improve and promote the health of individuals and communities.

As mentioned in Part I of this book, Lester Breslow, in his preface to the *Encyclopedia of Public Health*, described public health as one of the essential institutions of society existing to promote, protect, preserve, and restore the good health of all people. As will be seen in the next several chapters, there are many programs, services, organizations, and institutions devoted to public health. It is important to understand the nature of organizations since that is where most of the work is done. We live in an organizational society, and public health is no exception. It is equally important to be aware of the core functions of public health and the goals that keep moving it forward. As Breslow surmises, "Professionals engaged in the field regard it as an organized effort directed at improving the health of populations by assuring the conditions in which people can be healthy." In the next chapter we will be discussing professionalism and ethics with a specific focus on the drive to develop and promote core competencies for public health professionals and managers.

Public Health Leader Perspective

Amanda Parsons, MD, M.P.H., M.B.A., Deputy Commissioner, Primary Care Information Project, New York City Department of Health and Mental Hygiene

Dr. Amanda Parsons is the Deputy Commissioner at the New York City Department of Health and Mental Hygiene (DOHMH) as the Deputy Commissioner, overseeing all of the activities of the Primary Care Information Project. Previously, Dr. Parsons was the Director of Medical Quality in which position she was responsible for creating and leading the Quality Improvement, Billing, Consulting, and EMR Consulting teams deployed to PCIP's small physician-practices. She has her MD and M.B.A. from Columbia University and did medical post-graduate training in Internal Medicine at Beth Israel Medical Center. She completed her undergraduate studies at Boston College, where she was a Presidential Scholar. She serves on the Board of Directors of VIP Community Service and the New York eHealth Collaborative (NYeC). She is also on the Advisory Board of the Touch Foundation.

Interview by Scott Musch

Continues

(Q): Tell me about your position as Deputy Commissioner in New York City.

Dr. Parsons: I oversee the Primary Care Information Project which is a project, founded in 2005, within the Bureau of Health Care Access and Improvement. Our aim is to improve the care of NYC residents, particularly those who live in underserved areas, through the deployment of health information technology. We roll out electronic medical records to providers who work in low-income neighborhoods and treat low-income patients. We coach providers on how to use the electronic medical record [EMR] and do quality improvement work. We train them on how to use the EMR and provide a host of other services that affect people every day, such as screening for diseases like high blood pressure, high cholesterol, HIV, diabetes.

(Q): What are your main responsibilities?

Dr. Parsons: My role specifically is to run the program and make sure we continue to attract and retain talent at the organization. I also keep an eye on all the financial aspects of the organization to make sure we have enough money to meet the goals today, but also to think about what additional funding we should be seeking as it aligns with our strategic initiatives. I also think about ways we can improve the different programs we offer providers. We work with many private partners. About two-thirds (to three-quarters) of our budget is funded through a host of different grants and private foundations. I interface with those entities to advance our goals while at the same time preserving those of the granting agencies. We do a lot of stakeholder management, which means making sure that we have a seat at the table in conversations that would significantly impact us now or in the future. We make sure that we understand the issues and think about how to reflect the needs of NYC residents in those conversations. For instance, there are programs put into place by New York State around e-prescribing. We are very interested in having providers e-prescribe, so we work closely with the State to make sure the program is going well, that we understand what their program looks like, what they need from us, and how we can enhance their mission. We want to make sure our providers continue to receive incentives to e-prescribe. It involves working with stakeholders who might be partners, and recognizing that in partnering we can help each other. It can present a symbiotic relationship, so it's important to understand who's doing what in your space so you know the type of people you want at the table for joint programming and joint resource sharing. It's very similar to thinking about Porter's Five Forces.

(Q): Describe how health care information technology will improve public health.

Dr. Parsons: We firmly believe that health information technology [HIT] deployed correctly can improve public health. It requires learning how to use it appropriately. We understand that HIT has to be deployed in a context. It cannot just be throwing software at someone and saying, "Here, use this CD, improve your blood pressure, and get better." We understand the need to really help providers completely change from paper to electronic workflows. We need to show them how to use the tool correctly to do what they normally do day-to-day, as well as to do other things that HIT allows that they can't do in a paper setting. For instance, if you look at a wall of manila folders like in most offices and say, "I wish I knew how many of my patients had diabetes," it's not a question you can easily ask a wall of folders. It certainly is a question you can easily ask in an electronic medical record, but if you don't know how to do that, or you have never asked that question, or if you don't have a workflow around that, then you are not going to ask the question, so just because the electronic medical record can do it, if you

Continues

are not bringing the right questions or the right processes to that electronic medical record, you are not going to get out of it what you need. We work with providers to help them improve not only the care they deliver when seeing patients—electronic medical records can have flags, warnings, reminders, and prompts that help steer the provider in the right direction—but also to use the population health tools available in electronic medical records. These tools allow a provider to query questions like, how many patients do I have with diabetes, which ones have an A1c that is not in control, which ones haven't been seen in the last six months, and how many of those don't have an appointment in the next three months? Now the provider can actually contact those patients to bring them back in for care. These are the kinds of workflows that we try to embed in our processes. You see these workflows often in integrated settings, but you don't see them routinely in very small practice settings—one or two doctor practices. We bring care management/advanced care processes down to the single doctor in Harlem who otherwise wouldn't have access to these types of resources and thinking.

(Q): How is health information technology especially pertinent in a metropolitan area like New York City?

Dr. Parsons: We have many patients who suffer from chronic diseases, like diabetes. We have an obesity epidemic. HIT can have a lot of impact on chronic diseases where the screening process is well laid out and documented. I think what makes New York City in particular an interesting place to roll out HIT is that the health department has been very avant-garde. It has nationally acclaimed policies such as the Smoke-Free Air Act. This is a great synchronization of strategy when we are out talking with doctors and telling them that it is important to screen for smoking. The Health Department has been working with providers on a concerted strategy. We have ads on TV and in the trains that help send a message that smoking is dangerous. When doctors say, "What am I suppose to do about obesity?," we can say it is important to document that the patient is obese and it matters for drug dosing and a host of other things, but also you should counsel the patient as we are also counseling your patient by virtue of our campaigns, such as the "Pouring on the Pounds" ads where we talk about the impact of sodas on obesity. I think there is a really good partnership with the providers on chronic diseases that has been put in place by this Health Department for several years. It's not totally inconceivable to these providers that their local health department cares about chronic diseases because it is visible how the city has been tackling those issues for quite some time. New York City has a large density of population and most people are not too far from a provider. We are not dealing with rural health settings. Here on your way to work you probably trip over 12 different doctors' offices. There are economies of scale here when you are trying to roll out programs as you have not only a density of people but some 30,000 providers in New York City alone.

(Q): How many years have you worked in public health?

Dr. Parsons: I started working in global public health while I was at McKinsey & Company where I was a consultant for four years. I was doing private sector work, working for pharmaceutical clients and then eventually started to shift over to global health, which was my first foray into public health. Through this work, I became more interested in public health and then applied for a position with NYC DOHMH. In January 2008, I joined the PCIP.

(Q): Why did you choose to go into the field of public health?

Dr. Parsons: I'm a physician by training. Whenever I worked with patients, I loved it and felt like I could have a lot of one-on-one impact, but the appeal of being able to do the work on a

Continues

larger scale was very interesting to me. I have also been interested in programmatic approaches, thinking about how we can orchestrate the system in a different way to make good health a by-product of the system.

(Q): What are the most rewarding aspects about your job in public health?

Dr. Parsons: The most rewarding aspect is the mission-driven focus. We are not bottom line driven. This makes it easier to talk to providers as you have an aligned mission to provide good care for patients. I think the health department is a natural ally. This part is really rewarding as you don't have to spend so much time explaining why you care. It is self-evident and you can quickly get to work. Being in public health also helps to lend laser sharp clarity on the mission of why you do what you do. At the end of the day, you can look at a project and say, "Is this going to save lives?" And if it doesn't, then you shouldn't do it. Lastly, I think it is really energizing to be surrounded by people who feel very passionate about public health. There is a lot of self-reinforcing behavior in being with other people who are very mission-driven and really want to do the right thing. It is very energizing. I've been really lucky to work with a fabulous executive team that I work closely with on a day-to-day basis. Together, we help direct the work at PCIP.

(Q): What are some of the biggest management challenges you face as a leader in public health in general and within your organization in particular?

Dr. Parsons: One of the first challenges in public health is not being able to pay people what they are worth. This poses an extra challenge when you are trying to attract and retain talent. Society hasn't placed as much value on public health work as it does on other work like banking. This presents a day-to-day challenge as there is always a lot of work to do but not enough money to fund it. Another challenge is trying to get funding from grants and city and state budgets, all of which are subject to huge variations and changes in administrations that yield changes in priorities. It is really important to stay good at what you do and have a national impact and be able to show very quickly through metrics that your programs are worth having around no matter the budget situation.

(Q): What future trends do you see shaping the field of public health as a career opportunity?

Dr. Parsons: There has been a movement towards accountability and transparency in government; being able to say that a project met its goals and the data shows it. This is definitely shaping public health as a career. The field is becoming data driven and it's not enough to be just mission driven. You have to be able to show impact because people will know very quickly whether or not the idea made a difference. I think HIT is really going to revolutionize public health. In the past it has been hard to measure programs and understand what matters the most, what reduces hospitalizations, what reduces costs in health care? This data was locked up in handwritten patient charts and binders in storage facilities. There will be the opportunity, like in many other sectors, where you measure the impact of a specific project. Now in public health there will be an ability to focus resources on where they are needed the most. With this data comes the ability to say that this particular health system is not working very well, so let's deploy resources differentially there in order to get this health system up and running. There will

Continues

definitely be the need to increase the capacity to do data analysis, data mining, data warehousing, and business intelligence. We just have to put those processes in place, but I will never complain that there is too much data out there.

(Q): What advice would you have for a student interested in entering the field of public health?

Dr. Parsons: Early on, the road to public health will yield many things. It may yield fame, impact, mission, but it will not yield fortune. You need to embrace what it means to work in civil service. It's really quite a privilege to serve the public in this way. I think it is definitely important to understand if you want to work as a specialist or generalist, and find jobs that match those requirements. In addition, it is important to find leaders and mentors. There are professionals who have significant experience leading large health systems like hospitals and community health centers, and it's important to figure out how to connect with them. It is really important to reach out to them to foster mentoring relationships. I don't think it is easy to identify those people in public health without really sitting down and thinking about them. We don't tend to read about the public health "whizzes" in the newspaper every day. The spotlight doesn't shine as ubiquitously on leaders in public health as it does in the private sector. It is important to find those luminaries yourself and establish relationships.

End

Discussion and Review Questions

1. What is an organization? How is it similar to an "organism"? Give examples.

2. Why are organizations often understood as "complex systems"?

3. What are the seven functions of an organization? Briefly describe each.

4. Identify and describe pressures from the environment that are placed on public health organizations. Do they tend to adapt and respond to these pressures?

5. What are the general environmental conditions organizations exist in?

6. What values are especially important for public sector managers and/or public health organizations? Identify and discuss.

Action Learning and Critical Thinking

A. Do an Internet search and identify two organizations working in the health arena. One should be a public organization and the other a private (for-profit) organization. Read the mission statements and study the activities of each organization. What are the differences? Do you see different values at play? What is the primary purpose of each organization?

B. Watch the film *The Corporation* and discuss the overarching themes as they pertain to the structure and function of organizations. Discuss the role of corporate organizations from a values perspective.

Chapter 6

FEDERAL SECTOR PUBLIC HEALTH AGENCIES

Learning Objectives

Upon completion of this chapter, you should be able to:

1. Gain an understanding of the scope and scale of federal public health.
2. Identify the major federal agencies in public health.
3. Understand the mission and vision of federal agencies.
4. Know the duties of the Surgeon General and role of the USPHS.
5. Have a more thorough understanding of the CDC, NIH, and FDA.
6. Understand the inter-relatedness of agencies involved in public health.
7. Realize the incredible scope of public health responsibilities and activities of the federal sector.

Key Terms

Administration for Children and Families (ACF)

Administration on Aging (AoA)

Agency for Healthcare Research and Quality (AHRQ)

Agency for Toxic Substances and Disease Registry (ATSDR)

Centers for Disease Control and Prevention (CDC)

Centers for Medicare and Medicaid Services (CMS)

Food and Drug Administration (FDA)

Health Resources and Services Administration (HRSA)

Indian Health Service (IHS)

National Institutes of Health (NIH)

Substance Abuse and Mental Health Services Administration (SAMHSA)

Chapter Outline

INTRODUCTION

Every national government in the world has a department, ministry, or agency that has primary responsibility for the protection of the health and well-being of its citizens. This primary public health agency invariably must work with other units of the national government and in federalist countries, like the United States and Canada, the regional and local governments as well. National health agencies and ministries typically meet their responsibilities through the development of health promotion and prevention policies, the enforcement of health regulations, the direct provision of health services and programs, the funding of health and biomedical research, and support or funding of other government and nongovernmental agencies involved in public health.

This chapter describes the Department of Health and Human Services (HHS), which is the primary public health and social service agency of the United States. The Department has a long and rich history that began in 1789 with the passage by Congress of an act for the relief of sick and disabled seamen, thus establishing a network of hospitals for the care of merchant seamen. This became the forerunner of today's U.S. Public Health Service. In 1953 a Cabinet-level Department

(Health, Education, and Welfare) was formed and reported directly to the United States President. Later, in 1980, the education function became its own Department of Education and the health and welfare functions were organized under a newly formed Department of Health and Human Services.

As with the development of a consolidated health and social services agency in the United States, there are many variations in history and structure throughout the world. These typically parallel the development of political systems and institutional structures and often are shaped by major social events like wars and revolutions or by epidemics and health threats. A fascinating exploration of this history is provided in George Rosen's classic book, *A History of Public Health* (Rosen 1993 and 1958), and current descriptions and histories of national public health systems outside of the United States can be found in *Comparative Health Systems: Global Perspectives* by James Johnson and Carleen Stoskopf (2010).

Additionally, there are various United States agencies that work closely with HHS and some that provide their own public health services or have a role in health policy and regulation. These include the Environmental Protection Agency (EPA), the Department of Labor which houses the Occupational Safety and Health Administration (OSHA), the Department of Agriculture which does safety inspections and coordinates the Women, Infants, and Children (WIC) food program, the Department of Homeland Security (DHS), the Department of Veterans Affairs (VA), Department of Defense (DOD), Department of Transportation (DOT), and various other United States agencies and bureaus involved, at least partially, in public health.

DEPARTMENT OF HEALTH AND HUMAN SERVICES (HHS)

The Department of Health and Human Services (HHS) is the primary government agency for protecting the health of people in the United States. HHS provides essential human services, particularly to those in need of assistance.

> "A decent provision for the poor is a true test of civilization."—*Samuel Johnson, Eighteenth-century Philosopher*

HHS accounts for nearly a quarter of all federal expenditures, and it allocates more grant money than all other federal agencies combined. Medicare, which is operated by HHS, is the country's largest health insurer. Twenty-five percent of Americans receive health care coverage from Medicare or Medicaid.

HHS is comprised of 11 operating divisions, eight of which are in the U.S. Public Health Service and three that are human services agencies. With over 300 programs offering an array of services, HHS works with state and local governments as well as private sector grantees to deliver its services. Another important function of HHS is that it facilitates the collection of national health data.

The 11 operating divisions of HHS are as follows, in alphabetical order:

- Administration for Children and Families (ACF)
- Administration on Aging (AoA)
- Agency for Healthcare Research and Quality (AHRQ)
- Agency for Toxic Substances and Disease Registry (ATSDR)
- Centers for Disease Control and Prevention (CDC)
- Centers for Medicare and Medicaid Services (CMS)
- Food and Drug Administration (FDA)
- Health Resources and Services Administration (HRSA)
- Indian Health Services (HIS)
- National Institutes of Health (NIH)
- Substance Abuse and Mental Health Services Administration (SAMHSA)

HHS Mission and Goals

The mission statement for the Department is as follows:

> *The mission of the U.S. Department of Health and Human Services (HHS) is to enhance the health and well-being of Americans by providing for effective health and human services and by fostering sound, sustained advances in the sciences underlying medicine, public health, and social services. HHS accomplishes its mission through several hundred programs and initiatives that cover a wide spectrum of activities, serving the American public at every stage of life.*

The framework of strategic planning and goal setting for the Department is based on five over-arching strategic goals.

Goal 1: Transform Health Care

Goal 2: Advance Scientific Knowledge and Innovation

Goal 3: Advance the Health, Safety, and Well-Being of the American People

Goal 4: Increase Efficiency, Transparency, and Accountability of HHS Programs

Goal 5: Strengthen the Nation's Health and Human Services Infrastructure and Workforce

The HHS goals and objectives in the 2010–2015 Strategic Plan are interrelated, meaning that success in one goal area often facilitates or is necessary for success for another goal. For instance, strengthening the Department's workforce and infrastructure, as in Goal 5, will likely lead to increased efficiency, transparency, and accountability, which is Goal 4. As with the attributes of systems thinking discussed in Chapter 1, "Public Health Mission and Core Functions," the interconnections between these goals, their objectives, and the initiatives involved in accomplishing the mission of HHS are essential. In fact, each goal in this framework could also be considered a "critical success factor" for the achievement of this mission and the sustainability of the important role and contributions of HHS in American society and the world.

HHS Organization

Departmental leadership at the highest level for these 11 operating divisions is provided by the Secretary of HHS, who is appointed by and reports to the President. Also included in the Department is the Office of Public Health and Science, the Office of the Inspector General, the Office for Civil Rights, the Center for Faith-Based and Community Initiatives, and the Office of Global Health Affairs. Additionally, there is a Program Support Center to provide administrative services for HHS and other federal agencies. There are also several newer offices, including the Office of Consumer Information and Insurance Oversight (OCIIO), the Office of Recovery Act Coordination (ORAC) within the Office of the Assistant Secretary for Financial Resources (ASFR), and the Office of Health Reform (OHR). An organizational chart of the Department is provided in Figure 6-1.

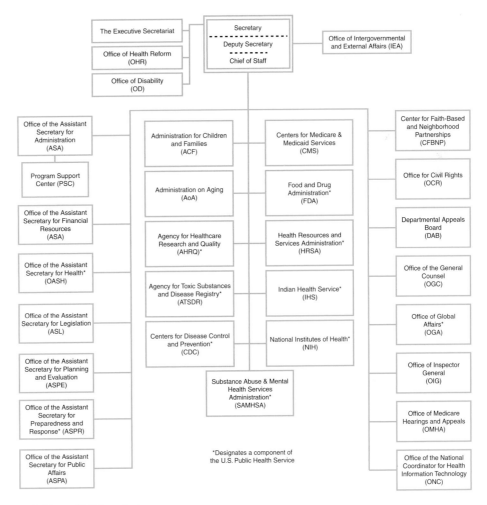

FIGURE 6-1 HHS Organization

Source: U.S. Department of Health and Human Services: http://www.hhs.gov/about/images/orgchart011912.jpg

The Office of the Assistant Secretary for Health directs many of the core public health offices, such as the Office of the Surgeon General and the U.S. Public Health Service Corps. The Office also oversees 10 regional health offices in the United States and 10 national advisory committees. The core public health offices and their functions are provided in Table 6-1.

Additionally, there are regional health offices and administrators who have delineated responsibilities.

TABLE 6-1 Core Public Health Offices of Assistant Secretary for Health

- **Office of Surgeon General (OSG):** Provides Americans the best scientific information available on how to improve their health and reduce their risk of illness and injury. The Office also manages the operations of the Commissioned Corps of the U.S. Public Health Service.

- **National Vaccine Program Office (NVPO):** Ensures collaboration among the many federal agencies involved in vaccine and immunization activities.

- **Office of Adolescent Health (OAH):** Coordinates adolescent health promotion and disease prevention initiatives across HHS.

- **Office of Disease Prevention and Health Promotion (ODPHP):** Provides leadership, coordination, and policy development for public health and prevention activities. Leads the Healthy People initiative for HHS.

- **Office of Healthcare Quality (OHQ):** Leads and coordinates cross-cutting issues that strengthen the health system and improve the quality of health care.

- **Office of HIV/AIDS Policy (OHAP):** Responsible for coordinating, integrating, and directing the Department's policies, programs, and activities related to HIV/AIDS.

- **Office of Human Research Protections (OHRP):** Supports, strengthens, and provides leadership to the nation's system for protecting volunteers in research conducted or supported by HHS.

- **Office of Minority Health (OMH):** Addresses health status and quality-of-life for minority populations.

- **Office of Population Affairs (OPA):** Advises on issues related to family planning and population affairs.

- **Office of Research Integrity (ORI):** Promotes integrity in research programs of the Public Health Service and responds to allegations of research misconduct.

- **Office of Women's Health (OWH):** Improves the health of American women by advancing a comprehensive women's health agenda throughout HHS.

Source: U.S. Department of Health and Human Services. Retrieved from http://www.hhs.gov

As mentioned earlier and as shown in the HHS organizational chart, there are 11 operating divisions. Each of these will be discussed in more detail later in this chapter and two of these, the Centers for Disease Control and Prevention (CDC) and the Food and Drug Administration (FDA), will be discussed at length with organizational charts provided. Meanwhile, it is important to better understand one of the core public health entities of HHS that overlaps many, if not all, of the other agencies and divisions. This is the U.S. Public Health Service Corps (USPHS) and the Office of the Surgeon General.

U.S. Public Health Service

The Office of the Surgeon General, under the direction of the Surgeon General, oversees the operations of the Commissioned Corps of the U.S. Public Health Service (USPHS). The Surgeon General is appointed by the President with the advice and consent of the United States Senate for a 4-year term of office. The duties outlined in Table 6-2 provide a good overview of the scope of this position

TABLE 6-2 Duties of the U.S. Surgeon General

- Protect and advance the health of the Nation through educating the public, advocating for effective disease prevention and health promotion programs and activities, and providing a highly recognized symbol of national commitment to protecting and improving the public's health.

- Articulate scientifically based health policy analysis and advice to the President and the Secretary of HHS on the full range of critical public health, medical, and health system issues facing the Nation.

- Provide leadership in promoting special Departmental health initiatives, e.g., tobacco and HIV prevention efforts, with other governmental and nongovernmental entities, both domestically and internationally.

- Administer the USPHS Commissioned Corps, which is a uniquely expert, diverse, flexible, and committed career force of public health professionals who can respond to both current and long-term health needs of the Nation.

- Provide leadership and management oversight for USPHS Commissioned Corps involvement in emergency preparedness and response activities.

- Elevate the quality of public health practice in the professional disciplines through the advancement of appropriate standards and research priorities.

- Fulfill statutory and customary HHS representational functions on a wide variety of Federal boards and governing bodies of non-Federal health organizations.

Source: U.S. Department of Health and Human Services. Retrieved from http://www.surgeongeneral.gov

Exhibit 6-1   U.S. Public Health Service Mission

The mission of the U.S. Public Health Service Commissioned Corps is to protect, promote, and advance the health and safety of our Nation.

As America's uniformed service of public health professionals, the Commissioned Corps achieves its mission through:

- rapid and effective response to public health needs;
- leadership and excellence in public health practices; and
- advancement of public health science.

Source: U.S. Public Health Services Commissioned Corps. Retrieved from http://www.usphs.gov

and range of responsibilities. The Surgeon General is a physician by training and often has public health or management experience as well. For example, the current Surgeon General, who is female, was previously a practicing family physician (MD) who also has a M.B.A. degree.

One of seven uniformed services, the USPHS Commissioned Corps is made up of over 6,500 highly dedicated public health professionals. Corps members work to provide medical services, promote health, prevent disease, and foster public health knowledge in the United States and abroad. The USPHS Commissioned Corps fills leadership and service roles within many Federal public health agencies. See Exhibit 6-1 for the mission statement of the USPHS Commissioned Corps.

The Corps has officers in a wide range of professions from fields such as medicine, nursing, public health management, epidemiology, health policy and economics, environmental sciences, dietetics and nutrition, engineering, behavioral health, veterinary medicine, biomedical sciences, dentistry, pharmacy, and allied health sciences.

HHS Operating Divisions

As mentioned previously, HHS programs are administered by 11 operating divisions, including eight agencies in the U.S. Public Health Service and three human services agencies. The Department includes more than 300 programs, covering an incredibly wide range of activities from research, to direct services, to regulation, and nearly any other health or human service improvement effort. A brief description of these major agencies along with their missions and goals is provided. Later in the chapter, a more detailed description will be provided for three of these: the Centers for Disease Control and Prevention, the Food and Drug Administration, and the National Institutes of Health because of their size and scope.

Exhibit 6-2 Mission and Goals of the ACF

The mission of the ACF is to be responsible for Federal programs that promote the economic and social well-being of families, children, individuals, and communities.

Its goals are:

- to empower families and individuals to increase their own economic independence and productivity;
- to promote strong, healthy, supportive communities that have a positive impact on the quality-of-life and the development of children;

- to form partnerships with front-line service providers, states, localities, and tribal communities, to identify and implement solutions that transcend traditional program boundaries;
- to improve needed access to services; and
- to develop a strong commitment to work with vulnerable populations including people with developmental disabilities, refugees, and migrants, to address their needs, strengths, and abilities.

Source: U.S. Department of Health and Human Services. Retrieved from http://www.acf.hhs.gov

Administration for Children and Families (ACF)

The **Administration for Children and Families (ACF)** funds programs that provide services to children and families through state, territory, local, and tribal organizations. These programs include family assistance, childcare, and child welfare, among others. In addition to funding, the AFC provides these organizations with technical assistance, information services, and policy direction. The agency's mission and goals are provided in Exhibit 6-2.

Administration on Aging (AoA)

The **Administration on Aging** mission is to help elderly people maintain their health and independence through a comprehensive system of home- and community-based services. The AoA awards grants to State government agencies on aging and Native American tribal organizations. AoA also awards grants to research organizations working on aging-related projects and engages in statistical activities in support of the research, analysis, and evaluation of programs to meet the needs of an aging population. Exhibit 6-3 includes the agency's mission and goals.

Agency for Healthcare Research and Quality (AHRQ)

The **Agency for Healthcare Research and Quality (AHRQ)** was established in 1999 by Congress to replace its predecessor agency, the Agency for Health Care Policy and Research. The AHRQ focuses on quality-of-care and medical care outcomes. It is responsible for conducting and sponsoring research to enhance the quality, appropriateness, and effectiveness of health care services. It supports research designed to improve the quality of health care, reduce its cost, and broaden access to essential services. The agency's mission and goals are provided in Exhibit 6-4.

Administration for Children and Families (ACF): The agency within the Department of Health and Human Services (DHHS) responsible for federal programs that promote the economic and social well-being of families, children, individuals, and communities.

Administration on Aging (AoA): The federal agency within the Department of Health and Human Services (DHHS) charged with serving the senior citizens of the United States.

Agency for Healthcare Research and Quality (AHRQ): The lead federal agency for research to improve the quality of health care, reduce its cost, and broaden access to essential services. A component of the Department of Health and Human Services (DHHS).

Exhibit 6-3   Mission and Goals of the AoA

The mission of AoA is to develop a comprehensive, coordinated, and cost-effective system of home- and community-based services that helps elderly individuals maintain their health and independence in their homes and communities.

Its goals are:

- to empower older people, their families, and other consumers to make informed decisions about, and to be able to easily access, existing health and long-term care options;
- to enable seniors to remain in their own homes with a high quality of life for as long as

possible through the provision of home- and community-based services, including supports for family caregivers;

- to empower older people to stay active and healthy through Older Americans Act services and the new prevention benefits under Medicare;
- to ensure the rights of older people and prevent their abuse, neglect and exploitation; and
- to maintain effective and responsive management.

Source: U.S. Department of Health and Human Services. Retrieved from http://www.aoa.gov

Exhibit 6-4   Mission and Goals of AHRQ

The mission of AHRQ is to support research designed to improve the quality, safety, efficiency, and effectiveness of health care for all Americans.

Its goals are:

- to reduce the risk of harm by promoting delivery of the best possible health care;
- to improve health care outcomes by encouraging the use of evidence to make informed health care decisions;

- to transform research into practice to facilitate wider access to effective health care services and reduce unnecessary costs; and
- to provide information that helps people make better decisions about health care.

Source: U.S. Department of Health and Human Services. Retrieved from http://www.ahrq.gov

Agency for Toxic Substances and Disease Registry (ATSDR): The ATSDR performs specific public health functions concerning hazardous substances in the environment. It works to prevent exposure and minimize adverse health effects associated with waste management emergencies and pollution by hazardous substances.

Agency for Toxic Substance and Disease Registry (ATSDR)

The **Agency for Toxic Substances and Disease Registry (ATSDR)** performs an important public health service by identifying and researching potentially harmful substances in the environment. It works to prevent exposure to and minimize the effects of toxic substances through projects such as the monitoring and assessment of waste sites, data collection and registries, and education and training regarding toxic substances. Exhibit 6-5 outlines the mission and goals of the ATSDR.

Exhibit 6-5   Mission and Goals of ATSDR

The mission of ATSDR is to serve the public through responsive public health actions to promote healthy and safe environments and prevent harmful exposures.

Its goals are:

- to protect the public from environmental hazards and toxic exposures;
- to promote healthy environments;
- to advance the science of environmental public health;
- to support environmental public health practice;
- to educate communities, partners, and policymakers about environmental health risks and protective measures;
- to promote environmental justice and reduce health disparities associated with environmental exposures; and
- to provide unique scientific and technical expertise to advance public health science and practice.

Source: U.S. Department of Health and Human Services. Retrieved from http://www.atsdr.cdc.gov

Centers for Disease Control and Prevention (CDC)

Centers for Disease Control and Prevention (CDC): An agency within the Department of Health and Human Services (DHHS), which is responsible for monitoring and studying diseases which are controllable by public health measures. The CDC is headquartered in Atlanta, Georgia.

The **Centers for Disease Control and Prevention (CDC)** with headquarters in Atlanta, Georgia, is the lead agency for the surveillance and identification of disease through epidemiological and laboratory investigations. The agency addresses a broad range of preventable health problems, from infectious disease to chronic diseases and risk factors to negative environmental effects on health. It is also the primary agency administering grants to support public health programs, such as HIV/AIDS, sexually transmitted diseases, injury protection, immunization, and cancer screening. Exhibit 6-6 outlines the goals and mission of the CDC.

Exhibit 6-6   Mission and Goals of CDC

Collaborating to create the expertise, information, and tools that people and communities need to protect their health—through health promotion, prevention of disease, injury and disability, and preparedness for new health threats.

Its goals are:

- to monitor health;
- to detect and investigate health problems;
- to conduct research to enhance prevention;
- to develop and advocate sound public health policies;
- to implement prevention strategies;
- to promote healthy behaviors;
- to foster safe and healthful environments; and
- to provide leadership and training for public health.

Source: Centers for Disease Control and Prevention. Retrieved from http://www.cdc.gov

It has personnel internationally and at every level of public health in each of the 50 states to facilitate data collection, analysis, and program implementation. Its organizational structure comprising centers, institutes, and offices allows it to be more responsive and effective when dealing with public health concerns. The organizational structure of the CDC and its range of functions and activities will be discussed in more detail later in this chapter.

Centers for Medicare and Medicaid Services (CMS)

The **Centers for Medicare and Medicaid Services (CMS)** headquartered in the Washington, D.C. area with 10 field offices operates from a consortia structure. Each consortium is led by a Consortium Administrator (CA) who serves as the Agency's national focal point in the field for their functional area and as such is responsible for consistent implementation of CMS programs, policy, and guidance across all 10 regions. CMS administers the three large HHS medical-care payment systems including **Medicare**, and in partnerships with the states, **Medicaid**, and the State Children's Health Insurance Program (SCHIP). CMS also engages in survey research, certification, and quality improvement, including technical assistance for the implementation of HIPPA. Within CMS is the Center for Consumer Information and Insurance Oversight (CCIIO), dedicated to helping HHS implement many of the provisions of the Affordable Care Act that address private health insurance. The office is responsible for ensuring compliance with the new insurance market rules, such as the prohibitions on rescissions and on pre-existing condition exclusions for children that take effect this year. The CCIIO will work closely with state insurance commissioners and governors, consumers, and stakeholders throughout the implementation process to ensure the new law best serves the American people. See Exhibit 6-7 for the CMS mission statement and goals.

> "Organization can never be a substitute for initiative and for judgment."—*Louis Brandeis, United States Supreme Court Justice*

Food and Drug Administration (FDA)

The **Food and Drug Administration (FDA)** is responsible for ensuring the safety, efficacy, and security of food, medicines, and products for use or consumption by the public (Exhibit 6-8 states the FDA's mission and goals). The FDA is also charged with regulating the manufacture, marketing, and distribution of tobacco products, advancing public health through innovations in food and medicine production, and providing information and education so that consumers can safely and effectively choose foods and medicines. The organizational structure of the FDA and its range of functions and activities will be discussed in more detail later in this chapter.

Health Resources and Services Administration (HRSA)

Created in 1982 with the merging of the Health Resources Administrations and the Health Services Administration, the **Health Resources and Services Administration (HRSA)** improves access to health care for people who are uninsured or medically vulnerable by providing financial support to health care agencies in states

---

Centers for Medicare and Medicaid Services (CMS): The agency within the Department of Health and Human Services (DHHS) which administers the Medicare, Medicaid, and the State Children's Health Insurance Program (SCHIP). CMS has three centers: Center for Medicare Management (CMM); Center for Beneficiary Choices (CBC); Center for Medicaid and State Operations (CMSO).

Food and Drug Administration (FDA): An agency within the U.S. Department of Health and Human Services (DHHS) responsible for protecting the health of the nation against impure and unsafe foods, drugs, cosmetics, biological substances, and other potential hazards. A major part of the FDAs activity is controlling the sale, distribution, and use of pharmaceutical drugs and medical devices, including the licensing of new drugs for use by humans.

Health Resources and Services Administration (HRSA): Improves access to health care for people who are uninsured or medically vulnerable by providing financial support to health care agencies in states and territories. The HRSA trains heath care professionals in rural communities and oversees organ donations and transplants, as well as maintains databases to protect against health care malpractice and health care waste, fraud, and abuse.

Exhibit 6-7   Mission and Goals of CMS

The mission of CMS is to ensure effective, up-to-date health care coverage and to promote quality care for beneficiaries.

Goals:
- Skilled, Committed, and Highly Motivated Workforce

- Affordable Health Care System
- High-Value Health Care
- Confident, Informed Consumers and Collaborative Partnerships

Source: Centers for Medicare & Medicaid Services. Retrieved from http://www.cms.gov

Exhibit 6-8   Mission and Goals of FDA

The mission of the FDA is protecting the public's health by ensuring the safety, efficacy, and security of human and veterinary drugs, biological products, and medical devices; ensuring the safety of foods, cosmetics, and radiation-emitting products; and regulating tobacco products.

Its goals are:
- to help speed innovations that make medicines and foods safer and more effective;

- to provide the public with the accurate, science-based information they need to use medicines and foods to improve their health;
- to regulate the manufacture, marketing, and distribution of tobacco products to protect the public and reduce tobacco use by minors; and
- to address the Nation's counterterrorism capability and ensure the security of the supply of foods and medical products.

Source: Food and Drug Administration. Retrieved from http://www.fda.gov

---

and territories. The HRSA trains health care professionals in rural communities and oversees organ donations and transplants, as well as maintains databases to protect against health care malpractice and health care waste, fraud, and abuse. Agency mission and goals are provided in Exhibit 6-9.

Indian Health Service (IHS)

The **Indian Health Service (IHS)** as an agency provides direct medical services and preventive measures involving environmental, educational, and outreach activities to American Indians and Alaska Natives who live on or near reservations or Alaska Villages. It also has programs that provide some access to care for American Indians and Alaska Natives who live in urban areas. Health services are provided directly by the IHS, through tribally contracted and operated health programs, and through services purchased from private providers. Exhibit 6-10 provides the IHS mission.

Indian Health Service (IHS): An agency within the Department of Health and Human Services (DHHS) whose goal is to ensure that comprehensive, culturally acceptable personal and public health services are available and accessible to American Indian and Alaska Native people. The IHS manages a comprehensive health care delivery system for more than 561 federally recognized Indian tribes in 35 states. IHS provides services to approximately 1.8 million members in urban areas as well as on reservations.

Exhibit 6-9 Mission and Goals of HRSA

The mission of HRSA is to improve health and achieve health equity through access to quality services, a skilled health workforce, and innovative programs.

Its goals are:
• to improve access to quality care and services;

• to strengthen the health workforce;
• to build healthy communities; and
• to improve health equity.

Source: Health Resources and Services Administration. Retrieved from http://www.hrsa.gov

---

Exhibit 6-10 Mission and Goals of the IHS

The mission of the IHS, in partnership with American Indian and Alaska Native people, is to raise their physical, mental, social, and spiritual health to the highest level.

Its goals are:
• to ensure that comprehensive, culturally acceptable personal and public health services

are available and accessible to all American Indian and Alaska Native people; and
• to uphold the Federal obligation to promote healthy Indian people, communities, and cultures and to honor and protect the inherent sovereign rights of Tribes.

Source: Indian Health Service. Retrieved from http://www.ihs.gov

---

National Institutes of Health (NIH)

National Institutes of Health (NIH): The nation's premier biomedical research organization. The NIH is an agency within the Department of Health and Human Services (DHHS). Based in Bethesda, Maryland, the NIH is comprised of 28 separate institutes and centers. The institutes carry out research and programs related to certain specific types of diseases, such as mental and neurological disease, arthritis, cancer, and heart disease. There is an institute for each of the categories of disease for which NIH has programs, and a number of other components not specific to any disease categories.

The **National Institutes of Health (NIH)** is headquartered in Bethesda, Maryland, and is composed of 27 different institutes and centers, including the National Institute of Environmental Health Sciences, located in North Carolina. The NIH funds biomedical research in its own laboratories, as well as in universities, hospitals, private research institutions, and private industry, to develop new knowledge that can potentially improve the health of the population, the quality of medical care, and the understanding of disease processes. It conducts and supports research in the causes, diagnosis, prevention, and cure of human diseases; the processes of human growth and development; the biological effects of environmental contaminants; the understanding of mental, addictive, and physical disorders; and it directs programs for the collection, dissemination, and exchange of information in medicine and health, including the development and support of medical libraries and the training of medical librarians and other health-information specialists. A more thorough description of the Institutes and Centers are provided later in the chapter; meanwhile, Exhibit 6-11 describes the overarching mission.

Exhibit 6-11   Mission and Goals of NIH

The mission of NIH is to seek fundamental knowledge about the nature and behavior of living systems and the application of that knowledge to enhance health, lengthen life, and reduce the burdens of illness and disability.

Its goals are:

- to foster fundamental creative discoveries, innovative research strategies, and their applications as a basis for ultimately protecting and improving health;
- to develop, maintain, and renew scientific human and physical resources that will ensure the Nation's capability to prevent disease;
- to expand the knowledge base in medical and associated sciences in order to enhance the Nation's economic well-being and ensure a continued high return on the public investment in research; and
- to exemplify and promote the highest level of scientific integrity, public accountability, and social responsibility in the conduct of science.

Source: National Institutes of Health. Retrieved from http://www.nih.gov

Substance Abuse and Mental Health Services Administration (SAMHSA): Provides grants and data collection activities to promote quality behavioral health services. Major activities include the improvement of the quality and availability of prevention, treatment, and recovery support services in order to help reduce illness, death, disability, and cost to society caused by substance abuse and mental illness.

Substance Abuse and Mental Health Services Administration (SAMHSA)

The **Substance Abuse and Mental Health Services Administration (SAMHSA)** provides grants and data collection activities to promote quality behavioral health services. Major activities include the improvement of the quality and availability of prevention, treatment, and recovery support services in order to help reduce illness, death, disability, and cost to society caused by substance abuse and mental illness. The agency mission and the goals of its current strategic indicatives are provided in Exhibit 6-12.

Exhibit 6-12   Mission and Goals of SAMHSA

The mission of SAMHSA is to reduce the impact of substance abuse and mental illness on America's communities.

Its goals are:

- to create prevention-prepared communities to promote emotional health and reduce the likelihood of mental illness, substance abuse including tobacco, and suicide;
- to reduce the pervasive, harmful, and costly health impact of violence and trauma;
- to support America's service men and women and veterans—together with their families and communities—to ensure needed behavioral health services are accessible and outcomes are successful; and
- to broaden health coverage to increase access to appropriate high-quality care, and to reduce disparities between the availability of services for substance abuse, mental disorders, and other medical conditions.

Source: Substance Abuse and Mental Health Services Administration. Retrieved from http://www.samhsa.gov

CENTERS FOR DISEASE CONTROL AND PREVENTION (CDC)

On July 1, 1946, the Communicable Disease Center (CDC) came into being on one floor of a small building in Atlanta, Georgia, under the direction of Dr. Joseph W. Mountin. In the CDC's early years, combating malaria was its chief priority. More than half of CDC staff was devoted to the pursuit of malaria, and there were only seven medical officers on staff in 1946, since entomologists and engineers were in higher demand at the organization. While the agency's first budget was under $10 million, it did expand its focus to include all communicable diseases and to provide practical help to state health departments when requested. Although medical social scientists and epidemiologists were scarce in those early years, disease surveillance eventually became the cornerstone of the CDC mission of service and over time changed the practice of public health in the United States and around the world. It changed its name from the Communicable Disease Center to the Center for Disease Control in 1970. Two decades later, in order to recognize the CDC's leadership role in prevention, the United States Congress changed the agency's name to the Centers for Disease Control and Prevention. The widely recognized acronym, CDC, has been retained and its 60th anniversary was celebrated in 2006.

CDC Today

Today, with nearly 20,000 employees worldwide and a budget approaching $10 billion, the CDC has become a world leader in the public health arena. Its workforce consists of 173 different occupations with over half of these having advanced degrees. With its proactive approach, the CDC is known worldwide for its research and investigations to control disease and curb environmental health threats. Building on its history and leadership record, the CDC keeps national health statistics and performs health surveillance to monitor and prevent disease outbreaks and implement disease prevention strategies. Furthermore, as part of its global mission and its increasing role in health security, the CDC guards against bioterrorism and international disease transmission, with personnel stationed in 40 foreign countries.

With its continuing evolution as an efficient, effective, high-impact organization, the CDC engages in strategic planning and responsible budget management. In his 2011 budget justification and message to Congress, the agency Director, Thomas Friedman, MD, M.P.H., described the budget and the strategic initiatives it supports, as allowing, the CDC "... to both fortify the nation's public health infrastructure as well as expand efforts to accelerate health impact, reduce health disparities, and respond to the public health challenges of the twenty-first century." He underscores this commitment and forward thrust by asserting the following priorities: "Strengthening our dedication to science, particularly in epidemiology and surveillance, improving support to state and local health departments, reducing the incidence of leading, preventable causes of death, intensifying our work in global health, informing the discussion on health reform, and building upon our gains in emergency preparedness." (CDC, 2011)

Organizational Values

As an organizational leader, the CDC adheres to a set of core values that drive its decisions and actions. One hallmark of organizations that accomplish their mission goals and become sustainable long-term is adherence to a set of socially responsible guiding values. Organizational values also help to assure responsibility to the members of the organization and to the communities they serve. The core values of the CDC are provided in Table 6-3.

Organizational Structure

With its many divisions, offices, centers, and institute, the CDC is a large and complex organization that addresses the widest array of public health functions and challenges (see Figure 6-2). While most of the employees are based in Atlanta, there are also regional offices in Anchorage, AK; Cincinnati, OH; Fort Collins, CO; Hyattsville, MD; Morgantown, WV; Pittsburgh, PA; Research Triangle Park, NC; San Juan, PR; Spokane, WA; and Washington, D.C.

TABLE 6-3 CDC Core Values

Accountability—As diligent stewards of public trust and public funds, we act decisively and compassionately in service to the people's health. We ensure that our research and our services are based on sound science and meet real public needs to achieve our public health goals.

Respect—We respect and understand our interdependence with all people, both inside the agency and throughout the world, treating them and their contributions with dignity and valuing individual and cultural diversity. We are committed to achieving a diverse workforce at all levels of the organization.

Integrity—We are honest and ethical in all we do. We will do what we say. We prize scientific integrity and professional excellence.

Source: Centers for Disease Control and Prevention. Retrieved from http://www.cdc.gov

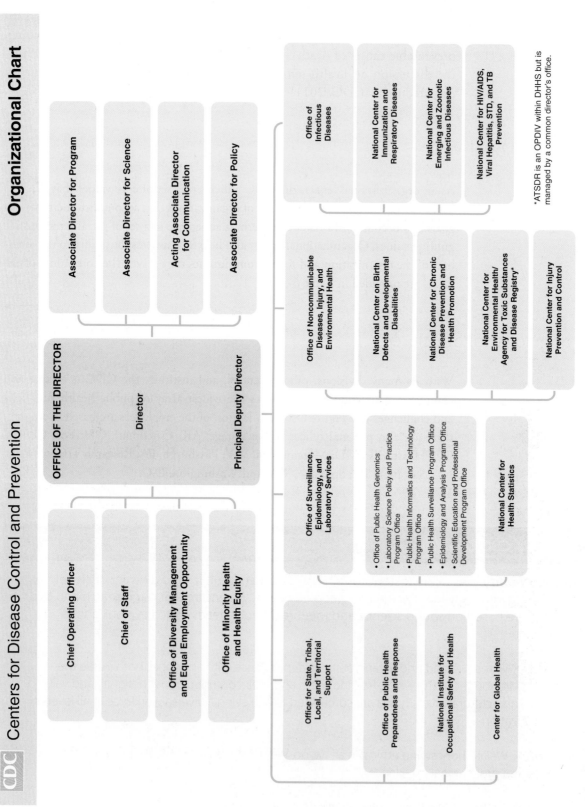

FIGURE 6-2 CDC Organization
Source: Centers for Disease Control and Prevention (CDC): http://www.cdc.gov/about/organization/orgChart.htm

FOOD AND DRUG ADMINISTRATION (FDA)

The FDA's beginnings can be traced back to around 1848 when the U.S. Patent Office hired Lewis Caleb Beck to perform chemical analyses of agricultural products. In 1906, the passage of the Pure Food and Drugs Act prohibited the commerce of adulterated and mislabeled goods, which began the FDA's function as a regulatory body as we know it today. The FDA, then known as the Bureau of Chemistry in the Department of Agriculture, led enforcement efforts offering basic elements of protection for consumers, a novel concept at that time. In July of 1930 the name was changed to the Food and Drug Administration (FDA), under the Department of Agriculture. The agency was transferred to HEW in 1953. Fifteen years later it became part of the Public Health Service and in 1980 became an operating Division of HHS. According to FDA historian John Swann, Ph.D., "To understand the development of this agency is to understand the laws it regulates, how the FDA has administered these laws, how the courts have interpreted the legislation, and how major events have driven all three." The responsibilities of the FDA have changed since 1906, just as the consumer environment has changed, but its core public health mission has remained the same.

The FDA Today

Today, with nearly 15,000 employees worldwide and a budget of approximately $4 billion, the FDA is responsible for ensuring the safety and effectiveness of products that Americans use every day. These products include, as stated on the FDA website, "human and animal drugs, 80 percent of the food supply, biological products, medical devices, cosmetics, radiation-emitting devices, and tobacco products." Ensuring the safety and effectiveness of these products requires a dedicated workforce, and the FDA has two major offices and seven product and research centers with employees working toward the FDA's primary goal, which is the public's health and safety. Many of the agency's employees are stationed outside of the Washington, D.C., area, staffing field offices and laboratories, regional and district offices, and international stations in other countries: China, India, the Middle East, Europe, and Latin America.

The agency is globally recognized for conducting research and investigations in its efforts to enforce food, drug, and product safety laws. Building on its history of consumer protection, the FDA works with states and other partners to provide a system of inspection and monitoring to prevent injury, harm, and illness. Investigators and inspectors visit thousands of facilities per year and work with state governments to help increase the number of facilities checked. Agency scientists evaluate applications for new human drugs and biologics, complex medical devices, food and color additives, infant formulas, and animal drugs. Additionally, the FDA monitors the manufacture, import, transport, storage, and sale of over $1 trillion worth of products annually.

In a 2011 report to Congress, Commissioner Margaret A. Hamburg, MD, described the context and challenges of the agency as follows:

> "Today, FDA is facing a critical set of public health challenges; challenges brought about by the unique demands of the twenty-first century. Science and technology are changing our world in dramatic ways; we are seeing an explosion of knowledge and capabilities emerging from many domains of research and from around the globe. In addition, we live in an increasingly globalized world, which has made ensuring the safety of food and drugs for the American people a global endeavor that integrates products and people across borders. It is clear that, today, FDA's job is fundamentally different—and far more complex—than it was even a few years ago. Although it will not be easy, we will address these challenges and aim to fulfill our mission by embracing innovation and actively pursuing partnerships with federal, state, and local agencies; international authorities; academia; nongovernment organizations; and the private sector." (FDA, 2011)

In its 2011–2015 Strategic Plan, the FDA outlines a path toward achieving a vision that includes: a transformed and integrated global food safety system, focused on prevention and improved nutrition; patients and families benefiting from decades of investment in medical science and technology; and a strong field of regulatory science so FDA can ensure the safety and effectiveness of new medical products throughout their life cycles.

Organizational Values

The FDA is a values-driven organization dedicated to excellence in the pursuit of its public health mission. It strives to be an effective national and international leader in protecting health and preventing illness. FDA planning, program implementation, and leadership are guided by these fundamental principles, as indicated on their website: "science-based decision making, innovation/collaboration, transparency, and accountability." These principles not only govern the actions of the FDA, but also govern FDA interactions within the organization, the scientific community, and the public. The agency values effective communication as the foundation for successful implementation of these principles. The FDA guiding principles are provided in Table 6-4.

NATIONAL INSTITUTES OF HEALTH (NIH)

The National Institutes of Health (NIH) was created in 1887, not as we know it today, but as a small laboratory in the Marine Hospital Service (MHS). Its purpose was to examine passengers of ships for cholera and yellow fever, which were serious public health concerns at the time. It was in this time period that scientists

TABLE 6-4 FDA Guiding Principles

Science-Based Decision Making—FDA has a solemn responsibility to protect and promote the public health. This responsibility requires that FDA base its policies, regulations, and enforcement decisions on sound science. For our decisions to have credibility, we must continue to seek the most current scientific understanding by supporting the work of agency scientists and scientific advisory committees. Strengthening FDA as a public health agency requires a culture that encourages scientific exchange, respects alternative viewpoints along the path of decision making, and protects the integrity of its scientific review processes.

Innovation/Collaboration—We cannot achieve our vision and address the challenges of the twenty-first century by working alone. To make rapid and efficient improvements in public health and drive innovation, we must harness the best ideas from a broad range of stakeholders and leverage resources through collaboration with other federal, state, and local regulatory and public health agencies; nongovernment organizations; consumer and patient organizations; academic medical centers and research universities; the private sector; and the public. For example, FDA is collaborating with state and local food safety authorities to develop standards and training that will establish a more integrated and coordinated national food safety system. The Critical Path Initiative (CPI), an agency effort to modernize the sciences for developing, evaluating, manufacturing, and using FDA-regulated products, has long recognized the importance of collaboration to leverage critical expertise and resources in driving scientific innovation.

Transparency—One of the most pressing FDA-wide goals is promoting transparency in FDA's operations, activities, processes, and decision making, as well as making information and data available in user-friendly formats while also protecting confidential and proprietary information. Transparency can enhance FDA's work and—more important—increase the trust and confidence of employees, policymakers, stakeholders, and the public. In response to a Presidential memorandum on transparency and open government, FDA established a Transparency Task Force to develop and implement recommendations for making useful and understandable information about FDA activities and decision making more readily available to the public in a timely and user-friendly manner. FDA will continue to engage the public in identifying ways to improve transparency at the agency.

Accountability—Consistent with our strong commitment to public service, we will maintain the highest degree of individual and professional accountability in the conduct of our work. Currently, we set measurable goals and openly monitor performance within the agency to make sure we continue to meet our commitments. We hold staff members and executives accountable for achieving organizational goals through annual performance plans that are aligned with our strategic priorities. And we monitor program performance by holding quarterly meetings with program managers and agency executives and sharing program performance data with the public through a new initiative called FDA-TRACK. We understand the importance of FDA's work to the health and welfare of our nation, and we will continue to hold ourselves accountable for delivering on that responsibility.

Source: Food and Drug Administration. Retrieved from http://www.fda.gov

in Europe were beginning to find that diseases could be caused by microscopic organisms transmitted from person to person. In response to this new evidence, the MHS assigned physician Joseph J. Kinyoun to operate the laboratory in 1887 in an attempt to curb the likelihood of cholera and yellow fever outbreaks. As described by NIH historian Victoria A. Harden, Ph.D., the Hygienic Laboratory, as it came to be called, was moved to Washington, D.C., in 1891, with Kinyoun remaining its sole full-time staff member for the next decade. In 1901, Congress legally recognized its function and funded the construction of a new laboratory charged with studying infectious diseases and similar public health matters. While the professional staff was previously limited to physicians, in 1902 the center was expanded to include divisions of pathology and bacteriology, chemistry, pharmacology, and zoology and authorization was given to hire Ph.D. scientists to head the divisions. Dr. Ida Bengtson, the first female bacteriologist, was hired in 1916. Then the influenza pandemic of 1918 struck Washington. Twelve years later, the Ransdell Act of 1930 changed the name of the Hygienic Laboratory to National Institute of Health (NIH) and authorized fellowships for biological and medical research. Following this by a few years, the National Cancer Institute was created, and by 1940 both agencies had moved to new facilities in Bethesda, MD, later to merge into a single organization. Following the 1944 Public Health Service Act, NIH went through a rapid growth in its funding and scope during the 1950s and 1960s with 15 institutes by 1970. During the next two decades NIH had grown to 27 institutes and centers, as well as specialized units such as the Office for Protection from Research Risks, the Office of AIDS Research, and the Human Genome Project which was completed in 2002.

Organizational Values

With nearly 6,000 scientists and many staff working at its 300 acre campus in Bethesda, MD, the NIH manages an annual budget of over $30 billion. This primarily supports projects through grants to over 325,000 researchers at over 3,000 universities, medical schools, and other research institutions in every state and around the world. In addition to its 27 Institutes and Centers, NIH has the Office of the Director which is responsible for setting policy and for planning, managing, and coordinating the programs and activities of all the NIH components. The Director provides overall leadership to NIH activities in both scientific and administrative matters. Although each institute within NIH has a separate mission, the Director plays an active role in shaping the agency's research agenda and outlook. With a unique and critical perspective on the mission of the entire organization, the Director is responsible for providing leadership to the institutes for identifying needs and opportunities, especially for efforts that involve several institutes. As a strategic leader, visionary, and biomedical scientist, Director Francis Collins, MD, Ph.D., has outlined five key themes for NIH:

1. Applying high throughput technologies to understand fundamental biology, and to uncover the causes of specific diseases

2. Translating basic science discoveries into new and better treatments

3. Putting science to work for the benefit of health care reform

4. Encouraging a greater focus on global health

5. Reinvigorating and empowering the biomedical research community

In a 2010 interview for the international journal, *Nature*, Dr. Collins summed up his forward thinking, action-oriented leadership style with this statement: "My job it seems to me is not to spend my time apologizing for being optimistic. But rather to try to take that optimism and turn it into reality." About two months later, he wrote in the same journal, while describing a new NIH initiative to get more young creative scientists into their own laboratories right after completion of their Ph.D.s, "We must develop ways to liberate our brightest minds to pursue high-risk, high-reward ideas during their most creative years…I fear that science may be suffering because of a failure to encourage the independence of the next generation of great minds." He concludes with, "I have been involved in the launch of many pilots, including that of the Human Genome Project, but I have a special affinity for this one: the future of biomedical research relies on the creativity and energy of its investigators. Unleashing that capability at all stages of a scientist's career should be a priority for us all."

The NIH Structure and Scope

There are more than 20 institutes and a library that comprise the core activities of the NIH organization, each described in Exhibit 6-13. Each institute has its own director and staff, mission, and budget, all under the broad umbrella of the NIH and HHS. In addition to the Institutes there is the Office of AIDS Research, Office of Research on Women's Health, Office of Disease Prevention, and Office of Behavioral and Social Sciences Research.

Exhibit 6-13   Institutes of the NIH

National Cancer Institute (NCI) leads a national effort to eliminate the suffering and death due to cancer. Through basic and clinical biomedical research and training, NCI conducts and supports research that will lead to a future in which we can prevent cancer before it starts, identify cancers that do develop at the earliest stage, eliminate cancers through innovative treatment interventions, and biologically control those cancers that we cannot eliminate so they become manageable, chronic diseases.

National Eye Institute (NEI) conducts and supports research that helps prevent and treat eye diseases and other disorders of vision. This research leads to sight-saving treatments, reduces visual impairment and blindness, and improves the quality of life for people of all ages. NEI-supported research has advanced our knowledge of how the eye functions in health and disease.

National Heart, Lung, and Blood Institute (NHLBI) plans, conducts, fosters, and supports an integrated and coordinated program of basic research, clinical investigations and trials, observational studies, and demonstration and education projects. It provides leadership for a national program in diseases of the heart, blood vessels, lung, and blood; blood resources; and sleep disorders. Since October 1997, the NHLBI has also had administrative responsibility for the NIH Woman's Health Initiative.

Continues

National Human Genome Research Institute (NHGRI) is devoted to advancing health through genome research. The Institute led NIH's contribution to the Human Genome Project, which was successfully completed ahead of schedule and under budget. Building on the foundation laid by the sequencing of the human genome, NHGRI's work now encompasses a broad range of research aimed at expanding understanding of human biology and improving human health. In addition, a critical part of the Institute's mission continues to be the study of the ethical, legal and social implications of genome research.

National Institute on Aging (NIA) leads a national program of research on the biomedical, social, and behavioral aspects of the aging process; the prevention of age-related diseases and disabilities; and the promotion of a better quality of life for all older Americans.

National Institute on Alcohol Abuse and Alcoholism (NIAAA) conducts research focused on improving the treatment and prevention of alcoholism and alcohol-related problems to reduce the enormous health, social, and economic consequences of this disease.

National Institute of Allergy and Infectious Diseases (NIAID) research strives to understand, treat, and ultimately prevent the myriad infectious, immunologic, and allergic diseases that threaten millions of human lives.

National Institute of Arthritis and Musculoskeletal and Skin Diseases (NIAMS) supports research into the causes, treatment, and prevention of arthritis and musculoskeletal and skin diseases, the training of basic and clinical scientists to carry out this research, and the dissemination of information on research progress in these diseases.

National Institute of Biomedical Imaging and Bioengineering (NIBIB) improves health by promoting fundamental discoveries, design and development, and translation and assessment of technological capabilities in biomedical imaging and bioengineering, enabled by relevant areas of information science, physics, chemistry, mathematics, materials science, and computer sciences.

National Institute of Child Health and Human Development (NICHD) research on fertility, pregnancy, growth, development, and medical rehabilitation strives to ensure that every child is born healthy and wanted and grows up free from disease and disability.

National Institute on Deafness and other Communication Disorders (NIDCD) conducts and supports biomedical research and research training on normal mechanisms as well as diseases and disorders of hearing, balance, smell, taste, voice, speech, and language that affect 46 million Americans.

National Institute of Dental and Craniofacial Research (NIDCR) provides leadership for a national research program designed to understand, treat, and ultimately prevent the infectious and inherited craniofacial-oral-dental diseases and disorders that compromise millions of human lives.

National Institute of Diabetes and Digestive and Kidney Diseases (NIDDK) conducts and supports basic and applied research and provides leadership for a national program in diabetes, endocrinology, and metabolic diseases; digestive diseases and nutrition; and kidney, urologic, and hematologic diseases. Several of these diseases are among the leading causes of disability and death; all seriously affect the quality-of-life of those who have them.

National Institute on Drug Abuse (NIDA) leads the nation in bringing the power of science to bear on drug abuse and addiction through support and conduct of research

Continues

across a broad range of disciplines and rapid and effective dissemination of results of that research to improve drug abuse and addiction prevention, treatment, and policy.

National Institute of Environmental Health Sciences (NIEHS) reduces the burden of human illness and dysfunction from environmental causes by defining how environmental exposures, genetic susceptibility, and age interact to affect an individual's health.

National Institute of General Medical Sciences (NIGMS) supports basic biomedical research that is not targeted to specific diseases. The Institute funds studies on genes, proteins, and cells, as well as on fundamental processes like communication within and between cells, how our bodies use energy, and how we respond to medicines. The results of this research increase our understanding of life and lay the foundation for advances in disease diagnosis, treatment, and prevention. NIGMS also supports research training programs that produce the next generation of biomedical scientists, and it has special programs to encourage underrepresented minorities to pursue biomedical research careers.

National Institute of Mental Health (NIMH) provides national leadership dedicated to understanding, treating, and preventing mental illnesses through basic research on the brain and behavior, and through clinical, epidemiological, and services research.

National Institute on Minority Health and Health Disparities (NIMHD) conducts and supports basic, clinical, social, and behavioral research, promotes research infrastructure and training, fosters emerging programs, disseminates information, and reaches out to minority and other health disparity communities to promote minority health and ultimately eliminate health disparities.

National Institute of Neurological Disorders and Stroke (NINDS) supports and conducts research, both basic and clinical, on the normal and diseased nervous system, fosters the training of investigators in the basic and clinical neurosciences, and seeks better understanding, diagnosis, treatment, and prevention of neurological disorders. The mission of the NINDS is to reduce the burden of neurological diseases, borne by every age group, every segment of society, and people all over the world.

National Institute of Nursing Research (NINR) supports clinical and basic research to establish a scientific basis for the care of individuals across the life span—from the management of patients during illness and recovery to the reduction of risks for disease and disability; the promotion of healthy lifestyles; the promotion of quality of life in those with chronic illness; and the care for individuals at the end of life. This research may also include families within a community context, and it also focuses on the special needs of at-risk and under-served populations, with an emphasis on health disparities.

National Library of Medicine (NLM) collects, organizes, and makes available biomedical science information to scientists, health professionals, and the public. The Library's web-based databases, including PubMed/Medline and MedlinePlus, are used extensively around the world. NLM conducts and supports research in biomedical communications; creates information resources for molecular biology, biotechnology, toxicology, and environmental health; and provides grant and contract support for training, medical library resources, and biomedical informatics and communications research.

Source: National Institutes of Health. Retrieved from http://www.nih.gov

Summary

"What we should be asking is not whether we need a big government or small government, but how we can create a smarter and better government."—*Barack Obama, 44th President of the United States of America and Nobel Laureate*

The federal sector, as has been seen, is very large and very broad in its scope. While it developed over many years there is a likelihood that the central role it plays in United States' society will continue to be deemed critical to the nation's well-being. It should be clear after reading this chapter that the federal sector offers many opportunities to work in public health at all levels. It also provides ample roles and occupations for leadership and management positions, some through the U.S. Public Health Service and others through an incredible range of programs and initiatives. In addition to the agencies described above there are many other federal sector initiatives being conducted by other departments that are engaged in public health activities, either directly or indirectly. Furthermore, the federal sector has a history of vigorously interacting with and engaging the state and local government public health agencies to help create a comprehensive system for public health.

Public Health Professional Perspective

Brandon Wood, Public Health Analyst/HRSA/CDR, Commander, U.S. Public Health Service

Interview by Dr. James Johnson

(Q): What is your own working definition of an effective manager?

Cmdr. Wood: I consider an effective manager to be one who is capable of balancing the responsibilities of his or her position while encouraging the development and growth of his or her subordinates in a productive, minimally stress-free, work environment. This by no means indicates that there will not be times a manager must challenge a subordinate to meet deadlines, but rather the subordinate enthusiastically is willing to go beyond the 100 percent required to accomplish the task at hand because the subordinate is confident that his or her manager has their best interest as the priority.

Continues

(Q): What are the biggest challenges you face on a daily basis?

Cmdr. Wood: The most challenging aspect of my position is meeting the constantly changing demands of delivering primary health care to the medically underserved communities within the United States. As our nation's health care system evolves into an entity no one yet knows, my job is to make sure that the least and the medically indigent of our communities have access to some form of primary care services. This becomes challenging under the auspices of performance-based outcomes, rising health care costs, increased incidence of chronic disease, and limited fiscal resources.

(Q): What skills are most essential for the work you do?

Cmdr. Wood: Flexibility, organization, patience, perseverance, enthusiasm, knowledge of government, knowledge of health care, knowledge of nonprofit operations, and assertiveness. Most of the skills are not technical or academic but rather interpersonal.

(Q): What is your favorite project or initiative you are currently working on? Please briefly describe.

Cmdr. Wood: I am currently assisting the Louisiana Primary Care Association and the 23 federally qualified community health centers in the state of Louisiana in preparing for its "Community Care Network" program. This program is a primary-care medical home model in response to the state's approved 1115 waiver for its Medicaid program. The concept promotes the risk sharing of the federally qualified health centers in providing managed care delivery to the centers' Medicaid population.

(Q): Do you consider yourself a "systems thinker"? If so, how or give an example.

Cmdr. Wood: I am very much a systems thinker. I am always aware that a decision I make can and potentially will affect something else. For example, when I am considering defunding a health center, I must be cognizant of the residual effects that the health center's closure will have on the surrounding community. Not only will the employees be affected, but their respective families and immediate community [too]. This is particularly salient in many rural communities of less than 5,000 residents. In many instances, the health center is one, if not the only, viable employer within the community. I am often reminded that we are all just a part of the whole; what affects one affects us all!

(Q): What advice do you have for students who plan a career in public health?

Cmdr. Wood: Health care in the United States is currently population based. With the advent on managed health care that focus on specific health outcomes and the rising concern of pandemics as a result of biological and chemical agents, public health care professionals need to be properly trained to respond to the needs of potential emergencies.

Finally, I would say from a personal development perspective that view every opportunity as means to learn, as each one of these opportunities will influence you into becoming a public health professional.

End

Public Health Professional Perspective

Maurice Davis, M.P.A., M.H.S.A., D.H.A., Health Scientist Administrator, Eunice Kennedy Shriver National Institute of Child Health and Human Development, National Institutes of Health

Interview by Dr. James Johnson

(Q): What is your own working definition of an effective manager?

Dr. Davis: An effective manager is one that must possess skills that are essential to keeping the organization moving in a forward direction while at the same time maintaining organizational operations and adhering to all internal and external regulations. The necessary skills or competencies includes being an effective communicator, controlling resources, staffing personnel, overseeing operations, and counseling employees.

(Q): What skills and values are most essential for the work you do?

Dr. Davis: In my current position, some of the most essential skills and values are being able to think analytically, being able to effectively communicate with others, and knowing that I am making an impact in the overall health of others.

(Q): What is a favorite project or initiative you are currently working on or have in the past? Please briefly describe.

Dr. Davis: My current favorite project is the "infant mortality" initiative. This initiative seeks to address the high rates of infant mortality, directly or indirectly, among African Americans specifically within the Washington, D.C., area. This initiative is charged with conducting biomedical and behavioral research aimed at exploring why the rates of infant mortality exceed those of similar geographic areas and populations. Over the past 17 years, this initiative has conducted 12 different research studies all focused on one health disparity issue—high rates of infant mortality among African Americans. There have been some very interesting findings from the research studies, some that include issues of health care accessibility, impact of new technology, lack of prenatal care, effects of racism, etc., that have all been essential for understanding issues effecting infant mortality among African Americans in Washington, D.C.

(Q): Do you consider yourself a "systems thinker"? If so, how or give an example.

Dr. Davis: I consider myself a "systems thinker" in that I try to view organizational interactions as a whole and how the subsystems interplay or impact the overall operation of the organization. This is really difficult to do in my current working environment due to the fact that it is a

Continues

government agency and there are many limitations due to regulations and laws that prevent the full spectrum of the systems thinking theory from being completely utilized. However, as much as possible, I do consider the systems thinking approach/techniques for those operations that are within my purview.

(Q): What advice would you give to students seeking careers in public health management?

Dr. Davis: Be diligent and seek opportunities that allow growth and creativity. Seek a career, not a job. Ask yourself "Is this something I can do for the rest of my life, grow from it, and make an impact of the overall health care system?" Oftentimes, the most rewarding careers are those in which you have the ability to gain a combination of extrinsic and intrinsic rewards. Your career should be something that you enjoy doing, not because it pays well, or provides flexibility, but because you enjoy doing it.

End

Public Health Professional Perspective

Deymon Fleming, M.P.H., Centers for Disease Control and Prevention, Atlanta, Georgia

Interview by Dr. James Johnson

(Q): What is your own working definition of an effective manager?

Mr. Fleming: An effective manager should be able to communicate the organization's direction, develop key relationships (internal and external), and provide a supportive growth environment for the development of employees.

(Q): What are the biggest challenges you face on a daily basis?

Mr. Fleming: Preparing staff for organizational change by ensuring smooth transitions during the change process.

(Q): What skills are most essential for the work you do?

Mr. Fleming: Planning, communication (oral/writing), organizing, coaching, flexibility, [being] team-oriented.

Continues

(Q): What is your favorite project or initiative you are currently working on? Please briefly describe.

Mr. Fleming: I am currently working on a newly formed committee for health disparities for infectious diseases. We are in the infancy stage and our mission is to promote efforts aimed at preventing and reducing infectious disease disparities. We are working to promote health equity and to identify and address the social determinants of infectious diseases and infectious disease disparities through research, surveillance, education, training, and program development. Populations with high infectious disease burdens and distinct infectious disease prevention needs, such as racial and ethnic minorities, immigrants, and women, are of major concern. Activities include work on vulnerable populations in preparedness, social determinants of infectious diseases, and neglected infections of poverty.

(Q): Do you consider yourself a "systems thinker"? If so, how or give an example.

Mr. Fleming: The principles that I find most challenging at this time are interconnected and all stem from my older conceptions of systems as rigid and oppressive, rather than as natural conditions of life and the universe as it is. Coming to systems with such preconceived notions, I have at times misperceived system purposes, not by inaccurately identifying some objectives, but by discounting the possibility of potentially conflicting ones. Thus, at times I have imagined that I got the *beat of the system*, but instead simply got the beat of part of it. It is important that I carry the explicit view that systems have multiple purposes and that I need to identify and name them, even if they appear to be in direct opposition to each other.

(Q): What advice do you have for students who plan a career in public health management?

Mr. Fleming: To always keep in mind that there are real people behind the data. Therefore, the decisions that are made at many levels can positively or negatively impact a "real person." Also, be willing to think outside of your comfort zone.

End

Discussion and Review Questions

1. What is the HHS? Identify its operating units.

2. Describe the duties of the Surgeon General.

3. Choose any three of the federal agencies described in this chapter and identify their organizational values. Are there similarities?

4. What is the role and purpose of the National Institutes of Health (NIH)? What are some of the research areas it is involved in? Describe at least five.

5. Where is the CDC located and what does it do?

6. What is the mission of the U.S. Public Health Service?

Action Learning and Critical Thinking

A. Visit the website of the CDC and identify at least three current initiatives it is involved in. Describe these and report to the class what you found.

B. Identify a disease or public health problem that has affected you or a family member. Look at the website of the NIH and determine which Institute is currently doing research in this area. Try to find out what new developments or breakthroughs there may be. Share this with your family or the class.

C. Visit the U.S. Public Health Service website or talk to a member of the USPHS and see what the requirements are for employment. Identify an area that you might be interested working in and learn as much as you can about it.

D. Search newspaper and magazine reports for timely articles on the FDA or CDC and share with classmates.

E. Identify and describe a federal agency that is doing public health work that is part of the core public health agencies like HHS. An example might be the Department of Defense (DOD) or Environmental Protection Agency (EPA). Go to their website and identify at least three public-health related initiatives they are involved in. Share this with the class.

Chapter 7

STATE AND LOCAL PUBLIC HEALTH AGENCIES

Learning Objectives

Upon completion of this chapter, you should be able to:

1. Understand the role of federalism in shaping state-level public health.
2. Identify examples of public health programs at the state and local levels.
3. Understand the functions and purpose of state and local public health.
4. Have greater knowledge about state public health law.
5. Understand the organization of public health at the state and local levels.
6. Identify a range of activities and services provided by state and local agencies.
7. Describe the responsibilities of a typical state or local health department.

Key Terms

block grants   federalism
categorical grants   fiscal federalism

Chapter Outline

INTRODUCTION

Before the United States became a country, public health was the responsibility of local villages and the colonies. Upon adoption of the U.S. Constitution the role of the state was further specified in the Tenth Amendment which states, "the powers not delegated to the United States by Constitution...are reserved to the States respectively." Subsequently, the States created their own constitutions, most of which provide for the protection of public health. In 1869, Massachusetts was the first state to create a board of health and by 1909 all states had health departments. At that time the primary functions were recording births and deaths and control of communicable disease. Over the next 100 years, state health departments expanded considerably and are now operational in all 50 states, the District of Columbia, and eight United States Territories. As described by Mary-Jane Schneider, at the State University of New York (located at SUNY-Albany), the states have the primary constitutional responsibility and authority for the protection of the health, safety, and general welfare of the population. The scope of this responsibility varies: some states have separate agencies for social services, aging, mental health, the environment, and public safety.

AUTHORITY AND FEDERALISM

From as far back as James Madison, the state governments have been characterized as "laboratories of experimentation" where prospective public health policies may be tried out on a smaller scale and where existing federal programs can be adapted to the conditions and needs of individual states. The cornerstone of this approach is fiscal federalism, the pattern of taxation and grants provided by the federal government. This involves **block grants** and **categorical grants**, typically emanating from the U.S. Department of Health and Human Services (HHS), as described in the preceding chapter. While the federal government often sets general goals and guidelines, individual states have a significant amount of discretion regarding the programs they implement. Most of the oversight, implementation, and enforcement of public health policy take place at the state level. Some states exceed federal requirements and often states have significant health programs and responsibilities of their own. One consequence of this type of state-based system is the wide variation in public health policy and organization we see in the United States. Concurrent with the influence of **federalism** on state public health policy and organizational structure, there are other factors that contribute to the differences among the states and territories. In the *Handbook of Health Administration and Policy*, Anne Kilpatrick and James Johnson identify these factors as "determinants of state policy variation":

- *Economic determinants:* One example is variation in per capita income. In 2010 the highest were Connecticut, New Jersey, Massachusetts, and Maryland while the lowest per capita incomes were in Mississippi, Utah, Idaho, and South Carolina.

- *Political determinants:* States with high citizen involvement and professional legislatures are more likely to support spending on public health programs. Examples of professional legislatures include California, Florida, and Massachusetts. Considerable grassroots citizen-initiated public health policies are seen in some states such as Oregon, Vermont, and California, but not others.

- *Interest Group determinants:* States may vary in interest groups due to their industries, religions, ethnicity, health patterns, and unique aspects of their local cultures. A dominant interest group in Arizona or Florida would be retirees; in heavy agriculture states like Kansas and Nebraska, it would be farmers; and in other states such as Texas and California there would be dominant Latino interest groups.

As shown in Exhibit 7-1, an example of state public health law resulting from all of the policy determinants is the one enacted in 1978 and amended several times until 2003 in the state of Michigan.

"No problem can be solved from the same consciousness that created it."
—*Albert Einstein, Physicist, Peace Activist, and Nobel Laureate*

fiscal federalism: The financial relations between and among units of government in a federal system. The theory of fiscal federalism, or multi-unit government finance, is one part of applied economics known as "public finance." The pattern of taxation and grants provided by the federal government.

block grants: A grant distributed in accordance with a statutory formula for use in a variety of activities within a broad functional area, largely at the recipient's discretion; grants that are allocated more broadly, with activities determined more by the grant recipient.

categorical grants: A grant that can be used only for specific, narrowly defined activities; grants that are very specific and targeted at selected public health programs and population groups.

federalism: A system of governance in which a national, overarching government shares power with sub-national or state governments.

STATE HEALTH DEPARTMENT ORGANIZATION

Given the variation in economic and political culture, the states and territories have developed different models of organizing their public health agencies. The Association of State and Territorial Health Officials (ASTHO) adopted the term *state health agency* as a term to describe any agency of the state that is vested with primary responsibility for public health within that state. Table 7-1 clarifies four different types of state health agency organizations.

Exhibit 7-1 Sample State Public Health Law

MICHIGAN PUBLIC HEALTH CODE

Act 368 of 1978

AN ACT to protect and promote the public health; to codify, revise, consolidate, classify, and add to the laws relating to public health; to provide for the prevention and control of diseases and disabilities; to provide for the classification, administration, regulation, financing, and maintenance of personal, environmental, and other health services and activities; to create or continue, and prescribe the powers and duties of, departments, boards, commissions, councils, committees, task forces, and other agencies; to prescribe the powers and duties of governmental entities and officials; to regulate occupations, facilities, and agencies affecting the public health; to regulate health maintenance organizations and certain third party administrators and insurers; to provide for the imposition of a regulatory fee; to provide for the levy of taxes against certain health facilities or agencies; to promote the efficient and economical delivery of health care services, to provide for the appropriate utilization of health care facilities and services, and to provide for the closure of hospitals or consolidation of hospitals or services; to provide for the collection and use of data and information; to provide for the transfer of property; to provide certain immunity from liability; to regulate and prohibit the sale and offering for sale of drug paraphernalia under certain circumstances; to provide for the implementation of federal law; to provide for penalties and remedies; to provide for sanctions for violations of this act and local ordinances; to provide for an appropriation and supplements; to repeal certain acts and parts of acts; to repeal certain parts of this act; and to repeal certain parts of this act on specific dates.

Source: Legislative Council, State of Michigan, 2009

TABLE 7-1 Types of State Health Agencies

Traditional public health agency: A type of state health agency that oversees public health and primary care only. Although it may also administer one other health-related program (i.e., environmental health, alcohol and drug abuse, etc.), its responsibilities are usually limited to improving or protecting the overall health status of the public.

Super public health agency: A type of state health agency that oversees both (a) public health and primary care and (b) substance abuse and mental health. This would likely include administering services supported by the federal Substance Abuse Prevention and Treatment (SAPT), Block Grant and the Community Mental Health Services (CMHS), and block grant programs.

Super health agency: A type of state health agency that oversees (a) public health and primary care and (b) the state Medicaid program.

Umbrella agency: A type of state health agency oversees (a) public health and primary care, (b) substance abuse and mental health, and (c) the Medicaid program, as well as (d) other human services programs.

Reprinted with permission from National Governors Association (NGA), *Transforming State Health Agencies to Meet Current and Future Needs*

Some states, about 26, have an agency specifically for public health, such as the Vermont Department of Health (see Figure 7-1) or the larger North Carolina Department of Health and Human Services. Other states, about 24, have super-agencies that combine many other functions, such as social services and/ or environmental protection, such as the Colorado Department of Public Health and Environment. See Exhibit 7-2 for the Michigan Department of Community Health, where the state agency has responsibility for public health, mental health, Medicaid, drug control, and aging services.

> "Vivacity, leadership, must be had, and we are not allowed to be nice in choosing. We must fetch the pump with dirty water, if clean cannot be had."—*Ralph Waldo Emerson, Poet and Public Health Activist*

The head of the state health agency is appointed by the governor, a board, or head of a larger umbrella agency, and will typically carry the title Director, Commissioner, or Secretary. In 26 states this is a cabinet-level position appointed by the governor. Access to the governor gives the agency head a greater opportunity to influence health policy. Many state health directors are physicians by training, with the MD or DO a requirement in 21 states. A recent report from ASTHO showed the following credentials among sitting state health directors:

- 33 MD/DO (medical degree)
- 21 MPH (master of public health)
- 16 MPA (master of public administration)
- 3 DrPH (doctoral degree)
- 5 JD (law degree)
- 1 DDS (dental degree)
- 1 RN (registered nurse)

The ASTHO described the state public health organizational landscape in their 2009 annual report as shown in Table 7-2.

STATE HEALTH AGENCY ROLES AND RESPONSIBILITIES

The core public health functions (assessment, policy development, and assurance) discussed in Chapter 1, "Public Health Mission and Core Functions," provide the overarching framework for public health policy in the state agencies. Each state health agency must assess the health status and needs of the population, set goals to improve the health status of its citizens, secure the funding necessary to implement strategies designed to achieve the goals, set standards and enforce regulations, and provide assistance to local health departments and other agencies. The Institute of Medicine reports from 1988 and the 2002 report *The Future of Public's Health in the 21st Century* serve as important yardsticks for states to compare against the conditions in their own areas. Furthermore, about 40 states use the *Healthy People 2010* report and *Healthy People 2020* when they are establishing their own goals and strategic plans.

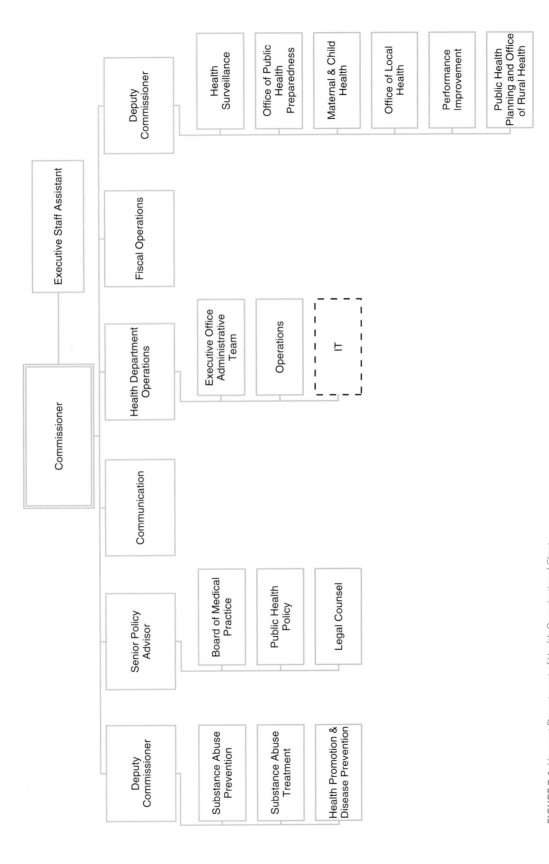

FIGURE 7-1 Vermont Department of Health Organizational Chart
Courtesy of Vermont Department of Health

Exhibit 7-2 Michigan Department of Community Health

The Michigan Department of Community Health (MDCH) is one of 18 departments of state government.

The department, one of the largest in state government, is responsible for health policy and management of the state's publicly-funded health service systems. About 2 million Michigan residents will receive services this year that are provided with total or partial support from MDCH.

The department was created in 1996 by consolidating the Department of Public Health, the Department of Mental Health, and the Medical Services Administration, the state's Medicaid agency. The Office of Drug Control Policy and the Office of Services to the Aging were later consolidated with MDCH.

MDCH has a 2010 gross appropriation of $13.1 billion and approximately 4,100 employees.

Services are planned and delivered through these integrated components:

- Medicaid health care coverage for people with limited incomes
- Mental health services for people who have a mental illness or a developmental disability, and services for people who need care for substance abuse
- Health needs assessment, health promotion, disease prevention, and accessibility to appropriate health care for all citizens
- Drug law enforcement, treatment, education, and prevention programs
- Promoting independence and enhancing the dignity of Michigan's older persons and their families
- Administering the Crime Victims Rights Fund, investigating and processing crime victim

compensation, and administering federal Victims of Crime Act grants

Medicaid provides health care coverage for more than 1.7 million Michigan residents who are eligible for Medicaid coverage under federal guidelines. Services covered include inpatient and outpatient hospital services, physician services, health screening for eligible children, maternity services, pharmacy, medical supplies and equipment, nursing, mental health care, community-based care, and other services.

The department's mental health services are primarily provided through contracts with 46 Community Mental Health Services Programs (CMHSP) and 18 Prepaid Inpatient Health Plans (PIHP). These programs provide community-based behavioral and mental health services and supports to persons with mental illness, developmental disabilities, and addictive disorders throughout Michigan. The CMHSPs are expected to serve more than 220,000 children and adults this year.

In addition, the department operates four adult state psychiatric hospitals for persons who have mental illnesses, one center for persons who have developmental disabilities, one children's psychiatric center, the state's Center for Forensic Psychiatry and, under a contractual agreement with the Department of Corrections, the Huron Valley Center, an inpatient program for prisoners. Substance abuse services are provided through 16 substance abuse coordinating agencies in various locations throughout Michigan.

The department's health administration component contracts with 45 local public health departments that serve all 83 Michigan counties. The local public health units assess health needs,

Continues

promote and protect health, prevent disease, and assure access to appropriate care for all citizens.

The office for services to the aging promotes independence and enhances the dignity of Michigan's older persons and their families through advocacy, leadership, and innovation in policies, programs, and services.

The crime victims' commission administers the Crime Victims Rights Fund, investigates and processes applications for crime victim compensation, and administers federal Victim of Crime Act grants.

Source: State of Michigan Department of Community Health

TABLE 7-2 ASTHO Report

- The majority of state public health agencies (28, or 55%) are structured as free-standing agencies, while the remaining 23 agencies (45%) are located within an umbrella agency structure in state government.

- In 13 states and the District of Columbia (28%), local health services are provided by the state public health agency (centralized or no local health departments).

- In 19 states (37%), local health services are provided by independent local health departments (decentralized states).

- The remaining 18 states (35%) function with some combination of the above arrangements (hybrid states).

- More than 82% of state health agencies have a quality improvement process in place, but only about 10% have it fully implemented department-wide.

- Over a third (18, or 35%) of state public health agencies operate with fewer than 1,000 full-time employees (or the equivalent).

- Six of the state public health agencies, however, have over 5,000 full-time equivalents. The median number of FTEs is 1,279.

Reprinted with permission from Association of State and Territorial Health Officials (ASTHO) Profile of State Public Health Volume 1. Retrieved from http://www.astho.org/Display/AssetDisplay.aspx?id=2882

Typical responsibilities performed by state health agencies serve the core functions of public health and address many of the goals and challenges outlined in the *Healthy People* reports. These are presented in Table 7-3.

Just as was shown in the last chapter at the federal level, many public health functions are carried out by other agencies within states. This requires close linkage between agencies and in some cases has led to duplication or fragmentation of

TABLE 7-3 Typical Responsibilities of a State Health Agency

Health Information

- Recording and issuing certified copies of birth and death certificates

- Publishing health statistics

- Birth defects registry

- Cancer registry

Disease and Disability Prevention

- Screening newborns for inborn errors of metabolism

- Immunization programs

- AIDS screening, counseling, and partner notification

- Tuberculosis control

- Screening children for lead exposure

- Investigating disease outbreaks

- Laboratory testing for infectious diseases

- Medical care for children with handicapping conditions

- Education on use of occupant restraints in vehicles

- Laboratory testing for weapons of mass destruction (biological, chemical, and radiological)

Health Protection

- Testing waters in which shellfish are grown

- Issuing permits for sewage disposal systems

- Monitoring drinking water systems

- Inspecting dairies

- License hospitals, nursing homes, and home health agencies

- Examining and certifying emergency medical personnel

- Inspecting clinical laboratories

(Continues)

TABLE 7-3 Typical Responsibilities of a State Health Agency *(Continued)*

Health Promotion

- Food vouchers for pregnant women, infants, and children (WIC)

- Prenatal care for low-income women

- Dental care for low-income children and adults

- School health education

- Family planning services

- Cholesterol and high blood pressure education programs

- Tobacco use cessation programs

Improving the Health Care Delivery System

- Scholarships for medical and nursing students

- Certificates of need for construction of health facilities

- Development of rural health policies and services

- Collecting and analyzing data on health care costs

© Cengage Learning 2013

public health services and policies. In order to meet these many responsibilities, states have chosen a range of organizational structures for their state health agencies. These fit broadly into four basic categories as described in Figure 7-2.

Just as with the federal government, there are other state agencies involved in public health or supporting public health efforts of the state health department. Table 7-4 provides some examples of public health services provided by other agencies at the state level.

An example of a state that combines many functions under a single umbrella or super-agency structure is Michigan.

Public Health Insurance

While it is not always a function of the state health department, as in the example of Michigan, all states do have responsibility for managing Medicaid insurance programs for people with limited means and certain disabilities. Most of the funding is provided by the federal government with oversight by the Centers for Medicare and Medicaid Services (CMS). However, states also contribute a large portion

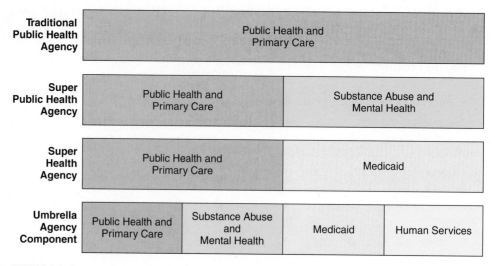

FIGURE 7-2 Common State Health Agency Organizational Structures
Reprinted with permission from National Governors Association (NGA), Transforming State Health Agencies to Meet Current and Future Needs

TABLE 7-4 Examples of Other State Agencies with Public Health Responsibilities

Public Health Function or Program	Agencies Reporting Full Authority	Agencies Reporting Partial Authority
Drinking Water Regulation	21	21
Environmental Health	25	23
Environmental Regulation and Management	11	28
Food Safety	31	17
Health Facility Regulation and Inspection	40	7
Health Professional Licensing	18	19
Medicaid	10	9
Medical Errors Reporting	17	11
Medical Examiner	12	4
Mental Health	9	10
Public Health Laboratories	47	3

(Continues)

TABLE 7-4 Examples of Other State Agencies with Public Health Responsibilities *(Continued)*

Public Health Function or Program	Agencies Reporting Full Authority	Agencies Reporting Partial Authority
Tobacco Prevention and Control	42	9
Substance Abuse Prevention	16	12
Vital Statistics Administration	49	2
WIC	47	3

Reprinted with permission from Association of State and Territorial Public Health Officials, 2005 Salary and Agency Infrastructure Survey

of Medicaid funding. The federal contribution varies based on state-per-capita household income relative to the national income average. The highest federal contribution of 83 percent goes to Mississippi.

Medicaid serves as the principle safety net for:

• low-wage working families and children;

• medicare-eligible beneficiaries with limited resources;

• blind or severely disabled children and adults; and

• uninsured pregnant women.

A breakdown by percentage of populations covered by Medicaid is provided in Figure 7-3.

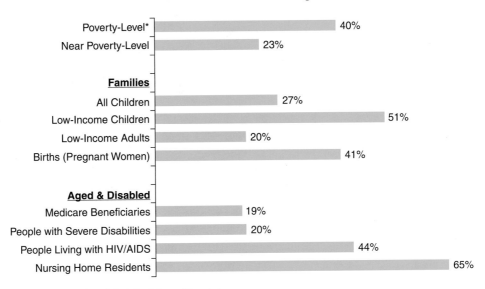

FIGURE 7-3 Medicaid's Role for Selected Populations
© Cengage Learning 2013

Environmental Protection

While only a few states have a specific agency, like the Colorado Department of Health and Environment, as the lead environmental agency, many states do have agencies which share the responsibility for a range of environmental services—usually food protection, safe drinking water, radiation control, health risk assessment, toxic substance investigation, and indoor air quality. Many states have also strengthened their capacity for surveillance and response in cases of biological and chemical terrorism.

Expanding Range of State-Level Initiatives

In 2010 the ASTHO described some of the many initiatives being undertaken by state public health agencies:

- Running efficient statewide prevention programs like tobacco quit-lines, newborn screening programs, and disease surveillance

- Assuring a basic level of community public health services across the state, regardless of the level of resources or capacity of local health departments

- Providing the services of professionals with specialized skills, such as disease outbreak specialists and restaurant and food service inspectors, who bring expertise that is otherwise hard to find, too expensive to employ at a local level, or involve overseeing local public health functions

- Collecting and analyzing statewide vital statistics, health indicators, and morbidity data to target public health threats and diseases such as cancer

- Providing statewide investigations of disease outbreaks, environmental hazards such as chemical spills and hurricanes, and other public health emergencies

- Monitoring the use of funds and other resources to ensure they are used effectively and equitably throughout the state

- Conducting statewide health planning, improvement, and evaluation

- Licensing and regulating health care, food service, and other facilities

State public health organizations also must engage in ongoing improvement; often this is done through embracing standards established by the federal government or external advisory groups. To varying degrees, state public health agencies have drawn from several tools developed to help them achieve higher standards in their organizations and programs. Among the most prominent:

- Turning Point, a network of 23 state partners and five National Excellence Collaboratives initiated by the Robert Wood Johnson Foundation to strengthen the public health system in the United States

- National Public Health Performance Standards Program (NPHPSP), a CDC National Partnership initiative that sets forth standards for state and local public health systems

LOCAL PUBLIC HEALTH DEPARTMENTS

The first governmental public health departments in the United States were established in urban areas, usually seaports and river ports, in response to health issues associated with population density and immigration. By the late 1800s, local health departments had been established along the east coast in Baltimore, Charleston, Philadelphia, Boston, Providence, and New York City and along inland waterways in Louisville, Indianapolis, New Orleans, and Chicago. The west coast port of San Francisco also had an early health department. The purpose then was primarily monitoring and addressing contagious diseases, enforcing quarantines, and eliminating environmental hazards through sanitation measures. As towns and cities grew between the two coasts so did the need for public health. Meanwhile, the scope of services expanded to reflect advances in science and the needs of diverse populations. Local health departments became involved in disease prevention by proving immunizations and health education. By 1950 there were over 1,200 health departments serving localities large and small, and by 2000 there were over 3,000 such agencies. These local government organizations retain most direct and immediate responsibility for performing public health activities at the community level. Given this large number of entities spread out across the country, it should be no surprise that the organizational structure and operational characteristics are even more diverse than what is seen at the federal and state levels. Likewise, the source of funds for local health departments varies widely among states. Some states provide most of the funding for local health departments while others provide very little. The federal government provides some funds to local health departments and often provides funding to the states to pass down to the local level. Local health departments can also receive funds from local taxes and fees collected for their services.

> "Public health must deal with short-term and longer-term issues. On a day-to-day basis, public health agencies are challenged to operate in a way that is proactive and anticipates public health issues before they become crises."—*Jan Carney, Vermont Public Health Commissioner and Public Health Scholar*

LOCAL HEALTH DEPARTMENT ORGANIZATION

Local health departments vary considerably by size and scope as well as jurisdiction, relationship with the state agency, and governance structure. The health departments serve different jurisdictions including cities, towns, counties, and regions (see Figure 7-4). Most local health departments serve the population of a county or a city-county jurisdiction. Many local health departments are governed by locally elected boards of health while others are governed by state agencies or local bodies such as a county commission or city council. Most states have at least some local boards of health since this is one of the earliest models of governance. However, a few states, Arkansas, Delaware, Hawaii, Louisiana, Mississippi, New Mexico, Rhode Island, and South Dakota, do not have any local boards of health.

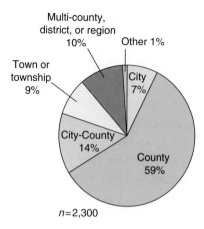

n=2,300

FIGURE 7-4 Type of Local Health Department Jurisdiction

Reprinted with permission from National Association of County and City Health Officials. (2006) 2005 National profile of local health departments. Washington, DC: NACCHO.

All local health departments work closely with state government and many are subsumed under the state public health agency. There are four basic models that explain the range of organizational relations between the local and state government in matters of public health.

- *Centralized:* The local health department is operated by the state health agency or board of health and the local department functions directly under the state's authority or the state health agency or board of health runs the local health department, which operates under the state's authority.

- *Decentralized:* Regardless of whether there is a board of health, in decentralized systems local governments have direct authority over health departments.

- *Shared Authority:* The local health department operates under the state health agency, board of health, and local government.

- *Mixed Authority:* In this kind of system, services are provided by a combination of the state agency, local government, boards of health, or health departments in other jurisdictions.

The variation of state-local relationships across the 50 states is shown in Figure 7-5.

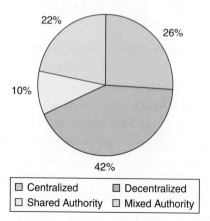

| ☐ Centralized | ☐ Decentralized |
| ☐ Shared Authority | ☐ Mixed Authority |

FIGURE 7-5 Types Local Public Health Organizational Relations

Reprinted with permission from Association of State and Territorial Health Officials

The Ohio Department of Public Health is one example of the close working relationships between state and local public health organizations. The 2011 Ohio policy statement on this topic is shown in Exhibit 7-3.

Exhibit 7-3   Ohio Policy on Local Health Department Support

The Office of Local Health Department Support, as well as many other offices and bureaus at the Department, work closely with local health departments to carry out the mission of public health in Ohio. The Office of Local Health Department Support works with local health departments by:

- serving as the agency liaison;
- administering public health minimum standards 3701-36-03 Ohio Administrative Code;
- drafting recommendations regarding approval of local health districts' contracts;
- serving on statewide committees, workgroups, and task forces; and
- providing technical assistance for program and policy support.

Good public health policies require dedicated champions and strong partnerships. The Ohio Department of Health (ODH) is fortunate to have both in the 127 local health departments which serve the citizens of Ohio. The public health system in Ohio is comprised of the ODH, local public health departments, and other partners, such as health care providers (public health associations) that work together to promote and protect the health of Ohioans. It is critical Ohio recognize the important role local public health serves in the state. In Ohio, local health departments—like school districts—maintain independent governance, but often work together, along with the state and federal public health agencies.

Depending on the type of health district (city, county or combined), funding for local public health departments comes from the support of their community through levies, city general operating funds, contracts, county government

and/or what is known as "inside millage." To help support local health departments, ODH receives funds from federal agencies, state general revenue, and other sources and distributes many of these funds through contracts and grants that contribute toward local public health programs and services. ODH also provides technical support, laboratory services, an IT communication network, and other critical services to aid local health department efforts.

As a profile of local health departments here are a few highlights:

- 58 urban health departments
- 71 rural health departments
- 22 city charters
- 61 combined health districts
- 24 counties with more than one health department
- Employs 5,574 individuals (2009)
- Total budget from federal, state, and local sources combined approximately $405,463,448.40 (2009)

Local health departments strive to promote health and the quality of life by preventing and controlling disease, injury, and disability. As was just recently seen, local health departments play a vital role in responding to public health issues like H1N1, providing significant public value in terms of dollars and lives saved. On a more day-to-day basis, depending on the size and budget of a local health department, services may include environmental health programs, immunization clinics, well-baby visits, prenatal, health screenings, dental, health promotion activities, and disease surveillance.

Source: State of Ohio Department of Health. Retrieved from http://www.odh.ohio.gov/localHealthDistricts/lhdmain.aspx

LOCAL HEALTH DEPARTMENT FUNCTIONS AND ACTIVITIES

A considerable amount of work has gone into assessment and the development of recommendations and guidelines by the Institute of Medicine, National Association of County and City Health Officials, the Centers for Disease Control and Prevention, and the Robert Wood Johnson Foundation. A summary of these functions and essential services is listed in Table 7-5.

TABLE 7-5 Ten Essential Functions of Local Public Health Departments

1. Monitor health status to identify community health problems:

a. Conduct or participate in community health assessments.

b. Obtain data that provide information on the community's health (e.g., provider immunization rates; hospital discharge data; environmental health hazard, risk and exposure data; etc.) to identify trends and population health risks.

c. Develop relationships with local providers and others in the community who have information on reportable diseases and other conditions of public health interest and help them report to the health department.

2. Diagnose and investigate identified health problems and health hazards in the community:

a. Using community health data, identify health problems and environmental health hazards.

b. Minimize, contain, and prevent adverse health events and conditions resulting from communicable diseases; food-, water-, and vector-borne outbreaks; chronic diseases; environmental health hazards; biological, chemical, and radiological threats; negative social and economic conditions; and public health disasters.

c. Receive and provide public health alerts to the general public, health care providers, emergency responders, and state and federal public health agencies.

d. Coordinate and facilitate public health emergency response activities with state and federal public health agencies in a manner consistent with the community's best public health interest.

e. Maintain access to laboratory capacity to help monitor community health status and diagnose and investigate public health problems and hazards.

3. Inform, educate, and empower people about health issues:

a. Work with individuals, community groups, other agencies, and the general public to share information to understand the social, economic, environmental, and other issues affecting the public's health.

(Continues)

TABLE 7-5 Ten Essential Functions of Local Public Health Departments *(Continued)*

b. Provide information, targeted to various audiences, to help those in the community understand what decisions they can make to be healthy.

c. Conduct health promotion activities to address public health issues.

d. Educate the public on policies and programs needed to improve the community's health.

4. Mobilize community partnerships to identify and solve health problems:

a. Lead, or participate in, a comprehensive planning process that engages the community in identifying, prioritizing, and solving problems affecting the community's health and establishing public health-related goals.

b. Lead and/or participate in partnerships of public and private organizations, state and local government agencies, businesses, schools, and the media to support and implement prevention strategies that address identified public health problems.

5. Develop policies and plans that support individual and community health efforts:

a. Serve as a primary resource to guide local, state, and federal elected and appointed officials to establish and maintain policies that support sound public health practice.

b. Lead and/or participate in policy development efforts to improve physical, social, and environmental conditions in the community as they affect public health.

c. Engage in an internal strategic planning process to develop and adhere to a vision, mission and guiding principles.

d. Promote social investments that sustain and improve community health.

6. Enforce laws and regulations that protect health and ensure safety:

a. Apply knowledge of public health law, ordinances, and regulations and the relationship between the law and public health practice to its ongoing operations.

b. Inform and educate individuals and organizations of the meaning, purpose, and benefit of public health laws, regulations, and ordinances.

c. Monitor the compliance of regulated organizations, entities, and individuals.

d. Conduct enforcement activities.

7. Link people to needed personal health services and assure the provision of health care when otherwise unavailable:

a. Lead efforts to increase access to culturally competent personal health services, including preventive and health promotion services.

(Continues)

TABLE 7-5 Ten Essential Functions of Local Public Health Departments *(Continued)*

b. Advocate for the development of systems that assure prevention and for the establishment of personal health services needed in the community.

8. Assure a competent public health and personal health care workforce:

a. Evaluate the local public health agency workforce on the demonstration of core public health competencies.

b. Address deficiencies in, and promote, public health competencies through continuing education, training, and leadership development activities.

c. Develop partnerships with academic institutions to provide educational experiences that address the public health workforce, including practice-based educational opportunities.

d. Recruit, train, develop, and retain a diverse staff.

e. Develop relationships with health care providers, community-based organizations, and others outside of the health department to promote the use of interventions appropriate for the prevention, containment, and/or remediation of public health problems.

f. Provide the public health workforce with access to support functions and tools needed to do their job.

9. Assess effectiveness, accessibility, and quality of personal and population-based health services:

a. Evaluate the effectiveness and quality of all local public health agency programs and activities against evidence-based criteria and use the information to improve performance.

b. Assess the effectiveness of strategies implemented through the comprehensive planning process to achieve the identified public health goals.

c. Review the effectiveness of interventions provided by those outside the health department for prevention, containment, and/or remediation of problems affecting the public's health.

10. Research for new insights and innovative solutions to health problems:

a. Using current data, develop evidence-based public health programs.

b. Work with researchers to actively involve the community in all phases of public health research.

c. Provide data and expertise to support research that benefits the health of the community.

d. Share results of program evaluations to contribute to the evidence base of public health.

Source: Institute of Medicine and Centers for Disease Control and Prevention

To demonstrate the relative effort in two important public health areas: 1) testing/screening and 2) population-based prevention activities, that local health departments manage, see Tables 7-6, 7-7, and 7-8.

TABLE 7-6 Local Health Department Provision of Testing and Screening Services

Disease or Condition	Percentage Providing
Tuberculosis	85%
High blood pressure	72%
Blood lead	66%
Other STDs	64%
HIV/AIDS	62%
Diabetes	51%
Cancer	46%
Cardiovascular disease	36%

© Cengage Learning 2013

TABLE 7-7 Local Health Department Population-Based Primary Prevention Activities

Condition or Behavior	Percentage Providing
Tobacco use	69%
Obesity	56%
Unintended pregnancy	51%
Injury	40%
Substance abuse	26%
Violence	25%
Mental illness	14%

© Cengage Learning 2013

TABLE 7-8 Local Health Department Activities and Services

Activity or Service	Percentage of LHDs
Adult immunization provision	91%
Childhood immunization provision	90%
Communicable/infectious disease surveillance	89%
Tuberculosis screening	85%
Food service inspection or licensing	76%
Environmental health surveillance	75%
Food safety education	75%
Tuberculosis treatment	75%
High blood pressure screening	72%
Tobacco use prevention	69%

© Cengage Learning 2013

Local health departments work closely with local schools, correctional facilities, public safety, law enforcement, and local community leaders. Examples from Boston; Orange County, FL; Nashville; and San Francisco are provided in Exhibit 7-4.

Exhibit 7-4   Examples of Local Initiatives

BUCKLE UP BOSTON!

Buckle Up Boston! is a child passenger safety program coordinated by the Boston Public Health Commission in collaboration with a host of public and private organizations. Their goal is to increase awareness about child passenger safety and increase usage rates of seats among low-income families in the city of Boston. According to the National Highway Traffic Safety Administration, motor vehicle crashes are the leading cause of unintentional injury-related death to children. Children age four

and under who ride unrestrained are at twice the risk of death and injury. Buckle Up Boston! provides car seats to families that might not otherwise have access to them and teaches parents about correct use of child passenger restraints.

THE WELLNESS CURRICULUM

The Wellness Curriculum, a collaborative project between the Orange County (FL) Health Department and the Orange County Corrections

Continues

Department, helps to address the health needs of inmates by providing information and education that is useful to them not only while they are in prison but, even more, as they are released into the community. Lack of adequate medical care prior to incarceration, combined with specific prison characteristics, places incarcerated people at higher risk for STDs, HIV, and hepatitis C, and also aggravates chronic conditions such as hypertension and diabetes. This program is targeted to a population that is hard to reach with traditional health education programs and uses surveys of the inmates to identify topics where education is most needed.

HEALTHY NASHVILLE 2010

MAPP provided the Metropolitan Nashville/Davidson County Health Department (TN) a way to reconnect with the community and engage them in a sustainable strategic health improvement planning process. Their process, called Healthy Nashville 2010, also offered the Nashville public health community the opportunity to integrate the work of various coalitions into one process, giving overarching direction for all existing health improvement initiatives in the county. Since the Mayor's announcement of the initiative, political support and strong momentum have sparked interest from a broad segment of the Nashville community. Healthy Nashville 2010 has given local public health system partners in Nashville the opportunity to collaborate and to coordinate their programs, decreasing duplication and competition among programs. A significant outcome of MAPP in Nashville has been rebuilding public health policy efforts. For example, Nashville's strategic plan for building sidewalks helped the Leadership Council foster relationships with other governmental agencies.

SAN FRANCISCO ASTHMA TASK FORCE

In 2002, the San Francisco Department of Public Health facilitated a process to address environmental health disparities in asthma, focusing on indoor air exposures of poor children. Published studies have related poor indoor air quality to the presence of substances frequently found in substandard housing: mites, cockroaches, and mold. The San Francisco Asthma Task Force, which included local public health and social service agencies, nonprofit and community-advocacy organizations, and community members, was formed to investigate the problem and develop recommendations for improving indoor air quality for lower-income tenants. The task force identified several major action strategies:

1. Establishing a cross-agency group to inspect public-housing properties and to create accountability mechanisms that rapidly brought conditions into compliance with the housing code.
2. Establishing standards and guidelines for comprehensive healthy housing, including roles for property owners—requiring government entities to strengthen the relationship between building codes and landlords' legal obligation to tenants to reduce housing-related health risks.
3. Instituting a legal housing-advocacy program for poor patients identified with asthma.

The health department was a key participant, but the project was broadly based in the community and led by community organizations. These recommendations addressed the social context of risk and incorporated nontraditional approaches for providing public health programs and services.

Local health departments also engage in planning based on population needs and demographics. The health status of each county is one measure that can be used in the planning and program design process. The Robert Wood Johnson Foundation has launched a national initiative to provide these data for every county in the United States. Working jointly with the University of Wisconsin, the initiative began with the state of Michigan and will continue until every state and county has been studied. See Exhibit 7-5.

Exhibit 7-5   Robert Wood Johnson Foundation, University of Wisconsin Population Health Institute—Michigan County Health Rankings

The Robert Wood Johnson Foundation in collaboration with the University of Wisconsin Population Health Institute released in February 2010 the first *County Health Rankings Report: Michigan 2010*. The *County Health Rankings* are a key component of the Mobilizing Action Toward Community Health (MATCH) project. This first-of-its-kind collection of 50 reports—one per state—helps community leaders see that where we live, learn, work, and play influences how healthy we are and how long we live. Each county receives a summary rank for its health outcomes and health factors and also for the four different types of health factors: health behaviors, clinical care, social and economic factors, and the physical environment. This report will be repeated for all states for at least three years.

Source: University of Wisconsin Population Health Institute. Retrieved from http://uwphi.pophealth.wisc.edu/

Summary

State and local health departments and agencies are central to the public health infrastructure of any country. This is especially so in a federalist system like the United States where there are 50 state governments, several territorial governments, and a vast number of local governments, such as counties and municipalities. The complexity and size of the United States demands a vast network of public health organizations, operating in a wide geographic area, with an incredible scope and range of services and activities. The interconnections between the various public health agencies provide a continuity that articulates with the federal sector to assure that public health needs are being addressed. Each state and locality shares some basic functions but also demonstrate considerable variability in the services they offer. Within this complex and diverse system there is ample opportunity for public health agencies to learn from each other. This has resulted in innovation and adaptation that ultimately benefits individuals and communities throughout the country.

Public Health Leader Perspective

Cathy Raevsky, Administrative Health Officer, Kent County Health Department, Michigan

In addition to her role as administrator in the Kent County Health Department, Ms. Raevsky is a Board member of the National Association of City and County Health Officers. She is also a leader in public health advocacy for Grand Rapids and the State of Michigan.

Interview by Dr. James Johnson

(Q): What is your own working definition of an effective manager?

Ms. Raevsky: Someone who can get the right things done efficiently and with grace.

(Q): What are the biggest challenges you face on a daily basis?

Ms. Raevsky: How to keep staff motivated to continue to work on ways to reduce costs, be more accountable and more data-driven while trying to function in an economic maelstrom.

(Q): What skills are most essential for the work you do?

Ms. Raevsky: Critical thinking skills and the ability to communicate to a wide variety of audiences both verbally and in writing (which surprisingly a lot of public health applicants don't seem to have anymore, no matter what their degree).

Continues

(Q): What is your favorite project or initiative you are currently working on? Please briefly describe.

Ms. Raevsky: Currently working on bringing five local hospital systems together (who are fierce competitors) to share the expense and results of a community health assessment required of all by health care reform. They are motivated to do an assessment together because it will cost much less than doing it individually, but my hope is that it will also lead to them developing their health care improvement plans together and community strategic plans together as that will be much better for the community.

(Q): Do you consider yourself a "strategic thinker"? If so, how or give an example.

Ms. Raevsky: Yes—my Board of Commissioners has to approve my fees, and many considered fees to be stealth taxes. It was painful for any department director to come before them to request a fee increase. Restaurant inspection fees had become extremely controversial, so I told them I would revisit the issue of how we came up with those fees. I took them all out on a restaurant inspection so they could see what the fee paid for and I explained how I planned to restructure my fees. I asked them if they had any problems whatsoever with my plan and if so, what would they recommend? I received no complaints about the plan, no recommendations, and only positive feedback when I went before them to request a total departmental fee increase of $450,000—much to the surprise and chagrin of my fellow department directors!

(Q): What advice do you have for students who plan a career in public health?

Ms. Raevsky: Begin your career at the state or federal level in order to establish networks and understand how state and federal systems work. When you have become accomplished at that level, seek a job at the local level because that is where public health actually happens. Don't start out local, because that will render you functionally and politically too naïve to be effective.

End

Discussion and Review Questions

1. What are the roles and responsibilities of local health departments?

2. What are the differences between state health agencies and local health agencies? What roles might be different? Discuss the difference in scope of activities.

3. Give an example of public health insurance. What purpose does it serve in public health?

4. Describe different types of state health agencies.

5. Discuss the range of relationships that exists between state and local health agencies.

Action Learning and Critical Thinking

A. Visit a local public health department (county or city) and tour the facility as a class or in small groups. Write down your observations and share with the class.

B. Interview a local public health official and ask them a series of questions pertaining to their organization and what it does. You are to design the questionnaire and have it approved by the course professor.

C. View the film *In Sickness and Wealth* and discuss what you learned about public health in Louisville, KY. What are your impressions of the public health director who is in the film?

D. Go to the website of your State Public Health Department. Look at its mission and organization chart. Identify its primary goals and objectives.

Chapter 8

NONGOVERNMENTAL AND GLOBAL HEALTH ORGANIZATIONS

Learning Objectives

Upon completion of this chapter, you should be able to:

1. Understand the importance of a global perspective in public health.
2. Better understand the range of international actors and agencies involved in global health.
3. Understand the importance and role of nongovernmental organizations.
4. Identify organizations in a wide range of global health sectors, including faith-based, nonprofit, foundations, and intergovernmental agencies.
5. Realize the significance of global health today and in the future.

Key Terms

effectiveness

efficiency

faith-based organizations (FBO)

Millennium Declaration

nongovernmental organizations

philanthropic organizations

social organizations

United Nations Organization (UN)

voluntary health organizations

World Health Organization (WHO)

Chapter Outline

INTRODUCTION

While most public efforts involve government at some level, much work is also done outside of government organizations or in partnership with government agencies. Within the United States alone there are over 100,000 voluntary health organizations, hundreds of health-related professional associations and societies, thousands of religious and faith-based health initiatives, and numerous large and small philanthropic foundations supporting and promoting public health. When we look globally, the number and variety of these kinds of organizations are even more considerable, plus there are large inter-governmental organizations like the United Nations that play a major role in public health.

BACKGROUND

While there had been considerable public health efforts in the old port cities of Alexandria, Athens, Rome, Constantinople (Istanbul), Venice, and Marseilles, as well as cities in Japan, India, and China, the focus was usually immediate and specific. In most of these locales there were problems with cholera, yellow fever, and plague, with quarantine being the dominant public health intervention. However, as the relationship between the environment and disease began to be better understood and the impact on trade came to be seen as profound, countries and city-states saw a need to work together to address concerns and share ideas. In 1851, the First International Sanitary Conference convened in Paris. This laid the foundations for international cooperation in health. Over the next 50 years, based on the work of

Louis Pasteur and Robert Koch, the germ theory of disease became widely accepted and new methods of disease prevention and mitigation were developed. Voluntary organizations established by churches and local citizens began to be established as part of the social justice and humanitarian mission of public health. One of the most notable private initiatives was the founding of the Rockefeller Foundation in 1909 and its International Health Commission in 1913. This Commission cooperated with many governments in campaigns against endemic diseases such as hookworm, malaria, and yellow fever. The Foundation provided essential financial support to establish medical schools in China and Thailand. Many foundations have been established since that time and have tackled some of the largest public health challenges in history.

After World War II, as countries rebuilt their infrastructure, there was an awareness of the need to invest in public health and the need for international cooperation. Specialized intergovernmental organizations (IGOs) representing most nations were formed under the umbrella of the United Nations. This included the United Nations Children's Fund (UNICEF) in New York City in 1946 and World Health Organization (WHO) in Geneva, Switzerland, in 1948, which led the effort to eradicate smallpox globally. Since then there have been global collaborative efforts involving IGOs, Foundations, governments, local nongovernmental organizations (NGOs), and the private sector to control and eventually eradicate infectious diseases such as malaria, polio, and tuberculosis.

TYPES OF NONGOVERNMENTAL PUBLIC HEALTH ORGANIZATIONS

A typology identifying the kinds of nongovernmental public health organizations is provided in Table 8-1, and a few examples are given to help foster an understanding of this important segment of public health.

TABLE 8-1 Typology of Nongovernmental Public Health Organizations
Voluntary Organizations (Example: American Cancer Society)
Nongovernmental Organization—NGO (Example: Partners for Health)
Social and Faith-Based Organizations (Example: Rotary Club—Campaign against Polio)
Professional Organizations (Example: American Public Health Association)
Philanthropic Foundations (Example: Robert Wood Johnson Foundation)
Intergovernmental Organizations (Example: World Health Organization)

© Cengage Learning 2013

VOLUNTARY HEALTH ORGANIZATIONS

Voluntary health organizations typically arise when a citizen or group of citizens identify a need that has not been met to their satisfaction. In the United States they are often called an association or society, such as the American Cancer Society and the American Heart Association. Sometimes they have taken a name that best captures the work or mission, for example March of Dimes or United Way. International examples of this type of organization are CARE and the International Diabetes Federation. Exhibit 8-1 offers a brief summary of some voluntary health organizations' mission statements. Most voluntary health organizations have local, national, and international headquarters since the health problems they focus on tend to be fairly universal. The primary objectives of these organizations are:

- raising money to fund programs;
- raising money to fund research;
- providing education to professionals;
- providing education to the public;
- advocating for public policy; and
- providing services to those with the disease or health problem.

> "The only ones among you who will be really happy are those who will have sought and found how to serve."—*Albert Schweitzer, Physician, Medical Missionary, and Nobel Laureate*

voluntary health organizations: When a citizen or group of citizens identify a need that has not been met to their satisfaction.

Exhibit 8-1   Examples of Voluntary Health Organization Missions

American Diabetes Association

The mission of this national association is to improve the lives of people with diabetes through prevention and research.

The organization embraces these guiding strategic principles:

- Funding diabetes research to prevent, cure, and manage the disease
- Providing services in hundreds of communities
- Offering accurate and reliable information about diabetes
- Defending the rights of those with diabetes

American Cancer Society

The American Cancer Society seeks to prevent and eliminate cancer through research, education, advocacy, and service. The Society also has a global mission that collaborates with other cancer-related organizations.

The organization embraces these guiding strategic principles:

- Supporting cancer research and programs to prevent, detect, and treat cancer
- Expanding access to quality cancer care, prevention, and awareness
- Reducing cancer disparities in minority and medically underserved populations

Continues

- Reducing and preventing suffering from smoking-related illnesses

Care

Based in Atlanta, Georgia, CARE is a humanitarian organization that fights global poverty by working with impoverished women. The organization maintains that, given the proper resources, women can lift their families and communities out of poverty. CARE is also active in delivering emergency aid to survivors of war and natural disasters.

The organization embraces these guiding strategic principles:

- Strengthening women's ability to help themselves and their communities
- Providing economic opportunity for women
- Delivering aid in emergencies and after natural disasters
- Influencing policy decisions
- Addressing discrimination

Sources: American Diabetes Association (http://www.diabetes .org); American Cancer Society (http://www.cancer.org); and CARE (http://www.care.org)

SOCIAL AND FAITH-BASED ORGANIZATIONS

social organizations: Like faith-based organizations, social organizations are formed to meet a social need.

faith-based organizations (FBO): A generic term covering all religious organizations, including nonprofit groups affiliated with a church or religion. Such organizations often address social issues by providing food, shelter, clothing, and health care to people in need. Began within a religion or group of religions that were established to meet the spiritual needs of a population.

Social organizations are typically formed to meet a social need and are not generally started with public health in mind. **Faith-based organizations (FBO)** begin within a religion or group of religions that were established to meet the spiritual needs of a population. Both social and religious organizations have existed from the beginning of human civilization. However, many have become involved in public health issues, either as fund raisers such as the Rotary Club for polio or the Lions Club for visually impaired people, or in the development of public health programs such as the sponsorship of food banks and shelters for the hungry, poor, and homeless. Religious organizations have a long history of volunteerism and generally see a relationship between spirituality and health. A Partnership Center has been established by HHS to lead efforts to build and support partnerships with faith-based and community organizations in order to better serve individuals, families and communities in need. Goals and focus areas of the faith-based initiatives are provided in Exhibit 8-2.

PROFESSIONAL ORGANIZATIONS

nongovernmental organizations: Legal entities created by private individuals, private organizations, publicly traded organizations, or in some combination where government influence, supervision, and management are removed, or at least greatly minimized, from the NGO's strategic and operational mission.

This category of **nongovernmental organizations** is comprised of a wide range of professional associations, societies, and federations representing health professions. The organizations typically support their members' interests and ideals, promote professional standards, and provide continuing education. Many also promote research and publish professional and scientific journals and reports. Professional organizations are typically supported by membership dues and donations. Many have developed the capacity to influence public policy at the state

Exhibit 8-2   About Faith-based and Neighborhood Partnerships

The HHS Center for Faith-based and Neighborhood Partnerships (The Partnership Center) is the department's liaison to the grassroots. The department recognizes that without the engagement of secular and faith-based non-profits, community organizations, neighborhoods, and wider communities, services will not reach people who need them most. The Partnership Center is a mechanism for the department to engage and communicate with the grassroots, ensuring that local institutions that hold community trust have up-to-date information regarding health and human service activities and resources in their area.

We work to build partnerships between government and community and faith-based organizations, which help HHS serve individuals, families and communities in need. The Partnership Center works in collaboration with HHS agencies, and our goal is to extend the reach and impact of HHS programs into communities.

The Partnership Center is committed to helping grassroots organizations access the necessary tools to reach those in need. While the center exists to supply information and resources, it is important to note that there is no "faith-based funding." Rather, the center works to enable community and faith-based organizations to

partner with the government through both non-fiduciary and fiduciary partnerships to achieve the goals of HHS and the specific goals put forward by President Obama for the Faith-based and Neighborhood Partnership Initiative. These are to:

Strengthen the role of community organizations in the economic recovery and poverty reduction.

Reduce unintended pregnancies and support maternal and child health.

Promote responsible fatherhood and healthy families.

Foster interfaith dialogue and collaboration with leaders and scholars around the world, and at home.

The priorities of the Partnership Center are carried out in a way that upholds and honors our Constitution-ensuring that both existing programs and new proposals are fully consistent with American laws and values. Our nation's Bill of Rights and important laws respecting both religious liberty and the non-establishment of religion protect not only our democracy, but also the plurality and vibrancy of America's religious and civic life.

Source: U.S. Department of Health and Human Services http://www.hhs.gov/

and national level through lobbying activities. Among the most influential are the American Medical Association, American Dental Association, American Nursing Association, and American Public Health Association. There is also the Association of State and Territorial Health Officials, National Association of City and County Health Officials, American Association of Health Education, American Association of Public Health Physicians, American Society for Public Administration, National Association for Public Health Policy, and hundreds of other health professions associations. In addition to their role nationally, these organizations often have an international association and kindred associations in other countries. In public health there is the World Federation of Public Health Associations representing about 70 country-level public health associations. Professional health organizations also have a state-level equivalent and often local chapters. Examples of this would be the Florida Public Health Association and Oregon Public Health Association.

Three very significant public health professional organizations, APHA, ASTHO, and NACCHO, are described in Exhibit 8-3.

Exhibit 8-3   Major Public Health Professional Organizations

APHA: Founded in 1872, the American Public Health Association brings together a diverse group of public health professionals who strive to improve the health of all Americans. APHA promotes community health and works to ensure that people throughout the United States have access to health care services and preventive health care. Acting as a collective voice for advocates of public health, APHA's mission is to protect funding for public health services, ensure broad access to health care, and eliminate health disparities, among other issues.

For more information go to their website at http://www.apha.org

ASTHO: Association of State and Territorial Health Officials is a national nonprofit organization that represents public health agencies in the United States and United States Territories. Many of the chief health professionals represented by ASTHO influence public policy, and the association provides support for policymakers. ASTHO's purpose is to monitor, assess, and advise on public health policies to improve health within states and territories.

For more information go to their website at http://www.astho.org

NACCHO: The National Association of County and City Health Officials is comprised of every health department across the country. NACCHO's mission is to provide support for local health departments in order to promote health and well-being in communities across the United States. Among other important issues, NACCHO focuses on community health, environmental health, public health infrastructure, and public health preparedness.

For more information go to their website at http://www.naccho.org

OTHERS: There are many professional societies and associations representing public health, such as the Society for Public Health Education, World Federation of Public Health Associations, and Health Section of the American Society for Public Administration. A list of these can be found at the CDC website at http://www.cdc.gov

Sources: American Public Health Association (http://www. apha.org); Association of State and Territorial Health Officials (http://www.astho.org); National Association of County and City Health Officials (http://www.naccho.org); and the Centers for Disease Control and Prevention (http://www.cdc.gov)

PHILANTHROPHIC FOUNDATIONS

Philanthropic organizations have made and continue to make significant contributions to public health in the United States and everywhere in the world. Foundations, starting with donations from wealthy individuals, families, or corporations, provide funding for health research, disease control and treatment, health promotion, and service delivery. There are local foundations that may restrict their funding to local challenges or populations, and there are national and international foundations with a larger mission. For many years the Rockefeller Foundation spearheaded research and initiatives in tropical disease control, health professions education, and family planning; the Ford Foundation has focused on education and poverty alleviation; Robert Wood Johnson Foundation has worked to improve access to care and lessen the impact of tobacco on health; and the largest foundation ever created, the Bill and Melinda Gates Foundation, has made unprecedented investments in global health and development (see Table 8-2). Other large foundations supporting public health are: the W.K. Kellog Foundation; Henry Kaiser Family Foundation; the Commonwealth Fund; Ted Turner Foundation, and the Clinton Foundation. See Exhibit 8-4 for a list of foundations promoting public health.

philanthropic organizations: Organizations and foundations that raise funds for research, disease control and treatment, health promotion, and service delivery.

Exhibit 8-4   Largest Foundation Endowments Promoting Public Health

1. The Bill & Melinda Gates Foundation

Believing that "every life has equal value," Microsoft cofounder Bill Gates and his wife, Melinda, established their foundation in 2000 with $106 million. The foundation's goals include improving health care and education, fighting extreme poverty, and providing increased access to information technology. The endowment now is about $35 billion.

2. The Wellcome Trust

The Wellcome Trust was founded in London in 1936 on the death of pharmaceuticals mogul Henry Wellcome. The mission of the Wellcome Trust is to promote research, improve human and animal health, and improve the understanding of science and medicine. Wellcome's endowment is approximately $25 billion, making it the largest charitable foundation in Great Britain and the second largest in the world.

3. The Howard Hughes Medical Institute

The Howard Hughes Medical Institute was founded in 1953 by aviator, moviemaker, and industrialist Howard Hughes to promote medical research and education. The initial endowment consisted of 75,000 shares of Hughes Aircraft. After Hughes' death in 1976, the endowment quickly grew from $4 million in 1975 to $15 million in 1978. During this time, the institute became more involved with genetics, immunology, and molecular biology. The endowment has since reached nearly $20 billion.

4. Lilly Endowment, Inc.

In 1937 the Lilly Endowment, Inc., was established by Josiah K. Lilly, Sr., and his sons with stock

Continues

from Eli Lilly pharmaceuticals company. While the endowment, which now totals $11 billion, is 13 percent of the company's stock, the foundation is separate from the pharmaceuticals company. The foundation's primary recipients are in community development and education. The Lilly Endowment is the largest private foundation in the United States to contribute mostly to local projects, especially in its home state of Indiana.

5. The Ford Foundation

Founded in 1936 by Edsel Ford and two Ford Motor Company executives, the purpose of the Ford Foundation was to fund scientific, educational, and charitable projects. Today, the foundation's mission includes promoting democracy, improving education, and reducing poverty. In its early years, the foundation supported National Educational Television, which was replaced by the Public Broadcasting Service (PBS) in 1970. The foundation's endowment is approximately $15 billion today.

6. The Robert Wood Johnson Foundation

The Robert Wood Johnson Foundation was established in 1936 by Robert Wood Johnson II, the son of Johnson & Johnson founder Robert Wood Johnson. The foundation focuses primarily on improving the health of all Americans by helping to provide quality health care at a reasonable cost, improving the quality of care for people with chronic illnesses, promoting healthy lifestyles, and reducing the problems caused by substance abuse and smoking. With an endowment estimated at $10 billion, the RWJ Foundation makes over $400 million in grants each year to support these causes and is the largest contributor to health improvement within the United States.

7. The W. K. Kellogg Foundation

Believing that "all people have the inherent capacity to effect change in their lives, in

their organizations, and in their communities," breakfast cereal magnate Will Keith Kellogg founded the W. K. Kellogg Foundation in 1930. Throughout his lifetime, Kellogg donated more than $66 million in Kellogg stock and other investments to the endowment, which today has assets of more than $7.8 billion. During 2006, the W. K. Kellogg Foundation funded $329 million in grants, including $39 million to areas devastated by Hurricane Katrina.

8. The William and Flora Hewlett Foundation

Hewlett-Packard cofounder Bill Hewlett and his wife, Flora, formed the William and Flora Hewlett Foundation in 1966 to address social and environmental issues. With more than $8 billion in assets, the Hewlett Foundation donates approximately $300 million annually. The foundation distributes grants worldwide in the areas of global development, education, performing arts, reproductive health, and environmental issues.

9. The Robert Bosch Foundation

The Robert Bosch Stiftung (Foundation) was established in Germany in 1964 to fulfill the philanthropic and social pursuits of Robert Bosch, founder of the automotive parts company Robert Bosch GmbH. Today, the foundation has an endowment of approximately $7 billion and distributes around $75 million in grants annually to promote education, international understanding, science and research, and health and humanitarian aid. The foundation also operates three health and research facilities in Germany.

10. The David & Lucile Packard Foundation

In 1964, David Packard, the other half of the Hewlett-Packard team, and his wife, Lucile Salter Packard, established the David & Lucile Packard Foundation. The foundation's mission

Continues

is "to improve the lives of children, enable the creative pursuit of science, advance reproductive health, and conserve and restore Earth's natural systems." The foundation's endowment is approximately $6 billion, and it awards about $200 million in grants each year.

Sources: Foundation Center (http://www.foundationcenter.org); Bill & Melinda Gates Foundations (http://www.gatesfoundation.org); Wellcome Trust (http://www.wellcome.ac.uk/); Howard Hughes Medical Institute (http://www.hhmi.org/); Lilly Endhowment Inc. (http://www.lillyendowment.org/); Ford Foundation (www.fordfoundation.org); Robert Wood Johnson Foundation (http://www.rwjf.org/); W.K. Kellogg Foundation (http://www.wkkf.org/); William and Flora Hewitt Foundation (http://www.hewlett.org/); Robert Bosch Foundation (http://www.bosch-stiftung.de); David and Lucile Packard Foundation (http://www.packard.org/).

TABLE 8-2 Rank Based on Number and Amount of Health Grants Given in U.S.

Foundation	Location
1. Robert Wood Johnson Foundation	Princeton, NJ
2. California Endowment	Los Angeles, CA
3. Susan Thompson Buffett Foundation	Omaha, NE
4. Duke Endowment	Charlotte, NC
5. Robert W. Woodruff Foundation	Atlanta, GA
6. Lincy Foundation	Beverly Hills, CA
7. Annenberg Foundation	Los Angeles, CA
8. Gordon and Betty Moore Foundation	Palo Alto, CA
9. California Wellness Foundation	Woodland Hills, CA
10. W.K. Kellogg Foundation	Battle Creek, MI
11. Kresge Foundation	Troy, MI
12. Eli & Edythe Broad Foundation	Los Angeles, CA
13. Moody Foundation	Galveston, TX
14. Starr Foundation	New York, NY
15. Silicon Valley Community Foundation	Mountain View, CA

(Continues)

TABLE 8-2 Rank Based on Number and Amount of Health Grants Given in U.S. *(Continued)*

Foundation	Location
16. Burroughs Wellcome Fund	Research Triangle Park, NC
17. Greater Kansas City Community	Kansas City, MO
18. David and Lucile Packard Foundation	Los Altos, CA
19. Blue Shield of California Foundation	San Francisco, CA
20. Donald W. Reynolds Foundation	Las Vegas, NV

Source: Foundation Center (http://www.foundationcenter.org)

INTERGOVERNMENTAL ORGANIZATIONS ON A GLOBAL SCALE

United Nations Organization (UN): Formed in 1945; multiple-nation body to promote health and humanitarian goals worldwide; headquartered in New York, NY.

Much of the work of public health occurs globally and often involves international organizations. Many of these exist under the auspices of larger governing- and decision-bodies that include governments from around the world. These entities are formed to benefit the global community in matters pertaining to public health, security, and other human needs and interests.

United Nations (UN)

Millennium Declaration: The Declaration asserts that every individual has the right to dignity, freedom, equality, a basic standard of living that includes freedom from hunger and violence, and encourages tolerance and solidarity. The Declaration also emphasizes the role of developed countries in aiding developing countries to achieve a "global partnership for development". These goals, referred to as the Millennium Development Goals (MDG), have served to guide global policy and many public health initiatives by foundations, governments, and nongovernmental organizations. There are eight goals with 21 targets, and a series of measurable indicators for each target.

The concept of multiple nations organizing to promote health and humanitarian goals began after World War II and was most substantially expressed with the formation of the **United Nations Organization (UN)** in 1945. In 2000 the UN adopted the **Millennium Declaration** with world development goals for 2015. The Declaration asserts that every individual has the right to dignity, freedom, equality, a basic standard of living that includes freedom from hunger and violence, and encourages tolerance and solidarity. The Declaration also emphasizes the role of developed countries in aiding developing countries to achieve a "global partnership for development." These goals, referred to as the Millennium Development Goals (MDG), have served to guide global policy and many public health initiatives by foundations, governments, and nongovernmental organizations. There are eight goals with 21 targets, and a series of measurable indicators for each target.

Goal 1: Eradicate extreme poverty and hunger

Goal 2: Achieve universal primary education

Goal 3: Promote gender equality and empower women

Goal 4: Reduce child mortality rate

Goal 5: Improve maternal health

Goal 6: Combat HIV/AIDS, malaria, and other diseases

Goal 7: Ensure environmental sustainability

Goal 8: Develop a global partnership for development

> "Living successfully in a world of complex systems means expanding not only time horizons and thought horizons; above all, it means expanding the horizons of caring…No part of the human race is separate either from other human beings or from the global ecosystem. It will not be possible in this integrated world for your heart to succeed if your lungs fail, or for your company to succeed if your workers fail, or for the rich in Los Angeles to succeed if the poor in Los Angeles fail, or for Europe to succeed if Africa fails…As so eloquently expressed by Dr. Meadows in this passage, we are all interconnected."—*Donella Meadows, Systems Scientist and MacArthur Fellow*

World Health Organization (WHO)

The **World Health Organization (WHO)** is the directing and coordinating authority for health within the United Nations system. It is responsible for providing leadership on global health matters, shaping the health research agenda, setting norms and standards, articulating evidence-based policy options, providing technical support to countries, and monitoring and assessing health trends. More than 8,000 people from more than 150 countries work for the Organization in 147 country offices, six regional offices, and at the headquarters in Geneva, Switzerland.

In addition to physicians, public health specialists, scientists, epidemiologists, nurses, engineers, and veterinarians, WHO staff includes people trained to manage administrative, financial, and information systems, as well as experts in the fields of health statistics, economics, and emergency relief.

World Health Organization (WHO): The division of the United Nations (UN) that is concerned with health. Headquartered in Geneva, Switzerland, the WHO came into being in April of 1948 when the United Nations ratified the WHO's Constitution. Its objective is the attainment by all peoples of the highest possible level of health. It is governed by the World Health Assembly which meets annually.

WHO has six core functions:

- Providing leadership and partnership in critical health matters

- Shaping health research and stimulating knowledge

- The implementation of public health standards and norms

- Generating policy options

- Aiding in the implementation of institutional infrastructure and capacity

- Monitoring and assessing health trends

WHO operates in an increasingly complex and rapidly changing landscape. The boundaries of public health action have become blurred, extending into other sectors that influence health opportunities and outcomes. WHO responds to these challenges using a six-point agenda. The six points address two health objectives, two strategic needs, and two operational approaches.

> "Go to the people. Learn from them. Live with them. Start with what they know. Build with what they have. The best of leaders when the job is done, when the task is accomplished, the people will say we have done it ourselves."—*Lao Tzu, Chinese Philosopher*

Promoting Development

During the past decade, health has achieved unprecedented prominence as a key driver of socioeconomic progress, and more resources than ever are being invested in health. Yet poverty continues to contribute to poor health, and poor health anchors large populations in poverty. Health development is directed by the ethical principle of equity: Access to life-saving or health-promoting interventions should not be denied for unfair reasons, including those with economic or social roots. Commitment to this principle ensures that WHO activities aimed at health development give priority to health outcomes in poor, disadvantaged, or vulnerable groups. Attainment of the health-related Millennium Development Goals, preventing and treating chronic diseases, and addressing the neglected tropical diseases are the cornerstones of the health and development agenda.

Fostering Health Security

Shared vulnerability to health security threats demands collective action. One of the greatest threats to international health security arises from outbreaks of emerging and epidemic-prone diseases. Such outbreaks are occurring in increasing numbers, fuelled by such factors as rapid urbanization, environmental mismanagement, the way food is produced and traded, and the way antibiotics are used and misused. The world's ability to defend itself collectively against outbreaks has been strengthened since June 2007, when the revised International Health Regulations came into force. Public health surveillance is the collection and analysis of data for global populations and the interpretation of that data for policymakers. Public health surveillance can warn public health officials of potential health emergencies, gauge the impact of implemented strategies, and track the occurrence of health problems.

Strengthening Health Systems

For health improvement to operate as a poverty-reduction strategy, health services must reach poor and underserved populations. Health systems in many parts of the world are unable to do so, making the strengthening of health systems a high priority for WHO. Areas being addressed include the provision of adequate numbers of appropriately trained staff, sufficient financing, suitable systems for collecting vital statistics, and access to appropriate technology including essential drugs.

Harnessing Research, Information, and Evidence

Evidence provides the foundation for setting priorities, defining strategies, and measuring results. WHO generates authoritative health information, in consultation with leading experts, to set norms and standards, articulate evidence-based policy options, and monitor the evolving global heath situation.

Enhancing Partnerships

WHO carries out its work with the support and collaboration of many partners, including UN agencies and other international organizations, donors, civil society, and the private sector. WHO uses the strategic power of evidence to encourage partners implementing programs within countries to align their activities with best technical guidelines and practices, as well as with the priorities established by countries.

Improving Performance

WHO participates in ongoing reforms aimed at improving its **efficiency**—the relationship of the amount of work accomplished to the amount of effort required—and its **effectiveness**—the degree to which the effort expended, or the action taken, achieves the desired effect, result, or objective—both at the international level and within countries. WHO aims to ensure that its strongest asset, its staff, works in an environment that is motivating and rewarding. WHO plans its budget and activities through results-based management, with clear expected results to measure performance at country, regional, and international levels. The WHO concept of a well-functioning health system has universal applicability and provides several critical success factors as delineated in it's definition, presented in Exhibit 8-5.

efficiency: The relationship of the amount of work accomplished to the amount of effort required.

effectiveness: The degree to which the effort expended, or the action taken, achieves the desired effect, result, or objective.

Exhibit 8-5   WHO Definition of Well-Functioning Health Systems

A well-functioning health system responds in a balanced way to a population's needs and expectations by:

- improving the health status of individuals, families and communities;
- defending the population against what threatens its health;
- protecting people against the financial consequences of ill-health; and
- providing equitable access to people-centered care.

Reprinted with permission from the World Health Organization. Retrieved from http://www.who.int

WHO Organizational Structure

The primary decision-making body of the World Health Organization is the World Health Assembly, which meets annually. Delegates from all 193 Member States meet to determine policies for the Organization and approve budgets. The Assembly is also responsible for appointing the Director-General, the head of the Organization, and for reporting to the Executive Board to advise on matters that need further study, investigation, or report.

The Executive Board consists of 34 health professionals who are elected for three-year terms. The Board meets twice per year, once before the Health Assembly and again afterward. The primary function of the Executive Board is to facilitate the work of the Health Assembly by enacting the decisions and policies set forth by the Assembly in their annual meeting.

The Secretariat of WHO, which is staffed on fixed-term appointments, is made up of health professionals, scientific experts, and support staff. They work at WHO headquarters, the six regional offices, and within countries.

Summary

The nonprofit and nongovernmental sector of health care is very large and universal. In public health this is especially so, and indeed much of the work of public health is carried out in these sectors. Often these agencies, organizations, and initiatives augment governmental public health and at other times they take the lead in addressing major health challenges. Within this sector there is incredible diversity of program and organization types. Some are over-arching and global, like the United Nations and its affiliates and agencies, while others are small and focused, such as an NGO working to mitigate diabetes in Belize or HIV/AIDS in Botswana. Furthermore, much of the funding for public health research and programs comes from the nonprofit sector, primarily through foundations and charitable organizations. Public health and global health could not accomplish their goals without the help and leadership of these groups.

The following case study in Chapter 16, "Cases in Public Health Management," is directly related to concepts and principles presented in this chapter:

- Case 22: Neglected Tropical Diseases—A Local NGO's Challenges

---

Public Health Professional Perspective

Dr. Omur Cinar Elci, MD, Ph.D., FRSPH, Director of Department of Preventive Medicine and Public Health, St. George's University, School of Medicine, Grenada, West Indies

Interview by Dr. James Johnson

(Q): What is your own working definition of an effective public health leader?

Dr. Elci: Public health is a discipline [that] interconnects population sciences, population dynamics, and medicine. An effective public health leader must have a robust understanding, knowledge, and experience in these disciplines as well as their interaction between each other. A successful public health leader should not limit her (him) self into one single sub-discipline or focus on an isolated interest. Issues in public health usually are multifaceted; multiple variables with complex relationships need to be successfully analyzed for a solution.

Continues

(Q): What skills and values are most essential?

Dr. Elci: Analytical thinking, leadership, problem solving, and flexibility are key skills for a successful and effective public health leader. Such person must value the cultural diversity, and have strong ethical and moral values.

(Q): Tell us a little about your current global projects.

Dr. Elci: Currently at St. George's University, we are on the process of establishing the first regional WHO Collaborating Center on Environmental and Occupational Health in the Caribbean. There are two related projects we are working on; one is to improve occupational health and working conditions of nutmeg productive workers and farmers, the other is to increase the use of renewable energy in the region. Another project aiming to hospital safety and needle stick injury is on the planning phase with our PAHO and CDC colleagues. There are various other global projects, such as investigation of cholera outbreaks in Kenya, continuing right now.

(Q): What advice do you have for students who want to work in international public health settings?

Dr. Elci: They need to prepare themselves by reading as much as they can before reaching their post. They need to remember that working with the people is the key element for the success; therefore; they need to be humble, respectful, and ready to serve. The preparation process must include intellectual, logistic, social, and mental preparation.

End

Public Health Professional Perspective

Evelyn Aako, M.P.H., Medical Case Manager, Pierce County AIDS Foundation, Tacoma Washington

(Previously Program Director, Community Health Outreach Work to Prevent HIV/AIDS, Honolulu, Hawaii)

Interview by James Allen Johnson III, M.P.H.

Continues

(Q): What is your own working definition of an effective policy leader?

Ms. Aako: An effective policy leader needs to possess the ability to take in information from diverse sources, sort and compare that information, and then use it to make informed decisions. This includes being open to information/knowledge from unconventional sources and analyzing issues from both micro and macro perspectives.

It is also vital to embrace a cooperative model of leadership that rejects the authoritarian idea that only leaders or those in the position to develop policy are the sole or best-qualified experts. Developing effective organizational policy requires the insights and knowledge of the entire organization, and while leaders are necessary to *guide* this process, they shouldn't be the only developers of policies which affect the staff and client population.

(Q): What are the biggest challenges you face on a daily basis?

Ms. Aako: My primary challenges include attempting to accomplish a lot with very little resources (i.e., time, funding, staff). On a related note, it is difficult to deliver services to populations struggling with multiple issues—chronic homelessness, substance abuse, past trauma, mental illness, etc. It can be a challenge to remain focused on the effective delivery of your organization's primary service when there are multiple problems facing the client population. I've had to accept that our organization does not have the time, resources, or expertise to address every issue faced by clients.

Another challenge I have encountered is hiring and managing staff members who are former peers of the client population. It is often helpful to employ former clients/peers; however, it can present complex issues around professional boundaries. Also, it can be a challenge to maintain staff that are adequately trained (especially in rapidly changing health fields such as HIV prevention) and equipped with the skills and knowledge to carry out frontline services.

(Q): What skills are most essential for the work you do?

Ms. Aako: It is essential to be excited about the work and passionate about delivering public health services, especially to marginalized and underserved populations, who are often most in need of public health interventions. An understanding and commitment to social change and social justice is vital.

It helps to have the ability to relate to and engage with broad ranging audiences: to work with street-based/homeless youth one day, and to give a presentation to Department of Health employees the next. Finally, my work requires flexibility and the ability to be creative with scarce resources.

(Q): What is a favorite project or initiative you are currently working on? Please briefly describe.

Ms. Aako: I developed a hepatitis A and B vaccination program which enabled homeless injection drug users (IDUs) to access free vaccinations at local methadone clinics. It was a wonderful project to work on because it was so firmly rooted in the model of harm reduction; increasing access to a necessary health service by implementing it in locations already frequented by IDU clients rather than expecting clients to visit the Department of Health clinic or a doctor's office (both very unlikely). That particular program felt like one of the best reflections of public health for all put into practice.

Continues

(Q): Do you consider yourself a "systems thinker"? If so, how or give an example.

Ms. Aako: Yes, I would consider myself a systems thinker, as I tend to analyze situations holistically and with an eye for how each part of the whole is interrelated. In terms of organizational management, I try to look at the health of the entire organization and the strengths that each part/individual contributes. I also tend to view dysfunction within one department (or exhibited by one employee) as a reflection of a larger organizational dysfunction and vice versa. Recognizing successes and failures is not about the actions of just one part of the system, but rather the interconnected workings of the system as a whole.

(Q): What advice do you have for students who plan a career in public health management or health policy?

Ms. Aako: I would advise spending some time working in the field providing direct public health services; that experience is invaluable to understanding how to best develop and implement public health policy. I don't think you can really effectively manage or develop policy if you don't know and understand the individuals/communities that are most affected. I also think it is important to integrate an understanding of social, political, and cultural factors into your work. This includes training in cultural competency and social justice studies of how class, race, gender, and sexuality affect people's lives and therefore how they might respond to different styles of management or forms of health policy.

End

Discussion and Review Questions

1. Discuss why global health organizations are important in public health.

2. Identify a public health organization involved in public health from each of these sectors: foundations, faith-based, nongovernmental, and intergovernmental.

3. Discuss the difference between nongovernmental and intergovernmental. Give examples.

4. What are the core functions of the World Health Organization (WHO)?

5. What is the WHO definition of a well-functioning health system?

6. What are the UN Millennium Development Goals (MDGs) and how are they used to promote public health?

7. What are the primary objectives of voluntary health organizations? Give some examples in addition to the ones provided in this chapter.

Action Learning and Critical Thinking

A. Watch the PBS series *Rx for Survival* and identify organizations from each of the sectors discussed in this chapter. Give examples of public health projects they are working on. Share your observation in class.

B. Go to the website of the United Nations and read about the MDGs and identify examples of where there are initiatives to address the goals. Try to find a success story for each one that pertains to health. Share this with the class or in a class paper.

C. Go to the World Health Organization (WHO) website and identify three initiatives to discuss and share with your class.

D. Visit a global public health organization and tour their facility and/or interview a senior staff member to better understand their purpose and activities. Some suggestions include CARE in Atlanta, GA; PanAmerican Health Organization in Washington, D.C.; Robert Wood Johnson Foundation in Princeton, NJ; United Nations in New York, NY; Kellog Foundation in Battle Creek, MI; Carter Center in Atlanta, GA; a local small NGO in your local area; or a faith-based initiative associated with a church.

PART III

PUBLIC HEALTH MANAGEMENT AND LEADERSHIP

This group of four chapters focuses on the inner workings of public health organizations and the many managerial and leadership processes necessary for effectiveness. Some of the processes and organizational dynamics addressed are strategy, human resources management, motivation, diversity management, conflict resolution, decision making, and workforce development. Many overarching themes and concepts are also discussed such as communications, systems thinking, innovation, healthy workplaces, and sustainability.

Chapter 9

MANAGEMENT, LEADERSHIP, STRATEGY, AND SYSTEMS THINKING

Learning Objectives

Upon completion of this chapter, you should be able to:

1. Distinguish between management and leadership.
2. Know the functions, roles, and responsibilities of managers.
3. Understand a range of leadership theories.
4. Determine which leadership approaches work well in public health and why.
5. Know the core competencies for leadership in public health.
6. Better understand systems thinking and strategic thinking.
7. Be able to see the relationship between leadership and sustainability.
8. Understand the process of decision making for managers.

Key Terms

adaptive leadership
conceptual skills
interpersonal skills
management

situational leadership
sustainability
systems theory
systems thinking

technical skills
transformational
  leadership
triple bottom line

Chapter Outline

INTRODUCTION

All organizations require managers and leaders. This is so in every sector—public, private, nonprofit—and in every kind of organization around the world. In fact, management is a universal element of the systems we design as organizations and is essential for their maintenance and sustainability. Whether it be the management of resources (people, money, buildings, technology) or strategy (vision, mission, goals, objectives) or behavior dynamics (motivation, conflict, politics, change, decision making) or values (fairness, responsiveness, accountability, social responsibility), the manager's role and effectiveness in that role are central to the organization's ability to exist and perform. In this chapter the functions of the manager are discussed along with the idea that managers are often leaders. Additionally, forces within the organizational culture and environment are discussed, with suggestions about ways to best address these. Public health managers are often leaders within their own professions, and many are leaders in their communities and in the world. In fact, public health, with its public service mission and global reach, is an ideal environment for managers who desire to have a positive and lasting impact. It is also a changing and sometimes demanding environment that offers many challenges and opportunities to grow professionally and personally.

MANAGERS IN PUBLIC HEALTH

In public health, the need for skilled and highly effective managers and leaders is great. The American Public Health Association (APHA), the Institute of Medicine (IOM), and the World Health Organization (WHO) have recognized the importance of management in public health systems, organizations, and programs. Furthermore, these groups have called for better management development and leadership if public health is to meet its greatest potential and achieve the goal of health for all. Exhibit 9-1 summarizes WHO's stance on modern public health management.

MANAGEMENT DEFINITIONS AND DOMAINS

management: A word that refers both to the people responsible for running an organization and to the running process itself; the use of numerous resources (such as employees and machines) to accomplish an organizational goal. Permeates all other functions and subsystems of the organization. It involves those in charge of all the other functions.

Management is the process of working with and through others to achieve organizational or program objectives in an efficient and ethical manner. From an organizational behavior and process perspective, the central feature of this concept of management is "working with and through others." From a resources perspective, efficiency is a key feature, and from a values perspective, managing in an ethical manner is central. Thus, the broad domains of management are: organizational behavior; organizational resources; organizational processes; and organizational values. Each of these requires different, sometimes overlapping, skill sets. Public health managers must be able to multitask as these domains are never exclusive and are highly interdependent. Because organizations are adaptive social systems, managers also must be well grounded in systems thinking and thus see both the micro-level effects and the larger macro perspectives, including unintended consequences

Exhibit 9-1   World Health Organization Perspective on Public Health Management

Public health practice is far more complicated in the twenty-first century than it was in the last century, when many important advances in public health were achieved. Public health is not merely a field devoted to technical and scientific research and practice; it is also a field that focuses on building effective partnerships to promote health and to manage organizations for the improvement of health.

The primary function of public health management is to provide leadership in the ever-changing environment of public health. Public health management is action oriented and should aim to effect positive changes in public health by building the capacity to facilitate policy implementation. Effective public health managers have both public health and management expertise.

Source: World Health Organization (WHO). Retrieved from http://www.who.int/chp/knowledge/publications/PH_management7.pdf

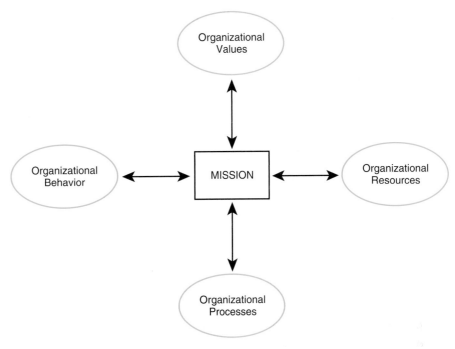

FIGURE 9-1 Management Domains
© Cengage Learning 2013

and organizational sustainability. The manager as systems thinker will be discussed further in this chapter (see Figure 9-1).

> "Management is efficiency in climbing the ladder of success; leadership determines whether the ladder is leaning against the right wall."—*Steven Covey, Leadership Scholar*

MANAGEMENT SKILLS AND BEST PRACTICES

Each domain requires certain knowledge, skills, and abilities that must be developed by the manager and continuously improved upon. Thus the manager, in a constantly evolving role, must engage in life-long learning and embrace change as a part of organizational life. Some skills that have been demonstrated to be useful across all four management domains can be grouped into three categories: technical skills, interpersonal skills, and conceptual skills. Social psychologist Robert Katz first identified these skill categories as technical, human, and conceptual.

> "The administrator needs: (a) sufficient technical skill to accomplish the mechanics of the particular job for which he is responsible; (b) sufficient human skill in working with others to be an effective group member and to be able to build cooperative effort within the team he leads; (c) sufficient conceptual skill to recognize the interrelationships of the various factors in his situation, which will lead him to take that action which is likely to achieve the maximum good for the total organization."—*Robert L. Katz, Harvard Business Review, 1955*

- **Technical skills** require knowledge about the procedures, regulations, policies, technology, tools, and techniques for conducting the activities of the manager's unit, division, or department.

- **Interpersonal skills** require an understanding of human behavior and interpersonal relationships; the ability to understand peoples' feelings, attitudes, and motivation; the ability to communicate in a clear and persuasive manner; the ability to foster cooperative relationships; and well-developed emotional intelligence.

- **Conceptual skills** involve analytical ability, systems thinking, logic, the ability to conceptualize complex situations and relationships, creativity, problem solving, anticipation of change, recognition of opportunities and problems, self-awareness, strategic thinking, intuition, and reasoning.

technical skills: Require knowledge about the procedures, regulations, policies, technology, tools, and techniques for conducting the activities of the manager's unit, division, or department.

interpersonal skills: Require an understanding of human behavior and interpersonal relationships; the ability to understand peoples' feelings, attitudes, and motivation; the ability to communicate in a clear and persuasive manner; the ability to foster cooperative relationships; and well-developed emotional intelligence.

conceptual skills: Involve analytical ability, systems thinking, logic, creativity, problem solving, anticipation of change and recognition of opportunity, self-awareness, and strategic thinking.

For the manager, technical skills are useful in training and directing employees in specialized activities. In public health some technical skills that are widely used include statistics, clinical procedures, informatics, quality improvement techniques, budgeting, and research methods. Interpersonal skills are essential to the manager because of the need to establish and enhance effective relationships with coworkers, organizational leaders, and people outside of the organization, including the public and professional peers. Lastly, conceptual skills are essential for effective planning, organizing, problem solving, decision making, innovating, and systems thinking. When considering management skills, it is important to realize skills can be developed through training and education. However, to achieve mastery in any skill, engagement and action is required. This is called *action learning*, and in some settings, *service learning* or *clinical learning*, where a skill can be put to the test and improved upon. It is also the opportunity to use mistakes as learning tools and to reflect upon choices, decisions, and behaviors as developmental insights. This approach to skill mastery is used widely with great success by athletic trainers, clinical instructors, art teachers, language coaches, research mentors, and individuals committed to all forms of self-improvement. The path to mastery of the skills associated with effective public health management often involves all four learning processes mentioned above: education, training, action learning, and reflection (Figure 9-2).

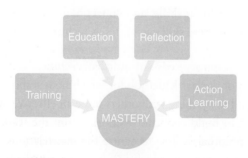

FIGURE 9-2 Management Skill Development
© Cengage Learning 2013

Another way to look at management skills is to consider *best practices.* According to Kiniki and Kreitner in their recent book, *Organizational Behavior: Key Concepts, Skills, and Best Practices*, the management best practices identified include:

- Clarifies goals and objectives for everyone involved

- Encourages participation, upward communication, and suggestions

- Plans and organizes for orderly workflow

- Has technical expertise and organization-related administrative expertise

- Facilitates work through team building, training, coaching, mentoring, and support

- Provides feedback honestly and constructively

- Keeps things moving with schedules, deadlines, and helpful reminders

- Controls details without being overbearing

- Applies reasonable pressure for goal accomplishment

- Empowers and delegates key duties to others while maintaining goal clarity and commitment

- Recognizes good performance with rewards and positive feedback

MANAGEMENT ROLES AND FUNCTIONS

Much of what public health organizations do is not determined by managers at all, but by external forces, events, and political leaders. From a systems perspective, organizations are open and cannot insulate themselves from the environment with which they interact nor from the larger global environment to which they belong, like every human being on the planet. *Interconnectedness* is a key concept in **systems theory**, and it is most applicable to public health managers and the organizations they work in. In public health there is a vibrant two-way interplay between organizations and environments. This includes the social, political, cultural, economic, and physical environment. As developed by Howard Zuckerman, and later presented in *Essentials of Health Care Management* by Steven Shortell at the University of California School of Public Health and Arnold Kaluzny at the University of North Carolina, managerial roles can be conceptualized as a triumvirate of three major roles: leader, designer, and strategist. Visually this can viewed as three interlocking triangles as shown in Figure 9-3. MIT systems scientist Peter Senge has made a strong case for the use of *mental models* in management as shown in this diagram.

This is a useful mental model to apply to public health managers since these managers often have to take an integrative approach and utilize all three perspectives. Furthermore, as systems thinkers, the need for design, strategy, and leadership become intertwined when dealing with complex problems as is often seen in public health.

systems theory: A view of an organization as a complex set of dynamically intertwined and interconnected elements, including all its inputs, processes, outputs, feedback loops, and the environment in which it operates and with which it continuously interacts.

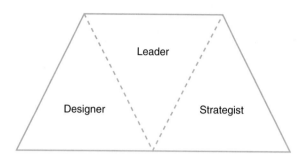

FIGURE 9-3 Mental Model of Managerial Roles
© Cengage Learning 2013

Public Health Manager as Designer

Public health managers must address such matters as organizational structure, innovation and change, informatics, service and research functions, operations, logistics, and myriad other aspects of the organization that require design. In designing public health organizations to meet future challenges, structures must be flexible and adaptive, while internal operating processes should also be malleable by design. Another concept of systems theory is uncertainty; this, along with the inevitability of change in the environment, necessitates a creative and innovation-embracing designer role for the public health manager. Figure 9-4 illustrates the various levels at which public health managers must be effective designers.

Public Health Manager as Strategist

Public health managers and leaders must be actively engaged in the process of strategic management (to be discussed more later in this chapter). As a strategist, the leader must articulate a vision for the organization and, working with managers, must develop plans and processes that establish goals to be achieved. This is all done in accordance with the organization's mission and values.

Public Health Manager as Leader

Many managers are leaders, but not all. In public health there is a responsibility for managers to be leaders by engaging staff and working to empower employees and communities to achieve desired goals and outcomes. The topic of leadership is expanded on later in this chapter, and its central importance to public health is emphasized.

In the next chapter we discuss motivation and the emphasis on the achievement motive in individuals, organizations, communities, and even nations. Not only is understanding motivation important to the manager's effectiveness in facilitating individual, team, and organizational performance, but it is also critical to his or her own level of achievement. In his research on managers, social psychologist Jay Hall, Ph.D.,

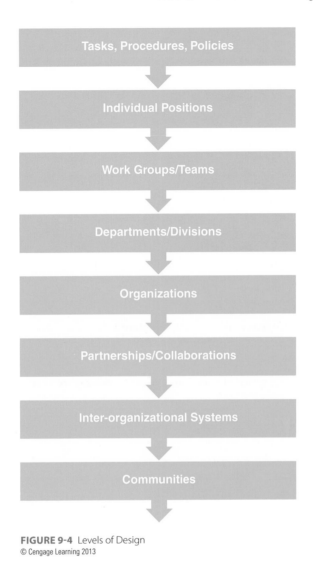

FIGURE 9-4 Levels of Design
© Cengage Learning 2013

has found a strong correlation between the achievement level of the manager and their ability to care for others and to communicate effectively. There is a marked difference between the way low- and moderate-achieving managers and high-achieving managers regard people. Low-achieving managers distrust the motives and the competence of their employees and generally have a pessimistic outlook. High-achieving managers, on the other hand, are generally more optimistic and tend to believe that their employees are both well-intentioned and competent.

OVERVIEW OF LEADERSHIP THEORY

There are many leadership theories as it is one of the most studied phenomena in all of human behavior. However, for the purposes of this book, it is best to identify the broad types of theories and then to expand upon a few that are most relevant to public health managers. Leadership theory can be categorized into eight different groups.

Each has elements that could be used to someday create a unified theory of leadership, but that is not likely to occur anytime soon.

- *Great Person theories* purport that leadership qualities are innate, that great leaders are born with certain qualities that make them great leaders and that these qualities are not learned. The term "Great Man" was originally tagged to these theories, since leadership was once thought of as being chiefly masculine. However, this changed considerably when female leaders, such as Elizabeth I of England, proved to be formidable military strategists as well as very effective leaders of their people.

- *Leader Trait theories* are similar to Great Person theories. They claim that a person possesses traits and attributes that make them suited to leadership roles. Trait theories often identify particular personality or behavioral characteristics shared by leaders. Traits might include such aspects as intelligence, good looks, or assertiveness.

- *Contingency theories*, as the name suggests, hold that leadership styles and qualities are dependent upon multiple external variables rather than innate traits of the leader. According to these theories, no single leadership style is the best fit for all situations because the reality is that situations are all unique. Success depends on many factors, such as the qualities of the leader, their subordinates, and the aspects of the situation. Thus the leader's approach or style is "contingent" on these variables.

- *Situational Leadership theories* maintain that leaders should alter their leadership styles based upon situational variables. These could include time, the nature of the task, urgency, or quality of information available. The kind of decision making required for a particular situation may require a particular kind of leadership. One situation might lend itself to delegating while another might require a more directive or participative approach.

- *Behavioral Leadership theories* are grounded in behavioral sciences and learning theory, implying that leaders can be made and are not necessarily endowed with innate qualities or inherited traits that make them good leaders. These theories focus on the actions of leaders as opposed to mental qualities or internal states. Through teaching and observation, people can learn to become great leaders.

- *Participatory Leadership theories* hold that leaders should take into consideration input from others. This is accomplished when leaders encourage participation and contributions from members of their subordinate group. This makes group members feel important to the decision-making process, which in turn makes them invested in the success of the group, organization, decision, action, or situation.

- *Transactional Leadership theories* rely on the role of management, organization, and performance and use a model that involves a system of punishment and reward. This approach to leadership is often used in business and industrial settings. Employees are rewarded for being successful (think of incentives to reach sales goals or production quotas) and punished or reprimanded for failure.

- ***Transformational Leadership theories*** focus on the relationship between leaders and their followers and the quality of that relationship. Transformational leaders help their subordinates see the importance of a task by motivating and inspiring them to achieve their greatest potential. Leaders reach goals and objectives by encouraging subordinates to reach their own goals and objectives. This kind of leadership is often associated with the embracing of high ethical standards and moral values.

SELECT MODELS OF LEADERSHIP FOR PUBLIC HEALTH

As was discussed earlier in the book when describing "servant leadership" in Chapter 2, "Public Health Professionalism and Ethics," public health has a great need for highly effective leaders. There are many resources utilized by the public health community and considerable accountability for responsible and effective use in the service of the public.

Additionally, public health organizations are very complex social systems that involve many people with a range of knowledge, skills, and abilities. Leadership is needed to create a common vision and to facilitate the achievement of goals and objectives. While there are many models of leadership styles and philosophies, several that are most applicable to public health are further described in the following sections.

> "Management is doing things right; leadership is doing the right things."
> —*Peter Drucker, Management Scholar*

Situational Leadership

situational leadership: Based substantially on aspects of a given situation, which in turn determines the style of leadership that is most likely to be effective.

As briefly described earlier, **situational leadership** is based substantially on aspects of a given situation, which in turn determines the style of leadership that is most likely to be effective. Figure 9-5 shows how this works on a continuum.

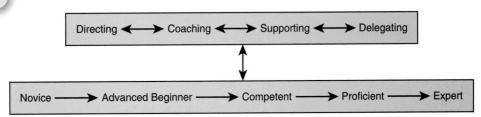

Novice does more directing and less delegating; expert does more delegating and less directing.

FIGURE 9-5 Situational leadership continuum
Source: Complied with information from Hersey & Blancahrd (1993) and Benner (1984)

Servant Leadership

This model of leadership was described in Chapter 2, "Public Health Professionalism and Ethics." However, it might also be useful, since this chapter focuses a great deal on management skills and leadership competencies, to look at the list of characteristics of a servant-leader as identified by the Greenleaf Center for Servant Leadership in Indiana (see Table 9-1.)

Transformational Leadership

transformational leadership: Leadership that strives to change organizational culture and directions. It reflects the ability of a leader to develop a values-based vision for the organization, to convert the vision into reality, and to maintain it over time.

Described previously under theories of leadership, **transformational leadership** places a major emphasis on vision. This is in part due to the "transformative" nature of this approach, which is very much about innovation and change (see Figure 9-6).

Adaptive Leadership

adaptive leadership: The practice of mobilizing people to tackle tough challenges and thrive. Adaptive leadership has three characteristics: 1) it preserves the DNA essential for continued survival; 2) it repels, reregulates, or rearranges the DNA that no longer serves current needs; and 3) it creates new DNA arrangements enhancing the ability to flourish in new ways and in new challenging environments. Successful adaptations enable a living system to take the best of its past into the future.

As described by Ronald Heifetz, MD, M.P.A., and colleagues at the Center for Public Leadership at Harvard University's Kennedy School of Government, **adaptive leadership** is the practice of mobilizing people to tackle tough challenges and thrive.

TABLE 9-1 Characteristics of Servant Leadership
1. Listening
2. Empathy
3. Healing
4. Awareness
5. Persuasion
6. Conceptualization
7. Foresight
8. Stewardship
9. Committment to the growth of people
10. Building community

Reprinted courtesy of Larry C. Spears, The Spears Center for Servant-Leadership.

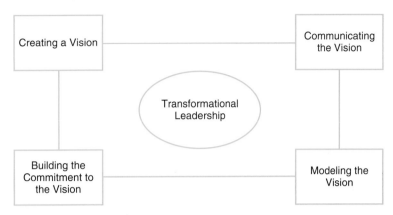

FIGURE 9-6 Transformational Leadership
© Cengage Learning 2013

Heifetz, who trained as a physician, draws from evolutionary biology to explain the concept of thriving as successful adaptation.

Adaptive leadership has three characteristics: 1) it preserves the DNA essential for continued survival; 2) it repels, reregulates, or rearranges the DNA that no longer serves current needs; and 3) it creates new DNA arrangements enhancing the ability to flourish in new ways and in new challenging environments. Successful adaptations enable a living system to take the best of its past into the future. Of course, new challenges always await, whether the system be an organism or an organization. In their recent book, *The Practice of Adaptive Leadership: Tools and Tactics for Changing Your Organization and the World*, Hiefetz and his coauthors offer six analogies from the organic world that can inform organizational leaders:

- Adaptive leadership is specifically about change that enables the *capacity to thrive*.

- Adaptive change *builds on the past*, being both conservative *and* progressive.

- Organizational adaptation occurs best when there is *experimentation*.

- Organizational adaptation relies on *diversity*, variation is central to system evolution.

- Innovations and new *adaptations displace*, reregulate, and rearrange old patterns.

- Organizational adaptation *takes time* and cultures change slowly.

LEADERSHIP COMPETENCIES FOR PUBLIC HEALTH

In addition to styles and philosophies of leadership, it is important to look at competencies. The public health leader and manager is in a very demanding position with many pressures placed upon him or her. Regardless of one's style of leadership, there are certain skills and knowledge bases that are needed to be effective. In their book *Principles of Public Health Practice*, Scutchfield and Keck place considerable emphasis on the acquisition of competencies demonstrated to be beneficial to individuals in leadership roles in public health, as shown in Table 9-2.

While competencies are an essential part of becoming an effective public health leader at any level of the organization, two areas—systems thinking and strategic leadership—require further explanation.

TABLE 9-2 Essential Public Health Services and Leadership

Essential Public Health Service	Leadership Activities
1. Monitor health status to identify community problems.	Use data for decision making.
2. Diagnose and investigate health problems and health hazards in the community.	Use data for decision making.
3. Inform and educate people about health issues and empower them to deal with the issues.	Engage in mentoring and training, social marketing, and health communication activities; empower others.
4. Mobilize community partnerships to identify and solve health problems.	Build partnerships; share power; create workable action plans.
5. Develop policies and plans that support individual and community health efforts.	Clarify values; develop mission; create a vision; develop goals and objectives.
6. Enforce laws and regulations that protect health and ensure safety.	Protect laws and regulations; monitor adherence to laws.
7. Link people to needed personal health services and ensure the provision of health care when otherwise unavailable.	Stress innovation; delegate programmatic responsibility to others; oversee programs.
8. Ensure a competent public health and personal health care workforce.	Build a learning organization; encourage training; mentor associates.
9. Evaluate effectiveness, accessibility, and quality of personal and population-based health services.	Support program evaluation; evaluate data collected; monitor performance.
10. Research for new insights and innovative solutions to health problems.	Utilize research findings to guide program development.

Reprinted with permission from Rowitz L. Public Health Leadership: Putting Principles into Practice. Sudbury, MA: Jones and Bartlett, 2001

SYSTEMS THINKING AND STRATEGIC LEADERSHIP

As described by Johnson and McIlwain in the *Handbook of Health Administration and Policy*, strategic planning and management are not a panacea for health care organizations, but instead a systematic approach to analyze an organization's situation and develop appropriate responses to improve. The **systems thinking** approach to strategy generally has four stages:

1. Situational analysis

2. Strategy formulation

3. Strategy implementation

4. Strategy control

The strategic leader as a systems thinker will deploy creativity, intelligence, and wisdom to assure success for each of these stages of the strategy process. Figure 9-7 provides a visual depiction of this.

> "Leadership is always dependent on the context, but the context is established by the relationships we value. We cannot hope to influence any situation without respect for the complex network of people who contribute to our organizations."—*Margaret Wheatley, Management Scholar*

In their book, *The Success Paradigm: Creating Organizational Effectiveness through Quality and Strategy*, Friesen and Johnson emphasize the importance of four cornerstones to any successful strategic planning process. These are: vision, focus, quality improvement, and organizational learning. Vision is essential in creating a mental model that can be articulated and shared with others to engage their support and participation. Focus is critical to concentrate the thought, energy, and resources

systems thinking: Generally has four stages: situational analysis, strategy formulation, strategy implementation, and strategy control.

- **creativity** to generate ideas,

- analytic **intelligence** to evaluate those ideas, and

- practical **intelligence** to implement the ideas and persuade others of their worth, and

- **wisdom** to balance the interests of all stakeholders and to ensure that the actions of the leaders seek the common good.

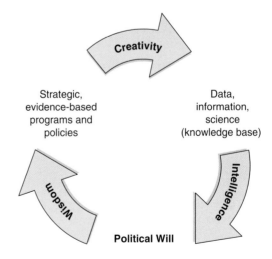

FIGURE 9-7 Systems Model of Strategic Leadership
Source: Sternberg RJ. "A Systems Model of Leadership." American Psychologist. 2007;62:34–42, and, Richmond-Kotelchuck. Oxford Textbook of Public Health. Oxford, England: Oxford University Press; 1991

needed for accomplishment of the mission and goals. Quality improvement ensures that the plan will use data in decision making, and organizational learning helps foster adaptation to a changing environment.

The skills a strategic leader will need are based on systems thinking since the organization is a complex adaptive social system as explained in Chapter 5, "Structure and Functions of Organizations." These skills and related competencies for different levels of staff, management, and leadership are presented in Figure 9-8.

Specific Competencies	Front Line Staff	Senior Level Staff	Supervisory and Management Staff
Creates a culture of ethical standards within organizations and communities	Knowledgeable to proficient	Proficient	Proficient
Helps create key values and shared vision and uses these principles to guide action	Aware to knowledgeable	Knowledgeable to proficient	Proficient
Identifies internal and external issues that may impact delivery of essential public health services (i.e., strategic planning)	Aware	Knowledgeable to proficient	Proficient
Facilitates collaboration with internal and external groups to ensure participation of key stakeholders	Aware	Knowledgeable to proficient	Proficient
Promotes team and organizational learning	Knowledgeable	Knowledgeable to proficient	Proficient
Contributes to development, implementation, and monitoring of organizational performance standards	Aware to knowledgeable	Knowledgeable to proficient	Proficient
Uses the legal and political system to effect change	Aware	Knowledgeable	Proficient
Applies the theory of organizational structures to professional practice	Aware	Knowledgeable	Proficient

FIGURE 9-8 Leadership and Systems Thinking Skills
Source: Public Health Foundation, Council on Linkages between Academia and Public Health Practice. *Competencies Project*

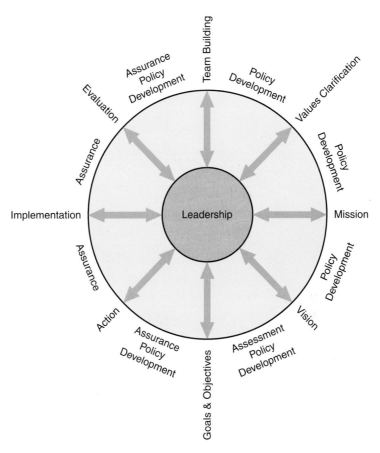

FIGURE 9-9 Systems Approach to Public Health Leadership and Core Functions
Reprinted with permission from Rowitz L. *Public Health Leadership: Putting Principles into Practice.* Sudbury, MA: Jones and Bartlett, 2001

The leader in their role as strategist and systems thinker must think globally and consider the interdependence of managerial processes, leadership responsibilities, public health competencies, and the elements of strategy such as mission, vision, values, goals, and objectives. In fact, the strategic leader is at the hub of a system of forces, influences, and responsibilities as depicted in Figure 9-9.

LEADERSHIP AND SUSTAINABILITY

In his book, *Public Health Leadership*, Rowitz advocates that public health leaders remain close to their communities, both internal and external. He provides a list of leadership practices that can be adopted to help with public health leader sustainability. These are provided in Exhibit 9-2.

Exhibit 9-2   Public Health Leadership Sustainability

1. Strengthen the infrastructure of public health by utilizing the core functions and essential public health services framework;
2. Improve the health of each person in the community;
3. Build coalitions for public health;
4. Work with leaders from culturally diverse backgrounds;
5. Collaborate with boards for rational planning;
6. Learn leadership through mentoring and coaching;
7. Commit to lifelong learning;
8. Promote health protection for all;
9. Think globally and act locally;
10. Manage as well as lead;
11. Walk the talk;
12. Understand the importance of community;
13. Be proactive and not reactive;
14. See leadership everywhere;
15. Know that leaders are born and made; and
16. Live our values.

Reprinted with permission from Rowitz L. Public Health Leadership: Putting Principles into Practice. Sudbury, MA: Jones and Bartlett; 2001.

---

sustainability: Creating and maintaining the conditions under which humans and nature can exist in productive harmony that permits fulfilling the social, economic, and other requirements of present and future generations; focuses on the organization's environmental practices in balance with fiscal and social responsibility to assure the long-term success of the organization and its programs.

triple bottom line: A new trend worldwide with a focus on sustainability, the triple bottom line focuses not only on the financial/economic bottom line, but includes social responsibility and the environment.

Another consideration for the leader is program **sustainability**. This is most likely to be assured by embracing a "**triple bottom line**." Instead of focusing only on the classic bottom line of finances, the leader attends to three concurrent ones: financial viability, social responsibility, and the environment. By doing so, a program or organization is more sustainable over a longer period of time. See a diagram of the triple bottom line in Figure 9-10.

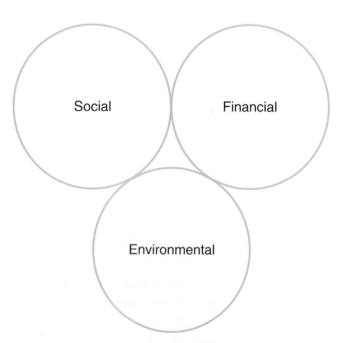

FIGURE 9-10 Triple Bottom Line and Sustainability
© Cengage Learning 2013

Summary

Management and leadership are closely related but as has been discussed, leaders can come from any part of the organization and can occupy any position. Leadership is not limited to the domain of managers. However, the public health manager is engaged in many activities that provide ample opportunity to engage in leadership. The style of leadership most compatible with public health values is transformational, adaptive, and based on the principles of servant leadership with a commitment to serve the public. Managers and leaders are most effective when they engage in systems thinking and embrace the full complexity of any public health challenge, program, or initiative. Furthermore, these leaders must think strategically and look for long-term effects as well as seek to assure organizational or program sustainability.

The following case studies in Chapter 16, "Cases in Public Health Management," are directly related to concepts and principles presented in this chapter:

- Case 3: The Anti-Vaccination Paradigm
- Case 7: Sick Building Syndrome
- Case 8: To Hear this Message in Korean, Press '9'
- Case 9: A *Giardia* Outbreak?
- Case 10: Zero-Tolerance for Smoking
- Case 11: Budget Cuts in Home Care Program
- Case 12: Don't Ask, But Tell
- Case 14: Collaborative Approach to Diabetes Prevention and Care
- Case 15: Toy Recall Prompts Attention to Lead Poisoning

Public Health Leader Perspective

Charles Green, MD, M.P.H., USAF Surgeon General, Washington, D.C., Public Health Background

Lt. Gen. (Dr.) Charles B. Green is the Surgeon General of the U.S. Air Force. After completing his medical degree at the Medical College of Wisconsin in Milwaukee, General Green entered active duty in 1978. He later completed a Master of Public Health (MPH) degree at Harvard University, School of Public Health. General Green is an expert in disaster relief operations and has planned and led humanitarian relief efforts after the Baguio earthquake in 1990 and the eruption of Mount Pinatubo in 1991. General Green also acts as functional manager of the

Continues

U.S. Air Force Medical Service, advising on matters pertaining to the medical aspects of the air expeditionary force and the health of Air Force service members. He has the authority to allocate resources worldwide for the Air Force Medical Service, make decisions that influence the delivery of medical services, and develop programs that support medical service missions.

Interview by Dr. James Johnson

Gen. Green: It is an honor and privilege to be interviewed as part of your new publication. Thank you! Before we begin, I would also like to share this honor with the 42,000 Air Force Medical Service men and women who I serve and their tremendous dedication and sacrifices which keep our great Country free. I would also like to thank our heroes who are no longer with us and our wounded warriors who have come home safely from the conflicts we are engaged in.

Little did I know 36 years ago when I first walked through the halls of the Medical College of Wisconsin my dreams of becoming a Family Physician would lead me to where I am today… serving as the Air Force Surgeon General.

(Q): What is your own working definition of a leader?

Gen. Green: As I reflect back and search for a common factor on leadership, I come up with one: being a lifelong student and learner and the desire to serve a higher calling have been essential ingredients of any successful endeavors. As soon as you close your mind to the possibility of another better reality, you are closing yourself off to other great opportunities. You're not serving to the greatest of your ability. My early work with pilots and their families inspired me to fully adopt the Air Force values of Integrity, Service before Self, and Excellence in all we do. I found myself continuously learning and looking for better ways to accomplish the mission and serve others. Further, the ability to be open to change and continue to improve oneself and one's organization is crucial to success in today's dynamic and rapidly changing environment. Challenging the status quo is the mark of a lifetime learner, a servant-leader, and a powerful vision worth pursuing.

My assignment to the Philippines reinforced the need for adaptability and demonstrated the value of continuous process improvement. My training really paid off in first response to 5 aircraft accidents, a flood, a coup, a typhoon, an earthquake, and ultimately the largest volcanic eruption of the twentieth century. Each event was different but the response was similar, and I found ways to improve each response. Later, these skills and expertise led to me being involved with development of smaller, modular response capabilities linked to air evacuation. Today, continuous learning, teamwork, [and] innovation have resulted in an integrated air-evacuation and casualty-care system to safely transport our wounded warriors from the front lines to world class care at our stateside facilities. This integrated system has led to an unprecedented died of wounds rate of less than 5 percent.

(Q): What are your ongoing challenges and what role does politics play in your decisions?

Gen. Green: People have and always will fear change and resist. However, if you succumb to this fear and never challenge the status quo, you will be destined to mediocrity, possibly even failure. In the hi-tech, hi-touch world of medicine this can be dangerous and deadly. In 2004, Dr. Don Berwick, CEO of Institute of Healthcare Improvement (IHI), challenged health care system CEOs to reduce medical errors and save 100,000 lives within 18 months. He rose above emotion, fear, and interests. He challenged the status quo. It was through our vision to challenge the status quo and harness the power of learning that led to improved health care outcomes and an increased focus on medical errors.

Continues

For me from day one, 'I don't know' became 'I don't know yet.' Let me explain. As a lifetime student, I continue to ask questions about the current state of the national and military health system. For the Air Force Medical Service creating a Medical Home involves challenging others to see the possibilities and transform a system of care whose focus is on healthier outcomes and continuity. Doing so will ultimately reduce system-wide costs and result in a healthier and more resilient nation. It won't be easy. We must confront fear and resistance to change by presenting the risk of complacency and the danger of inaction. As lifetime students and visionary leaders, we can shape our future, grow the next generation of critical thinkers, reduce fear and resistance, and ultimately save lives.

As the Air Force Surgeon General, I spend much of my time encouraging others to challenge the status quo and look for new innovations and ways to deliver care. As lifelong learners, this is where we get our fuel and energy. You inspired me then and continue to influence me today. You have helped transform an entire health care system to include the development of our expeditionary medical system. You have helped others see the possibilities of an Air Force Medical Home and shared the importance of prevention and patient-centered care. You made hope and healing a reality for thousands of victims of natural disasters through our humanitarian missions. You've inspired 42,000 medical personnel to go above and beyond.

(Q): What advice do you have for students who plan a career in public health management or public sector health management?

Gen. Green: Leaders are lifetime students and learners who help others see the possibilities. Success is not simply having the gift of intelligence; success is built upon a critical mind that never stops learning. We must continue to motivate ourselves and our next generation of public health leaders to become lifetime students. As a lifetime student there's a certain sharpness, an ability to absorb new facts; to ask insightful questions; to connect unrelated domains; and to help others to see the limitless possibilities of the future. My curiosity and probing questions inspire my team and encourages them to not only find answers, but [to] learn how to ask the right questions. I enjoy challenging my staff and myself to see the possibilities.

For me, no matter what you spend your time doing in life, you should never stop questioning, never stop learning, and never stop serving. It is only by increasing your understanding of the world around you [that you] are able to have a significant impact. For example, The Air Force Expeditionary Medical Systems (EMEDS) successfully responded to earthquakes in Indonesia, Haiti, and Chili. Air Evacuation has now moved over 70,000 casualties with only four losses in nine years from Afghanistan and Iraq. I am blessed that the Air Force has seen fit to promote me and let me continue to build my skills and expertise.

(Q): Any closing comment to share with the students?

Gen. Green: If you never stop learning, you will never stop seeing the possibilities. And you will continue to make a difference in the lives of those around you and inspire others to seek out and make new possibilities real.

End

Discussion and Review Questions

1. What are the domains of a public health manager and how do they relate to the agency's mission?

2. How do management and leadership differ? How are they similar? Can a non-manager be a leader? If so, how and give examples.

3. What are the characteristics of servant-leaders?

4. Describe transformational leadership and discuss how it is useful in public health.

5. Choose any leadership theory discussed in this chapter and describe how it best describes how you might be (or have been) as a leader.

6. Why is systems thinking so important to public health managers? Give an example of a public health challenge and explain it from a systems perspective.

7. What is meant by "sustainability" and what role does the manager have? Give an example.

Action Learning and Critical Thinking

A. Research the background, life, and accomplishments of a significant person in public health, medicine, or health policy history. Describe how they were a systems thinker and what they did that was transformational.

B. Read the book *Outliers* by Malcolm Gladwell and consider what this might mean for your own life and future. Discuss how you too might become an "outlier" who shapes public health in the future.

C. Watch the movie *Contagion* and identify examples of management and leadership. What theories of leadership seemed to be most-employed by which characters and when? Were all the leaders also managers? Give examples. Were there any instances of systems thinking? Strategic thinking? Discuss this film in class and see what different perspectives on leadership and management emerge during the discussion.

D. Do an online search for the U.S. Air Force Surgeon General and for the U.S. Surgeon General. How do their roles and responsibilities differ? From reading General Green's interview in this chapter, are there other differences or similarities you noticed? What leadership qualities would serve you best if you were someday in either of these positions?

Chapter 10

ORGANIZATIONAL BEHAVIOR, MOTIVATION, AND CONFLICT

Learning Objectives

Upon completion of this chapter, you should be able to:

1. Better understand human behavior in public health organizations.
2. Recognize elements of organizational culture.
3. Understand human motivation and the manager's role.
4. Compare varying theories of motivation.
5. More effectively manage conflict and understand its place in the organization.
6. Gain an appreciation of organizational values important to public health.

Key Terms

Alderfer's ERG model
bureaucracy
equity theory
expectancy theory
goal setting
knowledge, skills, and abilities (KSAs)

Maslow's hierarchy of needs
McClelland's Acquired Needs model
motivation
organizational behavior

organizational culture
organization theory
reinforcement
scientific management

Chapter Outline

INTRODUCTION

organizational behavior:
The study of individual and group behaviors in organizations, analyzing motivation, work satisfaction, leadership, work-group dynamics, and the attitudes and behaviors of the members of organizations.

As described earlier in this book, organizations are complex, multifaceted, adaptive social systems. Those involved in public health have overarching values and an overriding mission to improve and promote health of individuals and communities. Public health managers, in order to be effective in helping their organizations accomplish their missions and in turn serve the public, must have a solid understanding of human behavior and how it is manifested in the organizational setting. At its most fundamental level, the study of **organizational behavior** is the study of human behavior. Fortunately, there is extensive research on human behavior in organizations and considerable insights provided by the fields of psychology, sociology, systems science, behavioral economics, political science, anthropology, and many other social sciences.

STUDYING BEHAVIOR IN ORGANIZATIONS

The roots of this area of study in the modern era can be traced back to the early 1900s with the work of German sociologist Max Weber and his theories of **bureaucracy**, the organizational structure based on the sociological concept of rationalization of collective activities, and American management engineer Frederick Winslow Taylor and his principles of **scientific management**, a systematic approach to managing that seeks the "one best way" of accomplishing a task by discovering the fastest, most efficient, and least fatiguing methods. Both of these perspectives saw organizations as closed systems that sought to maximize efficiency. Later, theorists began to look at organizations differently; organizations began to be seen as social systems. American social worker Mary Parker Follett argued that management must be grounded in "our cognition of the motivating desires of the individual and of the group." Studies by Harvard anthropologist Elton Mayo and colleagues, now called the *Hawthorne Studies*, demonstrated the importance of human relationships on motivation and behavior in organizations. Carrying these ideas further, economist Chester Barnard, who later served as President of the Rockefeller Foundation, wrote *Functions of the Executive* in 1938 to emphasize the importance of human cooperation on organizations. Deriving them from his conception of cooperative systems, Barnard summarized the functions of the executive as follows:

- Establishing and maintaining a system of communication
- Securing essential services from other members
- Formulating organizational purposes and objectives

The study of collaboration as a central theme of organizational behavior was further underscored by the work of German social psychologist Kurt Lewin and American anthropologist Margaret Mead in their experiments on cooperation in food rationing. Lewin identified three basic work environments:

- Authoritarian
- Democratic
- Laissez-faire

Another important book was published in 1960 by MIT management professor Douglas McGregor, titled *The Human Side of Enterprise*, in which he identified two basic types of organizations based on the leaders' approach to command and control. He described these as follows:

- *Theory X* is based on assumptions that employees dislike work, lack ambition, and resist change.
- *Theory Y* is based on assumptions that employees are willing to work and accept responsibility, are capable of self-direction, and are able to make their own decisions.

Today the study of human behavior in organizations continues in all of the social sciences previously mentioned. Exciting new research is emerging from the fields of information science, systems science, and neuroscience along with increasing awareness of the importance of social justice, multiculturalism, and sustainability. Going even further, **organization theory**—sociological approach to the study of organizations focusing on topics that affect the organization as a whole, such as organizational environments, goals and effectiveness, strategy and decision making, change and innovation, and structure and design—is beginning to embrace the science of quantum physics as it sees characteristics not unlike those seen at

bureaucracy: A termed coined by Max Weber to represent an ideal or completely rational form of organization. The organizational structure is based on the sociological concept of rationalization of collective activities. The key features Weber believed were necessary for an organization to achieve the maximum benefits of ideal bureaucracy include: 1) a clear division of labor to ensure that each task preformed is systematically established and legitimized by formal recognition as an official duty; 2) positions are arranged in a hierarchy so that each lower position is controlled and supervised by a higher one, leading to a chain of command; 3) formal rules and regulations uniformly guide the actions of employees, eliminating uncertainty in the performance of tasks resulting from differences among individuals; 4) managers should maintain impersonal relationships and should avoid involvement with employees' personalities and personal preferences; 5) an employment should be based entirely on technical competence and protection against arbitrary dismissal. The term is now usually associated with large public-sector organizations to describe undesirable characteristics such as duplication, delay, waste, low morale, and general frustration.

scientific management: A systematic approach to managing that seeks the "one best way" of accomplishing a task by discovering the fastest, most efficient, and least-fatiguing methods.

organization theory: A sociological approach to the study of organizations focusing on topics that affect the organization as a whole, such as organizational environments, goals and effectiveness, strategy and decision making, change and innovation, and structure and design.

the micro and macro levels of physical reality. An insightful statement from organizational theorist Margaret Wheatley, author of *Leadership and the New Science*, captures the essence of this perspective:

> We live in a time of chaos, rich in potential for new possibilities. A new world is being born. We need new ideas, new ways of seeing, and new relationships to help us now. New science—the new discoveries in biology, chaos theory, and quantum physics that are changing our understanding of how the world works—offers this guidance. It describes a world where chaos is natural, where order exists "for free." It displays the intricate webs of cooperation that connect us. It assures us that life seeks order, but uses messes to get there.

- Relationships are what matters—even at the subatomic level.
- Life is a vast web of interconnections where cooperation and participation are required.
- Chaos and change are the only route to transformation.

ORGANIZATIONAL VALUES AND BEHAVIOR

Many scholars have distinguished public organizations from those of business organizations and further set apart health service organizations as being different in various ways. Johnson's book *Health Organizations: Theory, Behavior, and Development* provides a thorough description of health service organizations and their unique characteristics and different organizational cultures. However, health service organizations exist in all sectors: public, nonprofit, and for-profit, with each sector imposing varying demands. Many health service organizations are also public health organizations; examples include county health departments, federal community health centers, and Indian Health Service clinics. Most public health organizations, whether engaged in research, prevention, direct services, or regulation, are operated by federal, state, or local governments. Thus they are primarily public institutions with a mission to serve citizens and communities. As discussed in Chapter 8, "Nongovernmental and Global Health Organizations," there are also many nongovernmental public health organizations, yet again, the mission is typically one of public service. While the public service mission doesn't necessarily change the applicability of various organizational theories, it does change some of the underlying assumptions upon which these organizations were established. In *Managing Human Behavior in Public and Nonprofit Organizations*, Denhardt identifies five critical assumptions important to understanding organizational behavior in today's public service organizations. These assumptions are especially important to public health managers as they view human behavior in their workplaces:

- *Assumption 1*: Human behavior is purposeful. Much of what people do in organizations is intended and goal directed.

- *Assumption 2:* Behavior is not random—it is caused. By looking at the causes of behavior in organizations, including patterns, insights can be gained about the behavior of others.

- *Assumption 3:* Behavior can be changed through learning. When people change how they think, they typically change how they act. Furthermore, behavior that has favorable consequences will more likely be repeated.

- *Assumption 4:* People should be valued simply as humans aside from their contributions to organizational goals. Treating people with respect and dignity is a value in its own right.

- *Assumption 5:* Public service is about serving others. The needs of others take precedence. The desire is to make a difference in the lives of others and in the communities being served.

As discussed previously, professionalism and ethics are part of the foundation for individual behavior in organizations, especially in public health. A good example of how one local health department, the Mahoning District Board of Health in Ohio, chooses to state their expectations is their Code of Organizational Ethics. Furthermore, the core assumptions about human behavior in organizations and its relationship to the public service mission are expressed by the Santa Barbara County Health Department in its statement of organizational values shown in Exhibit 10-1.

Exhibit 10-1   Santa Barbara County Department of Health Organizational Values

OUR VALUES

We value our clients and patients.

Valuing clients and patients means we recognize we are here to serve. We do all we can to identify and meet their needs. We treat each person with respect, dignity, courtesy, and understanding. We deliver culturally-sensitive, respectful service in a friendly and helpful manner.

We value teamwork.

Teamwork means all divisions within the department cooperate, communicate, and respect each other's needs in working to achieve our common goals. Teamwork allows us to combine energy and creativity to benefit our organization and those we serve.

We value quality.

We strive for excellence. We value doing it right the first time, accepting responsibility for and learning from our mistakes. We focus our work on making the department better. We value providing the best services to our clients and patients based on available resources.

We value communication.

We recognize the two-way nature of communication and know the value of listening as well as the importance of expressing ourselves. We value each individual's point of view. We focus on issue-oriented communication with clients, vendors, staff, and the public.

Continues

We value integrity.

Integrity means we value principles over personal interests. We interact with coworkers, clients, and patients in the spirit of respect and professionalism. We treat people in an open, fair, and ethical manner.

We value respect.

Respect means treating everyone with whom we interact with the same dignity and consideration we would want ourselves. We value each individual's unique personal, cultural, and professional qualities.

We value the public's health.

Public health addresses the needs of the population as a whole. Our department plays an essential role in providing leadership and policy direction to promote the health and well-being of individuals and communities and to protect them from illness, injury, and environmental hazards.

Reprinted with permission of County of Santa Barbara. Retrieved from http://www.countyofsb.org/phd/default_all.aspx?id=23554&menu2id=1310

ORGANIZATIONAL CULTURE

Just like every organization has a structure, it also has a culture which is comprised of attitudes, values, behavioral norms, expectations, and assumptions shared by members of an organization. Some of these were discussed in Chapter 2, "Public Health Professionalism and Ethics," with the discussion of professionalism and ethics. Likewise, in Chapter 1, "Public Health Mission and Core Functions," we discussed core values and beliefs important to public health. All of this, in addition to the individual experiences brought into the workplace, contribute to shaping an organization's culture. Not unlike the culture of a community, the organization takes on unique characteristics that can be seen and felt by employees, visitors, and the clients being served. An **organizational culture** is the pattern of shared values, beliefs, and norms—along with associated behaviors, symbols, and rituals—that are acquired over time by members of an organization. There are strong cultures and weak cultures. A weak organizational culture is one in which there is limited agreement on the core elements of culture, giving these factors limited influence on how people behave. Strong organizational cultures are those in which there is widespread agreement with respect to the core elements of culture and it is demonstrated in the behavior of the organization's members. Some examples of core cultural values are:

- Sensitivity to the needs of others
- Interest in new ideas and innovation
- Willingness to take risks and learn from mistakes
- Value placed on people
- Open and available communication
- Friendliness toward one another

organizational culture: The pattern of shared values, beliefs, and norms—along with associated behaviors, symbols, and rituals—that are acquired over time by members of an organization.

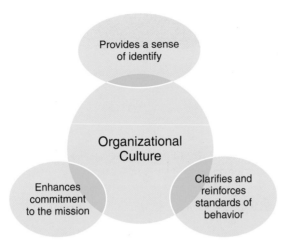

FIGURE 10-1 Organizational culture and its effect on individuals within the organization
© Cengage Learning 2013

The role of organziational culture is quite profound. It has an impact on peoples' sense of identity with the organization, facilitates commitment to the organization's mission, and it clarifies and reinforces standards of behavior (Figure 10-1).

It is important to realize that organizations do have a dominant culture, but because of size, specializations within the organization, and geography, there are often subcultures. People generally have attitudes and values more in common with others in their own field of work or profession or within a given location. A large organization, such as the U.S. Department of Health and Human Services (HHS), is likely to have many subcultures, each with norms and behaviors. This is further reason why a commitment to core values and the organization mission is so important. Within public health, organization cultures tend to be very performance-oriented. For example, within HHS each division would focus on its own performance goals, for CDC this might cluster around disease surveillance, and for HRSA it might focus more on the quality of care provided by federally funded community health centers. Regardless of the specific performance focus, public health organizations typically have organizational culture characteristics that lead to high performance. Table 10-1 identifies several of these characteristics.

MOTIVATION IN ORGANIZATIONS

motivation: An amalgam of all of the factors in one's working environment that foster or inhibit productive efforts. Defined as the set of processes that drive, direct, and maintain human behavior toward attaining some goal or meeting a need.

Motivation is a significant aspect of human behavior and critical to any understanding of organizational behavior. Drawing from various social sciences, **motivation** can be defined as the set of processes that drive, direct, and maintain human behavior toward attaining some goal or meeting a need. There are two broad categories of theories about motivation: 1) *content theories* and 2) *process theories*. Content theories are concerned with what energizes (drives) behavior, and process theories focus on how behavior is energized and directed.

TABLE 10-1 Characteristics of High-Performance Organizational Cultures

High-Performance Organizations

- Value people as human assets, respect diversity, and empower individuals to use their talents to advance personal and organizational performance

- Mobilize teams that build synergy from the talents of their members and are empowered to use self-direction and personal initiative to maximize performance

- Successfully bring people and technology together in a performance context

- Thrive on learning, encourage knowledge sharing, and enable members to continuously grow and develop

- Are achievement oriented, sensitive to the external environment, and focused on total quality management to deliver outstanding and sustainable results

Content Theories of Motivation

The most widely recognized theory of motivation is the one developed by psychologist Abraham Maslow in 1943 and published in his classic work, *A Theory of Human Motivation.* Previously, in the late 1800s, Austrian neurologist (and later psychoanalyst) Sigmund Freud first identified motivational needs and drives as mostly hidden from human awareness. He called this the *subconscious* and developed a theory based on the need to avoid pain and the need to seek pleasure (or satisfaction), with both needs influencing human behavior, often without self-awareness.

> "Thus every action must be due to one or other of seven causes: chance, nature, compulsion, habit, reasoning, anger, or appetite."—*Aristotle*

The concept of subconscious processes shaping behavior became an important building block in many later theories of motivation, including that of Abraham Maslow. While Freud used an iceberg metaphor, with the small tip above the water representing awareness and the large body of the iceberg below the surface representing the unconscious, Maslow choose a different imagery to represent his theory of motivation, that of a pyramid. Structurally, this represented a hierarchy of needs. The theory gained wide acceptance in management and organizational science, which had already embraced the concept of hierarchy, as described by German social scientist Max Weber at about the same time Freud was developing his theories. While Maslow was not as concerned as Freud about the interplay between conscious and unconscious processes, he did share the premise that people cannot be healthy and well adjusted in life unless their needs are met. To Freud, and later the medical community in general, unmet needs were seen as contributing to psychosomatic disorders and neurosis, but for Maslow, a humanistic psychologist, unmet needs were seen primarily as barriers to becoming a fully functioning member of society or an organization.

Maslow's Theory of Motivation

Specifically, Maslow identified five universal human needs, which he claimed are activated in a particular order and must be satisfied sequentially. Following the order of hierarchy, the needs begin at the lowest, most basic level, and work upward to higher-level needs, known commonly as **Maslow's hierarchy of needs**. As shown in Figure 10-2, at the base are physiological needs, then security needs, social (belonging) needs, esteem needs, and finally at the top are self-actualization needs. As one need is met, the next need becomes dominant. In regards to motivation, the theory claims that although no need is ever fully gratified, a substantially satisfied need no longer motivates. So, from this perspective, if a manager wants to motivate someone, they must understand which needs must be met and work toward fulfilling them. Each level of need is identified in Figure 10-2 and subsequently described.

Physiological Needs

Maslow's hierarchy of needs: Abraham Maslow's five sets of basic human needs arranged in a hierarchy of prepotency: physiological needs (food, water, shelter, etc.), safety needs, affiliation needs, esteem needs, and self-actualization.

Air, food, water, warmth, sleep, and sex are examples of basic physiological needs. They are the essentials for sustaining human life. According to Maslow, no other motivating factors can operate until these basic physiological needs are met. In the organizational setting, such needs are satisfied by providing adequate wages and healthy work environments. In public health, the needs that fall into this category are especially salient in health promotion and healthy communities.

Security or Safety Needs

The next step in Maslow's hierarchy is the need to be free of physical and emotional harm. The feeling of safety and security is very important at this level. Organizations

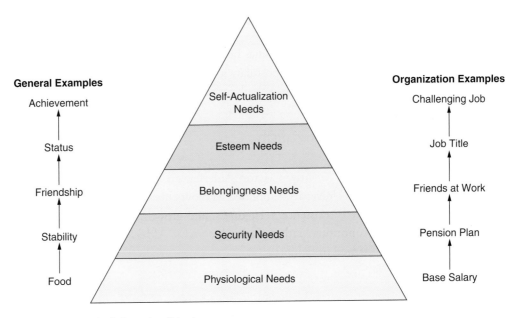

FIGURE 10-2 Maslow's Hierarchy of Needs
Source: Based on Maslow, A.H. (1943), A theory of human motivation. *Psychology Review 50*, 370–396

help address this need through retirement plans, job security, health insurance, and psychologically safe work climates. In public health, programs that provide vaccinations to prevent illness or inspections that assure food security are just two examples of ways this level of needs can be addressed in the community.

Social or Belonging Needs

Humans are social beings who need to be accepted by others. We seek out affection and friendship. For most this need is met by family, friends, and community. Within organizations, the need is often met at the level of the team or work group, as well as friendships. In public health, efforts such as community organizing, support groups, and community-based participatory research all help to address this need.

Esteem Needs

Following the need for acceptance is the need for self-esteem and the need to be held in esteem by others. Thus there are two concurrent needs: the need for a positive self-image or self-respect and the need for recognition and respect from others. Managers can address these needs through praise and recognition of accomplishments or through employee empowerment and challenging assignments. In public health the values of social justice, women and minority empowerment, and health education all serve to meet this need.

Need for Self-Actualization

This is the highest need in Maslow's hierarchy. Self-actualization involves achieving one's full potential and finding personal fulfillment and satisfaction in doing so. In public health this concept comes close to the WHO definition of health, "a state of complete physical, mental, and social well-being." The U.S. Army uses another motto that is instructive, "Be all that you can be." Maslow further elaborates on the process and identifies characteristics of individuals who are functioning at this level, as listed in Table 10-2.

> "This process has been phrased by some as the search for 'meaning'. We shall then postulate a desire to understand, to systematize, to organize, to analyze, to look for relations and meanings."—*Abraham Maslow*

Alderfer's Theory of Motivation

Alderfer's ERG model: Clayton Alderfer's idea of advanced needs that motivate people. Like Maslow, he believed that needs motivate people to take certain actions, and once lower-level needs are met, new needs can be sought. Alderfer stated three levels of needs: existence, relatedness, and growth.

More recently, Clayton Alderfer, an organizational psychology professor at Rutgers University, simplified Maslow's hierarchy of needs and identified three broader needs: existence, relatedness, and growth. Alderfer conceptualizes these needs as a continuum rather than a hierarchy. **Alderfer's ERG model** of motivation is presented in Exhibit 10-2.

TABLE 10-2 Characteristics of Self-Actualized People According to Maslow
• Clearer perception of reality
• Acceptance of self, others, and nature
• Spontaneity and openness to experience
• Problem-centered as opposed to ego-centered
• Ability for detachment and healthy objectivity
• Autonomy and a firm identity
• Continued freshness of appreciation
• Transcendence and peak experiences
• A feeling of kinship with others
• Deeper and more profound interpersonal relations
• Democratic principles
• Discernment between means and ends
• Non-hostile sense of humor
• Creativeness
• Ability to love

Source: Based on Maslow, A.H. (1943), "A Theory of Human Motivation," Psychology Review 50, 370–396

McClelland's Theory of Motivation

A third content theory of individual motivation, based on specific needs, developed by psychology professor David McClelland at Harvard University, was published in two seminal books, *The Achievement Motive* and *The Achieving Society* in the 1950s. Primary theoretical constructs of his theory came from colleagues, medical physiology professor Henry Murray at Harvard and organizational psychology professor John Atkinson at the University of Michigan. McClelland further developed his *acquired needs theory*, sometimes called a *learned needs theory*, at Boston University

Exhibit 10-2   Alderfer's ERG Model

Need for Existence

The need for existence, similar to Maslow's physiological and safety needs, is the need to stay alive and safe. When the need for existence is met, we feel physically and mentally well and secure.

Need for Relatedness

The need for relatedness is the need for social interaction and relationships. Encompassing Maslow's esteem needs and belonging needs, the need for relatedness is our concern with

our own identity and where we fit into our community.

Need for Growth

The need for growth is the need to be creative and learn. Growing results in a sense of completeness, fulfillment, and personal achievement. The need for growth is similar to self-actualization in Maslow's hierarchy of needs.

Source: Alderfer, C. P., Existence, Relatedness, and Growth; Human Needs in Organizational Settings, New York: Free Press, 1972

in the 1990s by applying its constructs to the study of nations and cultures around the world. During this time he also became a pioneer in the field of competency assessment and development, which is widely used in in many professions, including medicine, nursing, and public health. His work is continued today at the McClelland Center for Research and Innovation in Boston, where post-doctoral fellowships are awarded for the study of human motivation, competencies, organizational performance, leadership, and the physiological correlates of motives as they relate to health and wellness issues.

McClelland's theory proposed that needs are acquired over time and are shaped by life experiences and cultural background. Most of the needs expressed in organizations and other communities can be classed as *achievement, affiliation,* or *power.* A person's motivation and effectiveness in a certain job or profession is influenced by these three needs. See Exhibit 10-3 for **McClelland's Acquired Needs model**. The importance of each of these needs will vary from one person to another. If a manager can determine the importance of each of these needs to an individual, it will help decide how to most effectively influence that individual or what type of work-setting might be most conducive. A person's motivation and effectiveness can be increased through an environment that provides them with their ideal mix of each of the three needs.

All individuals have each of these three motivating needs to some degree. However, since this is a learned/acquired needs theory, the idea is that through life experience, educational and professional socialization, cultural and family influences, personality characteristics, and neurophysiological factors, people will have varying levels of each need. There is a general tendency, though, to have a "preferred" need domain. In a public health organization, the director (manager) might be highest in nPwr, especially socialized power, with his or her lowest need being one of the

McClelland's Acquired Needs model: David McClelland's theory that needs are learned through life experiences. These needs develop throughout a person's life. He stated three levels of needs: achievement, power, and affiliation.

> ## Exhibit 10-3   McClelland's Acquired Needs Model
>
> ### Need for Affiliation (nAff)
>
> This reflects a desire for friendly relationships and human interaction, to feel liked and accepted by others. People with a high need for affiliation work well in teams and thrive in participative work environments. They typically enjoy interacting with the public. Individuals with a high degree of this need are often well suited for critical staff and professional positions in public health that involve interaction with others, but not necessarily managing them. Many community-based health programs and health-education initiatives provide highly conducive work environments.
>
> ### Need for Power (nPwr)
>
> This comes from the desire to influence others' behavior or to control one's environment. It can also be a desire to make an impact or to control others. The need for power can exhibit itself in two ways. The need for *personal* power, which may be detrimental, is the need to have control over others. However, the need for *socialized* power is a desire to direct the efforts of a team for the benefit of the workplace, organization, or community. This need for power can be very beneficial. Power used in the service of others is an example often seen with public health managers, public policy advocates, and leaders involved in crisis management, such as disaster response or pandemic control.
>
> ### Need for Achievement (nAch)
>
> This is the need to achieve, excel, accomplish complex tasks, solve problems, and succeed. A person whose dominant need is for achievement will thrive in a challenging environment. This type of individual sets challenging but realistic goals and finds that the achievement of the goal is an incentive for hard work. People with a high need for achievement will often work well alone or with other achievers. Many thrive in complex and stimulating environments, like the science-driven organizational cultures at NIH and CDC.

© Cengage Learning 2013

other two. Often in public health, this individual will also be a scientist or physician, so their need ratios could likely be nPwr first, nAch second, and nAff third. Yet at another time in their career they might return to research, as their primary engagement and the ratios shift, with nAch becoming dominant again as it perhaps was when they started their career after completing their Ph.D. or medical degree. In public health there are numerous opportunities for individuals to work in environments that support any or all of these needs.

Some organizations use psychological testing to determine the proportional ratios of nAch, nPwr, and nAff, along with other factors, to help guide staffing and other human resource decisions. A medical center in Irvine, California, has been very successful using this approach to develop a collaborative, achievement-oriented culture with shared values among the employees. The Hay Group, a large international consulting firm based in Philadelphia, also uses McClelland concepts to help clients worldwide, including public health organizations, ministries of health, and health delivery systems, achieve better organizational performance.

Herzberg's Theory of Motivation

Another well-known content perspective on motivation in organizations was developed by Frederich Herzberg, who founded the Department of Industrial Mental Health at Case Western Reserve University. In agreement with Maslow's needs hierarchy is Herzberg's theory of needs and motivation. Herzberg found that people are not content with the minimum provisions of employment, such as minimum salaries and safe working conditions. Instead, people seek gratification from higher-level psychological needs associated with success in the work place, such as responsibility, achievement, and advancement. Going beyond Maslow, Herzberg added a new dimension to motivation theory by proposing a two-factor model of motivation whereby certain factors lead to satisfaction at work while others lead to dissatisfaction. Working from this two-factor model, Herzberg developed the *motivation-hygiene theory* to demonstrate that motivation factors are needed to motivate an employee to higher performance while hygiene factors are needed to ensure an employee is not dissatisfied. The motivation factors he identified are intrinsic, while the hygiene factors are more extrinsic in that they have to do with the work environment. Examples of each type of factor can be seen in Figure 10-3 along with comparisons to Maslow, Alderfer, Herzberg, and McClelland.

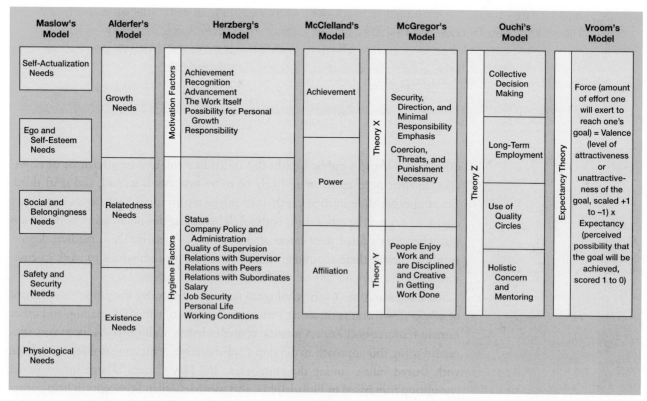

FIGURE 10-3 Comparison of Content Theories of Motivation

Source: Compiled with information from *Health Care Management* (5th Ed.) by S.M. Shortell and A.D. Kaluzny. 2006, Clifton Park, NY: Delmar Cengage Learning; and Leadership and Management by L.S. Leach, from *Nursing Leadership & Management* (2nd ed.) by P. Kelly, 2008, Clifton Park, NY: Delmar Cengage Learning

Process Theories of Motivation

There are many theories of motivation that focus on different processes instead of content (needs). Two of these will be discussed; one based on the processes associated with expectations, called **expectancy theory**, and the other focusing on perceptions of fairness and justice, called **equity theory**. Two other processes with implications for motivation are **reinforcement**, to reward or punish an action or response so that it becomes more or less likely to occur, and **goal setting**, the cognitive process through which conscious goals, as well as intentions about pursuing them, are developed and become primary determinants of behavior. These will be discussed in other chapters, as invaluable tools for managers, both of which are used widely in public health.

Expectancy theory was first developed by Victor Vroom at the Yale University School of Management. It is based on the idea that people make decisions based on the expected outcomes. Individuals estimate how well the results of a given behavior will coincide with desired results and act accordingly.

> "This theory emphasizes the needs for organizations to relate rewards directly to performance and to ensure that the rewards provided are those rewards deserved and wanted by the recipients."—*Victor Vroom*

The theory was further developed by Lyman Porter, Ph.D., organizational behavior professor at the University of California-Irvine, and Edward Lawler, Ph.D., then Director of the Institute for Social Research at the University of Michigan to describe the intrinsic and extrinsic elements of rewards. Their model also claims that a person's perception of the value of a reward will affect motivation, as would the person's perception of the task and their ability to perform it. Lawler, now Director of the Center for Effective Organizations at the University of Southern California, has added to the growing understanding of expectancy theory by offering the following four basic points concerning human motivation:

1. People have preferences among the various outcomes that are potentially available to them.

2. People have expectancies about the likelihood that an action on their part will lead to the intended behavior or performance.

3. People have expectancies about the likelihood that certain outcomes will follow their behavior.

4. In any situation, the actions a person chooses to take are determined by the expectancies and the preferences that person has at the time.

Equity theory, as developed by John Stacy Adams in its application to work motivation, assumes that individuals value and seek fairness, or *equity*, in their relationships in the organization. Building on the content theories discussed earlier, Adams acknowledges the many variables that affect each individual's perception of their relationship with the organization. However, perception of the wider situation, especially comparison, is more central to equity theory than many other earlier motivational models. In this way equity theory goes beyond the individual and incorporates others in determining what motivates people. Adams claims that people look at others, perhaps friends and colleagues, in determining what is fair or equitable. Therefore, when people feel that they are being treated fairly, say in terms of wages, they are more likely to be motivated. However, when people feel that they are being treated unfairly, they are prone to feelings of demotivation. Using the language of systems theory, Adams referred to work effort as *inputs* and rewards as *outputs*. To get desirable outcomes (motivation, performance, satisfaction) there must be a balance, which in turn reinforces a sense of fairness or equity.

Outside of the organizational setting, equity theory is used by leaders and policymakers to promote social justice, empowerment, and community development. The kinds of inputs and outputs may vary in the community setting or at the state and national level, but the concept of balance and perceived fairness remains the same. Public health organizations tend to embrace workplace equity, public health practice emphasizes equity in its professional norms, and public health policy uses equity theory for planning and resource allocation.

MOTIVATION AND PERFORMANCE

There is a strong link between motivation and performance. While performance at the individual level has certain inputs like **knowledge, skills, and abilities (KSAs)**, it is most certainly energized or stymied by motivation. Thus, KSAs and other input factors (i.e., mental and physical well-being) are more likely to lead to desired performance when motivational factors or needs have been addressed effectively. This process of inputs being energized by motivation leading to desired performance is the path to the achievement of results or outcomes and thus accomplishing goals.

> **knowledge, skills, and abilities (KSAs):** Performance-related inputs. KSAs are more likely to lead to desired performance when motivational factors or needs have been addressed effectively.

A similar process can occur at the group level, discussed more in Chapter 13, "Groups, Teams, and Working with the Community." Furthermore, motivational problems can become a barrier to individual performance and should be addressed by the manager or in the case of a group by the team leader. Table 10-3 describes common employee-motivation problems and potential solutions.

CONFLICT IN ORGANIZATIONS

Given the complexity and scope of public health organizations, conflict in the workplace is inevitable. As described in the section on organizational behavior and culture, there are many interpersonal relations and dynamics including organizational politics, values differences, power differentials, and varying motivational factors. Each of these dynamics and myriad more increase the potential, and likelihood, of conflict arising. Ideally, conflict is addressed openly and resolved in a timely and appropriate way. Some conflict, if channeled effectively, can be a constructive part of organizational change and development. However, as with our own personal lives, conflict is not always utilized in a constructive and developmental way.

TABLE 10-3 Motivation Problems and Potential Solutions	
Motivational Problems	**Potential Solutions**
1. Inadequate performance definition (i.e., lack of goals, inadequate job descriptions, inadequate performance standards, inadequate performance assessment)	• Well-defined job descriptions • Well-defined performance standards • Goal setting
2. Impediments to performance (i.e., bureaucratic or environmental obstacles, inadequate support or resources, poor employee-job matching, inadequate information)	• Feedback on performance • Improved employee selection • Job redesign • Enhanced hygiene factors (i.e., safe and clean environment, salary and fringe benefits, job security, staffing, time off job, equipment)
3. Inadequate performance-reward linkages (i.e., inappropriate rewards, inadequate rewards, poor timing of rewards, low probability of receiving rewards, inequity in distribution of rewards)	• Pay for performance • Enhanced achievement or growth factors (i.e., employee involvement-participation, job redesign, career planning, professional development opportunities) • Enhanced esteem or power factors (i.e., autonomy or personal control, self-management, modified work schedule, recognition, praise or awards, opportunity to display skills or talents, opportunity to mentor or train others, promotions in rank or position, information concerning organization or department, preferred work activities or projects, preferred work space) • Enhanced affiliation (i.e., work teams, task groups, social activities, professional and community group participation, personal communication or leadership style)

© Cengage Learning 2013

Conflict Styles

Most people tend to embrace one or two of the following conflict styles and stick with them in nearly all situations. This has to do with life experiences, early socialization, and temperament. Sometimes in a conflict situation one individual resorts to one style and the other person resorts to another style. The one approach that addresses this incongruence directly is the conflict style referred to as "problem solving." The most common conflict styles in the organizational setting are:

- Accommodating
- Avoiding
- Collaborating
- Competing
- Compromising
- Problem solving

Table 10-4 provides situational contexts and objectives that lend themselves to each of the six conflict styles.

TABLE 10-4 Conflict Styles, Contexts, and Objectives

Accommodating

- Helps to satisfy others in order to maintain a spirit of cooperation

- Often used to better achieve harmony and stability

- This allows others to develop by learning from their mistakes

Avoiding

- Allows people time to get emotions in check and regain perspective

- Sometimes need to gather further information instead of making immediate decisions

- Can serve to allow others to resolve the conflict without your involvement

Collaborating

- Fosters creativity by merging insights from people with different perspectives

- Helps to gain commitment by building consensus and integrative solutions

- Helps resolve interpersonal issues and foster learning

Competing

- Best for quick decisive or emergency situations that need your expertise

- Sometimes used to address unpopular but necessary actions

- Should be used with caution in the organizational setting

(Continues)

TABLE 10-4 Conflict Styles, Contexts, and Objectives *(Continued)*

Compromising

- Important for addressing mutually exclusive goals

- Can be used to achieve temporary agreement on complex issues

- Helps to arrive at expedient solutions under time constraints

Problem Solving

- Focuses on solving the problem, not on accommodating differing views

- Based on a realization that many solutions have positive and negative aspects

- This maximizes each person's skills, abilities, and knowledge

© Cengage Learning 2013

An individual who has the opportunity and skill to choose their own style of approaching conflict must take into consideration two key factors: 1) the importance of the relationship and 2) the importance of the desired outcome. Different conflict styles and negotiation strategies align themselves according to these two factors (see Figure 10-4).

Conflict Management

The public health manager has an important role in managing conflict in the organization. How leaders and managers resolve their own conflict issues sends a powerful message throughout the organizations. Thus the manager has an opportunity to model behaviors and desired approaches for conflict resolution or prevention.

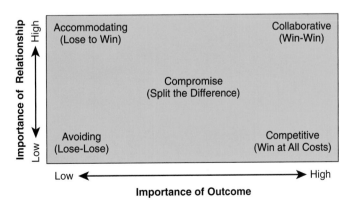

FIGURE 10-4 Negotiating Strategies
© Cengage Learning 2013

Ultimately, as Northern Kentucky University nursing leadership professors Kristine Pfendt, M.S.N., and Margaret Anderson, Ed.D., have stated, "Open, honest, clear communication is the key to successful conflict management." There are several approaches to effective management of conflict, each of which has advantages and disadvantages (see Table 10-5).

TABLE 10-5 Summary of Conflict Management Techniques

Conflict Management Technique	Advantages	Disadvantages
Avoiding—ignoring the conflict	Does not make a big deal out of nothing; conflict may be minor in comparison to other priorities	Conflict can become bigger than anticipated; source of conflict might be more important to one person or group than to others
Accommodating—smoothing or cooperating; one side gives in to the other side	One side is more concerned with an issue than is the other side; stakes not high enough for one group, and that side is willing to give in	One side holds more power and can force the other side to give in; the importance of the stakes are not as apparent to one side as to the other
Competing—forcing; the two or three sides are forced to compete for the goal	Produces a winner; good when time is short and stakes are high	Produces a loser; leaves anger and resentment on losing side
Compromising—each side gives up something and gains something	No one should win or lose, but both should gain something; good for disagreements between individuals	May cause a return to the conflict if what is given up becomes more important than the original goal
Negotiating—high-level discussion that seeks agreement but not necessarily consensus	Stakes are very high, and solution is rather permanent; often involves powerful groups	Agreements are permanent, even though each side has gains and losses
Collaborating—both sides work together to develop the optimal outcome	Best solution for the conflict and encompasses all important goals of each side	Takes a lot of time; requires commitment to success
Confronting—immediate and obvious movement to stop conflict at the very start	Does not allow conflict to take root; very powerful	May leave impression that conflict is not tolerated; may make something big out of nothing

Summary

Public health organizations, just as all organizations in modern society, have many challenges that result from human behavior dynamics. To best understand this and effectively manage in these settings it is important to study organizational culture and its influences. Furthermore, future managers in these organizations must have an appreciation and understanding of the role of motivation in order to assure the effectiveness needed to accomplish the work and goals of the organization. Within these settings, conflict is inevitable, yet can be managed in ways that help instead of ways that are harmful. Conflict can be successfully managed, and there are numerous techniques and approaches that can be utilized in public health organizations.

The following case studies in Chapter 16, "Cases in Public Health Management," are directly related to concepts and principles presented in this chapter:

- Case 3: The Anti-Vaccination Paradigm
- Case 7: Sick Building Syndrome
- Case 10: Zero-Tolerance for Smoking
- Case 11: Budget Cuts in Home Care Program
- Case 12: Don't Ask, But Tell
- Case 13: Senior Cyber Café
- Case 15: Toy Recall Prompts Attention to Lead Poisoning
- Case 22: Neglected Tropical Diseases—A Local NGO's Challenges

Public Health Professional Perspective

Anthony V. Drautz, M.P.A., Administrator of Environmental Health, Oakland County, Michigan

Interview by Scott D. Musch

Anthony Drautz is the Administrator of Environmental Health for the Oakland County Health Division in Oakland County, Michigan. Prior to this position, Mr. Drautz served as the Chief for the Land, Water and Technology Programs in Environmental Health for Oakland County. He has over 20 years of experience working in Environmental Health. Mr. Drautz received a

Continues

Bachelor of Science degree in Environmental Health Science from Eastern Kentucky University and a Master of Science degree in Health Services Administration from Central Michigan University. He holds credentials as a Registered Sanitarian with the State of Michigan and a Registered Environmental Health Specialist with the National Environmental Health Association. He is a Certified Hazardous Materials Technician and serves as Administrator on the Oakland County Radiological Response Team for the Oakland County Department of Health and Human Services.

(Q): Tell us about your position at Oakland County Health Division as the Environmental Health Administrator.

Mr. Drautz: The Oakland County Health Division is the largest health department in Michigan and serves approximately 12 percent of the population of the state. As the Environmental Health Administrator, I work closely with an administrative team that includes the Manager/Health Officer for the Health Division as well as a Medical Director, Administrator for Finance/Administrative Services, Personal and Preventive Health Services Administrator, and an Administrator for Community Health Promotion and Intervention Services. As administrators, we are each responsible for running the day to day operations and managing the budget of our individuals units.

(Q): What are your main responsibilities?

Mr. Drautz: I am responsible for the oversight of all Environmental Health Programs in Oakland County. This includes successful management of an approximately $7 million budget, 66 professional staff that includes two Program Chiefs, eight Supervisors, 52 Program Staff, and four interns. In addition, there are 12 clerical support staff, four in each of the three Health Division offices.

I administer all Land, Water, Technology, Food Safety, Shelter, and Prevention Programs and staff within the Environmental Health Unit of the Health Division. We have successfully met minimum program requirements and contractual obligations with the Michigan Department of Environmental Quality, the Michigan Department of Agriculture, and the Michigan Department of Community Health since inception of the local health department accreditation process. Our Division is fully accredited with commendation.

I am the liaison between the health division and federal, state, and local agencies related to environmental health issues. I serve on numerous committees to draft and/or revise legislation, administrative rules, and policy at the state and local level. I also participate in numerous professional organizations and serve on the Board of Directors of the Michigan Association of Local Environmental Health Administrators. Finally, I plan and monitor the annual operating budget and complete and submit mandatory reporting requirement documentation for all Environmental Health Services Programs.

(Q): Why did you choose to go into the field of public health?

Mr. Drautz: I was introduced to the field of environmental health from a classmate in a zoology course during my freshman year in college. He was in his second year in the environmental health program and recommended that I take the Introduction to Environmental Health course. Prior to enrollment in this course, I was not aware of the importance of public health and how it impacted individuals and populations each day. After declaring my major in environmental health, I completed internships that allowed me to gain practical public health experience in rural eastern Kentucky. Our ability to make a difference in the conditions in

Continues

which people lived to improve their quality of life was captivating. As a result, I knew that I would pursue a career in public health.

(Q): I noticed that you oversee the operating budget for all Environmental Health Services Programs for Oakland County. What are some of the management challenges you face working in a climate of limited funding and budget cuts, yet no corresponding reduction in health services?

Mr. Drautz: We have never been faced with a more uncertain future regarding funding and the sustainability of public health programs since the recent downturn in the economy. Many environmental health programs are funded by the state or federal government grants. With budget deficits and strains on public health resources, our funding reductions have been minimal in relation to other public health services. Environmental health programs are often regulatory in nature and mandated in state statute or local codes and ordinances for the general health, safety, and welfare of the citizens of the state. Local units of governments have the ability to charge fees to cover the reasonable costs for services. Many local environmental health units have survived on the fees collected for services such as water well and onsite sewage disposal permits and inspections, water sample collection and analysis, surface and groundwater food service establishments inspections and investigations, institutional inspection (child care centers, foster care homes, schools), public swimming pool inspections, and public campgrounds.

Before the current recession, we recognized that we were in a position to fund the development and implementation of an electronic program management tool. We have realized the projected return on investment; improved quality, efficiency, and workload management. In addition, Oakland County has prepared three-year budgets [three-year, rolling, line-item budgets] for several years. This approach is unique for a County government from others across the nation. We were able to forecast and amend budgets as necessary to absorb the reductions in funding while maintaining the level and quality of services expected by our citizens.

(Q): One of the distinguishing features about your career in Environmental Health is your experience serving as a liaison to local and state governments on behalf of the County. What have been some of the most challenging aspects of working with different levels of governments?

Mr. Drautz: At times, agencies come to the table with interests unique to their organizations. Often, questions of authority, jurisdictional boundaries, oversight, and funding produce the most challenges. Most local units of government would rather request assistance from state and federal authorities than have mandates, sometimes unfunded, forced upon an already resource-thin agency. Many of the programs funded by state and local governments require periodic audits. There continues to be much debate on agency accreditation review and compliance with minimum program requirements and with federal voluntary standards. The questions revolve around the audit and the intent of the funding agency. Is the audit to assess program quality and quality improvement or is it to assess contract and minimum program requirement compliance? With less funding expected in years to come, program review and oversight will continue to be a challenge and source of debate.

Continues

(Q): Could you share with us some management or general considerations that might be useful for new professionals in the field who will interface with different levels of government?

Mr. Drautz: Many decisions are driven by politics and seem to progress at a very slow rate. This is not unusual when you have a large number of stakeholders that provide input and have interests unique to their situation. These colleagues are your partners. There is strength in numbers. Developing an ability to negotiate, compromise, and come to some mutual agreements and consensus are rewarded with progress. Generally, I would encourage a new professional to network and develop relationships with the various agencies. In our county, there are 61 separate cities, villages, and townships. Each has established units of government and elected officials. It is important to build relationships and partnerships. You should consider yourself a liaison between the local jurisdiction and public health.

(Q): What advice would you have for a professional who is a member of a public health agency at the county level working with a team at the state or federal level?

Mr. Drautz: Be flexible and listen. Depending on the initiative, this can be an opportunity to build relationships, develop partnerships, and establish collaborative efforts to address environmental health issues. Often state and federal agencies can provide resources not available to local units of governments. This is critically important during public health emergencies. The time to introduce yourself to your colleagues from state and federal agencies is not at the onset of a crisis.

(Q): We noticed you have worked in both technical (as a Sanitarian) and administrative roles during your career in Environmental Health. What are some of the different skill sets required to be successful in each type of role?

Mr. Drautz: From the technical side, you will need to possess a strong academic background in the natural sciences—specifically coursework in biology, chemistry and physics—as well as calculus and environmental and public health. Often technical staff will possess professional credentials including state or national registration as a sanitarian and/or an environmental health specialist. You may be employed as an environmental health generalist or a program specialist. Most local health departments and state and federal agencies that hire new sanitarians provide extensive training and standardization of staff related to the program(s) as assigned.

As a supervisor or administrator you should possess leadership skills and be able to motivate your staff. As a new administrator, you will face numerous challenges from your subordinates who prior to your promotion may have been your peers. You will be tested and should be able to lead by example. Motivating staff to meet the goals and objectives of your department will lead to fulfillment of the desired outcomes of your organization.

(Q): What are some of the major challenges shifting from a technical to administration position?

Mr. Drautz: Many of [the] challenges I have witnessed for technical staff shifting into administrative positions relate to the lack of management and leadership skills. I would strongly encourage staff that desire to transition into an administrative role as their careers progress to consider

Continues

graduate coursework specific to organizational leadership and management. Those in the public health field would benefit from a concentration in public policy and/or administration. Another challenge for some new supervisors involves human resource issues and the discipline and evaluation of staff. For some, this reality is not something they are prepared to overcome, and there have been staff that has returned to field positions as a result.

(Q): Could you share with us some management or general skills that might be useful for professionals looking to make the transition?

Mr. Drautz: Organizational leadership plays a critical role in the development of staff and the successful implementation of change in any organization. The professional workforce within a public health agency is no different. Both management and leadership skills are necessary to be an effective administrator. A new supervisor or administrator will quickly realize the challenges of increasing employee turnover and retention. Generational considerations must also factor into decisions of an effective Health Administrator. Institutional coaching and leadership skills can be acquired through successful implementation of training and continuing education of not only supervisory staff, but senior staff as well.

(Q): What advice would you give to a student studying public health who wants to enter the field?

Mr. Drautz: Take advantage of all the opportunities to participate in internships and/or study abroad. In addition, volunteer work and community service can open many doors. There are many specializations and disciplines in public health and specifically, environmental health. Choosing a broad curriculum when selecting coursework in your major and electives can further expose you to the vast possibilities that may provide you direction when deciding on a career. I would also recommend that a student seek membership in professional organizations. Student memberships are affordable and offer discount rates to attend professional trainings and conferences. Networking with professionals in public health can further reveal opportunities for employment and graduate study. A career in public health is very rewarding!

End

Discussion and Review Questions

1. Why should we study human behavior and how does it help us better understand organizations?

2. What is organizational culture? Give examples in class from different organizations you are familiar with, either through work or those you have seen in the media.

3. What would most likely motivate you as an employee? Please explain and be willing to share with the class. Which theory of motivation best describes this for you? Why?

4. Do you think the culture and values of public health organizations differ from that of other kinds of organizations, (i.e., business)? What are some contrasts?

5. Which conflict management style best describes you? What are the advantages and disadvantages of this approach? What would be an alternative style you might also be comfortable with? Which approach would make you least comfortable?

6. Discuss how Mr. Drautz has to engage in "systems thinking" in order to accomplish his wide range of responsibilities and how it helps in a complex area such as environmental health.

Action Learning and Critical Thinking

A. In class, identify a controversial topic or issue to discuss. Have two sides offer their perspectives. A third group of students should serve as "conflict management experts" and offer suggestions about how to best resolve the issue.

B. Watch the movie *Damaged Care* and describe: 1) three different organizational cultures; 2) three different conflict situations and how they were resolved; 3) the motivation elements of at least three of the primary characters. Compare and contrast each of the three foci culture, conflict situations, and motivational elements and discuss in class.

C. Ask your friends and family what motivates them and compare that to your own motivational factors. Spend an hour reflecting upon your conversations with others and identify two things you learned about yourself.

Chapter 11

WORKFORCE DEVELOPMENT, DIVERSITY, AND HUMAN RESOURCES

Learning Objectives

Upon completion of this chapter, you should be able to:

1. Appreciate the complexity of the public health workforce.
2. Know about and gain knowledge of the settings and roles of the public health workforce.
3. Understand the concept of diversity and its importance to public health.
4. Be familiar with employment law and regulations.
5. Know the functions of human resource management.
6. Understand the processes of job analysis, recruitment, and selection.
7. Conduct a performance evaluation.
8. Know about and gain knowledge concerning health workplaces and environments.

Key Terms

discrimination

Doctor of Health
Administration
(D.H.A.)

Doctor of Medicine
(MD)

Doctor of Public Health
(Dr.P.H.)

Doctor of Science
(Sc.D.)

human resources
department

human resources
management

Master of Business
Administration
(M.B.A.)

Master of Health
Administration
(M.H.A.)

Master of Public
Administration
(M.P.A.)

Master of Public Health
(M.P.H.)

Master of Science
in Administration
(M.S.A.)

Occupational Safety
and Health Act of
1970

performance appraisal

recruitment

selection

Chapter Outline

Introduction
Public Health Workforce
Professional Development
Public Health Management and Administration
Diversity in the Workplace
Workplace Laws and Regulations
Human Resource Management Functions
Human Resource Management Processes
  Recruitment and Selection
  Performance Measurement and Improvement
The Healthy Workplace
Summary
Public Health Professional Perspective
Discussion and Review Questions
Action Learning and Critical Thinking

INTRODUCTION

human resources management: The function of an organization where the focus is on job analysis, performance appraisal, recruitment, and selection. The human resources domain of public health management ultimately serves to promote healthy workplaces, thus keeping with the foundations and fundamentals of public health.

The public health workforce is comprised of over a half-million workers and an even larger number of volunteers and associated professionals and staff in various governmental agencies and private organizations. The accomplishment of the core public health goals of disease prevention and health improvement depends upon an effective and committed workforce that is aligned with the populations and communities being served. Furthermore, as society's needs and characteristics change, so must the public health workforce. This involves workforce planning, development, and human resource management. It also necessitates an evolving fund of knowledge and skills that must be addressed by educational programs involved in public health training and continuing professional development provided by organizations and associations. As this chapter demonstrates, public health is multidisciplinary and public health management must be attuned to that reality. Managers must also embrace the need for workplace diversity and value the many benefits it brings to the organization. Finally, public health managers must be aware of labor laws and personnel regulations as well as the mechanisms of **human resources management**,

sis, performance appraisal, recruitment, and selection. The human
[...] public health management ultimately serves to promote healthy
[...]ng with the foundations and fundamentals of public health.

[...] chapters in this book, public health organiza-
[...] and most can best be understood from a systems
[...] public health practice is very relational, involving
[...]nities, policymakers, and many more stakeholder groups.
[...] connection between systems and relationships in the public
[...]ce, Patricia Sweeney, J.D., M.P.H., R.N., at the University of Pitts-
[...]s it up well in her statement, "Systems and relationships can only be
[...] and maintained by individuals; thus a competent workforce is essential. If
[...]e connections made are to serve the health of the public, those making them
must understand what public health is, and how it might be achieved." Over a
decade ago the U.S. Department of Health and Human Services, in their report
The Public Health Workforce: An Agenda for the 21st Century, provided the following conclusive definition:

> The public health workforce is composed of individuals whose major
> work focus is delivery of one or more of the essential services of public
> health.

Thus, the public health workforce is defined more by what it does and the services
that are provided, as shown in Table 11-1. The report went on to state this definition applies regardless of the organizational setting: public, nonprofit, voluntary, or
private sector.

A joint effort between the Department of Labor, the Bureau of Health Professions, and Columbia University developed a classification system for public health
professionals in a study titled *The Public Health Workforce, Enumeration 2000.* This
helps employers, policymakers, educators, and human resource managers to better
track employment numbers and trends. It also helps you, the student, better understand the wide range of occupations represented in the public health workforce (see
Exhibit 11-1).

PROFESSIONAL DEVELOPMENT

The public health workforce participates in professional development in several ways. As with other professions and occupations, there is skills training, education, and lifelong learning. Sometimes there is certification, such
as Certified Health Educator (CHE) or Certified in Public Health (CHP),
and for some professions, such as public health nursing or medicine, there is
licensure. Central to most training and educational approaches to professional
development is the focus on core competencies for public health practice.

TABLE 11-1 Essential Public Health Services

- Monitor health status to identify community health problems.

- Diagnose and investigate health problems and health hazards in the community.

- Inform, educate, and empower people about health issues.

- Mobilize community partnerships to identify and solve health problems.

- Develop policies and plans that support individual and community health efforts.

- Enforce laws and regulations that protect health and ensure safety.

- Link people to needed personal health services, and assure the provision of health care when otherwise unavailable.

- Assure a competent public health and personal health care workforce.

- Evaluate effectiveness, accessibility, and quality of personal- and population-based health services.

- Research for new insights and innovative solutions to health problems.

© Cengage Learning 2013

Exhibit 11-1   Columbia University Center for Health Policy and U.S. Bureau of Health Professions Classification of Public Health Occupations

(1) Epidemiologist Investigates and describes the determinants and distribution of disease, disability, and other health outcomes and develops the means for their prevention and control.

(2) Environmental Engineer (e.g., Water Supply/Waste Water Engineer, Solid Waste Engineer, Air Pollution Engineers, Sanitary Engineer) Applies engineering principles to control, eliminate, ameliorate, and/or prevent environmental health hazards.

(3) Environmental Engineering Technician and Technologist (e.g., Air Pollution Technician, Water/Waste Water Plant Operator and Testing Technician) Assists Environmental Engineers and other environmental health professionals in the control, elimination, amelioration, and/or prevention of environmental health hazards. May collect data and implement procedures or programs developed by Environmental Engineers and other environmental health professionals.

Continues

(4) Environmental Scientist and Specialist (e.g., Environmental Researcher, Environmental Health Specialist, Food Scientist, Soil and Plant Scientist, Air Pollution Specialist, Hazardous Materials Specialist, Toxicologist, Water/Waste Water Solid Waste Specialist, Sanitarian, Entomologist) Applies biological, chemical, and public health principles to control, eliminate, ameliorate, and/or prevent environmental health hazards.

(5) Environmental Science Technician and Technologist (e.g., Air Pollution Technicians, Vector Control Workers) Assists Environmental Scientists and Specialists and other environmental health professionals in the control, elimination, and/or prevention of environmental health hazards.

(6) Occupational Safety and Health Specialist (e.g., Industrial Hygienists, Occupational Health Specialists, Radiologic Health Inspectors, Safety Inspectors) Reviews, evaluates, and analyzes workplace environments and exposures and designs programs and procedures to control, eliminate, ameliorate, and/or prevent disease and injury caused by chemical, physical, biological, and ergonomic risks to workers.

(7) Occupational Safety and Health Technician and Technologist Collects data on workplace environments and exposures for analysis by Occupational Safety and Health Specialists. Implements programs and conducts evaluation of programs designed to limit chemical, physical, biological, and ergonomic risks to workers.

(8) Health Educator (e.g., Public Health Educator, Community Health Educator, School Health Educator) Designs, organizes, implements, communicates, provides advice on and evaluates the effect of educational programs and strategies designed to support and modify health-related behaviors of individuals, families, organizations, and communities.

(9) Public Health Policy Analyst Analyzes needs and plans for the development of health programs, facilities, and resources; analyzes and evaluates the implications of alternative policies relating to health care.

(10) Health Service Manager/Health Service Administrator Plans, organizes, directs, controls, and/or coordinates health services, education, or policy in establishments such as hospitals, clinics, public health agencies, managed care organizations, industrial and other types of businesses, or related entities.

(11) Public Health and Community Social Worker (e.g., Community Organizer, Outreach and Education Social Worker, Public Health Social Worker) Identifies, plans, develops, implements, and/or evaluates programs designed to address the social and interpersonal needs of populations in order to improve the health of a community and promote the health of individuals and families.

(12) Mental Health and Substance Abuse Social Worker (e.g., Alcoholism Worker, Clinical Social Worker, Community Health Worker, Crisis Team Worker, Drug Abuse Worker, Marriage and Family Social Worker, Psychiatric Social Worker, Psychotherapist Social Worker) Provides services for persons having mental, emotional, or substance abuse problems. May provide such services as individual and group therapy, crisis intervention, and social rehabilitation. May also arrange for supportive services to ease patients' return to the community.

NOTE: Social Worker occupations proposed (#11 and #12) are distinct from, and in addition to, social worker occupations already proposed, including "Medical Social Worker"; "Child, Family, and School Social Worker"; and "Social Worker, other."

Continues

(13) Psychologist, Mental Health Provider (e.g., Clinical Psychologist, Counseling Psychologist, Marriage Counselor Psychologist, Psychotherapist) Diagnose and treat mental disorders by using individual, child, family, and group therapies. May design and implement behavior modification programs. (Requires doctoral degree.)

NOTE: Psychologist occupation proposed (#13) is distinct from, and in addition to, Psychologist occupations already proposed, including "School Psychologist"; "Industrial/Organizational Psychologist"; and "Psychologists, except Mental Health Providers."

(14) Alcohol and Substance Abuse Counselor, including Addiction Counselor (e.g., Substance Abuse Counselor, Certified Substance Abuse Counselor, Certified Alcohol Counselor, Certified Alcohol and Drug Counselor, Certified Abuse and Drug Addiction Counselor, Drug Abuse Counselor [Associates Degree or higher], Drug Counselor [Associates Degree or higher], Alcoholic Counselor [Associates Degree or above] Assesses and treats persons with alcohol or drug dependency problems. May counsel individuals, families, or groups. May engage in alcohol and drug prevention programs.

(15) Mental Health Counselor (e.g., Clinical Mental Health Counselor, Mental Health Counselor) Emphasizes prevention and works with individuals and groups to promote optimum mental health. May help individuals deal with addictions and substance abuse; family, parenting, and marital problems; suicidal tendencies; stress management; problems with self-esteem; and issues associated with aging,

and mental and emotional health. Excludes psychiatrists, psychologists, social workers, marriage and family therapists, and substance abuse counselors.

- **Public Health Physician** (e.g., General Preventive Medicine/Public Health, Occupational Medicine, Epidemiologist, Physician Executive, Clinician)
- **Public Health Nurse** (e.g., Occupational Nurse, School Nurse, Community Health Nurse, Nurse Practitioner, Clinician)
- **Public Health Dentist** (e.g., Dental Public Health Clinician)
- **Public Health Dental Worker** (e.g., Dental Hygienist, Dental Assistant)
- **Public Health Veterinarian**
- **Public Health Nutritionist** (e.g., Community Nutritionist, Registered Dietician, Nutrition Scientist, Clinician)
- **Public Health Pharmacist**
- **Public Health Laboratory Scientist** (e.g., Microbiologist, Chemist, Physicist, Entomologist)
- **Public Health Laboratory Technician and Technologist** (e.g., Medical Laboratory Technician, Medical Technologist, Histologic Technician and Technologist, Cytotechnologist)
- **Public Health Attorney or Hearing Officer**
- **Health Information System/Computer Specialist**
- **Public Relations/Public Information/ Health Communications/Media Specialist**
- **Biostatistician**

Source: HHS, Bureau of Health Professions. Retrieved from http://www.health.gov/phfunctions/pubhlth.pdf, pages 23–25

As discussed in earlier chapters of this book, these competencies are deemed necessary to the delivery and monitoring of essential public health services as defined by the Council on Linkages between Academia and Public Health Practice. Many universities and colleges involved in graduate and undergraduate public health education use these core competencies as part of their curriculum design. This is especially the case for Master of Public Health (M.P.H.) programs. Additionally, there are core areas of knowledge and skill needed by currently employed public health workers. These are best summarized by Kristine Gebbie, Dr.P.H., formerly of Columbia University, and others in a document they referred to as the Charleston Charter presented in Table 11-2.

In addition to educational institutions that provide public health education and training, most health organizations and government agencies have their own continuing education and professional development programs and departments. Both the individual worker and the organization they work in have a shared responsibility for competency and new skill development. Through a collaborative effort led by the Centers for Disease Control and Prevention (CDC), other federal agencies and several public health professional associations, a strategic plan for the development of the public health workforce is being implemented. An outline of the plan is presented in Figure 11-1.

TABLE 11-2 Charleston Charter: Knowledge Areas for Current Public Health Professionals

The nine core curriculum areas for currently employed public health workers are:

1. Public health values and acculturation

2. Epidemiology/quality assurance/economics

3. Informatics

4. Communication

5. Cultural competency

6. Team building/organizational effectiveness

7. Strategic thinking and planning/visioning

8. Advocacy/politics/policy development

9. External coalition building/mobilization

Source: Gebbie KM, Hwang I. Preparing Currently Employed Public Health Professionals. New York: Columbia University School of Nursing; 1998

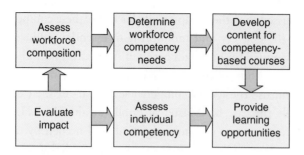

FIGURE 11-1 Strategic Elements for Public Health Workforce Development
Source: U.S. Department of Health and Human Services, Centers for Disease Control and Prevention. Strategic Plan for Public Health Workforce Development. Atlanta, GA: CDC, Public Health Practice Program Office, 1999

PUBLIC HEALTH MANAGEMENT AND ADMINISTRATION

Master of Public Administration (M.P.A.): Master of Public Administration degree or sometimes Master of Public Affairs degree. Many offer concentrations in health administration and health policy. This is a commonly held degree for public-sector managers and administrators, including many in federal public health organizations and state and county health departments.

Master of Public Health (M.P.H.): Students can specialize in health administration and health policy or other areas of focus such as environmental health, community health, epidemiology, etc. The Council on Education in Public Health is a strident advocate.

Master of Health Administration (M.H.A.): A management and administration degree for health care that is prevalent in hospitals and health delivery settings. It sometimes requires a postgraduate residency in health administration.

Master of Science in Administration (M.S.A.): A management and administration degree for health care that is used in hospitals, government agencies, the military, and health delivery settings.

Master of Business Administration (M.B.A.): This may have a concentration in health administration or multi-sector health management. An advanced college degree, earned by those who successfully graduate from their college or university's MBA program. A typical MBA program deals with multiple aspects of business, including finance and management skills.

The role and functions of public health managers and administrators is a primary focus of this book, and students should gain considerable knowledge about the many processes and dynamics involved in these careers. However, it is important also to be aware of the various educational pathways that are common to this subset of the public health workforce. Typically public health managers have at least an undergraduate degree in fields such as public or business management; behavioral and social sciences; accounting; engineering; or life sciences. However, as managers progress up the organizational ladder into higher-level administrative and leadership positions, they will almost always acquire a graduate degree. Most often this will be a **Master of Public Administration (M.P.A.)** degree with a specialization in health administration and policy or a **Master of Public Health (M.P.H.)** degree with a specialization in administration. To a lesser extent, other public health administrators acquire management focused degrees such as **Master of Health Administration (M.H.A.)**; **Master of Science in Administration (M.S.A.)** or management; and the **Master of Business Administration (M.B.A.)**. However, the largest number of senior administrators in public health agencies have either the M.P.A. or M.P.H. degree. A few universities offer joint degrees where the student graduates with both, such as the M.P.H./M.P.A. program at the University of Alabama-Birmingham (UAB). The learning objectives and curriculum reflect the kind of depth and scope needed by public health administrators in an increasingly complex organizational world (see Exhibit 11-2).

In addition to undergraduate education, masters' degrees, and continuing education training, a few public health administrators go further and pursue doctoral education. This is especially the case for those in executive leadership and policy positions. However, it has not yet become essential or expected. In fact, the highest placed public health official in the United States, the Secretary of Health and Human Services, Kathleen Sebelius, has a M.P.A. degree. For those who do seek doctoral-level education, often seen in federal agencies such as the CDC, NIH, and FDA, there are a couple of options that have been most embraced. The primary doctoral-level credential in public health is the **Doctor of Public Health (Dr.P.H.)** degree. For senior administrators there is typically a track offered in leadership or policy.

> ## Exhibit 11-2   UAB Coordinated MPH/MPA Learning Objectives
>
> - Describe the economic, legal, organizational, and political underpinnings of the United States health system (both tracks).
> - Apply skills required to work effectively in an administrative position in the government sector based on public health principles and programs (both tracks).
> - Apply the principles of management and strategic planning in health care organizations (management track).
>
> - Apply basic planning and management skills necessary for administration of health care organizations (management track).
> - Critically evaluate health policy research studies and resulting recommendations (policy track).
> - Design and implement health policy studies and draw appropriate conclusions (policy track).
>
> *Source: State of Alabama, Department of Education. Retrieved from http://www.soph.uab.edu*

Doctor of Public Health (Dr.P.H.): An advanced practice degree for public health leaders and professionals. This is sometimes offered with specializations such as epidemiology, community health, environmental health, outcomes research, and public health leadership.

Some programs, such as the Executive Dr.P.H. in Public Health Leadership at the University of North Carolina-Chapel Hill, are designed to meet the needs of working public health professionals. Additionally, a few universities, such as Central Michigan University, offer a **Doctor of Health Administration (D.H.A.)** in a similar executive format, and there is a **Doctor of Science (Sc.D.)** in health systems management offered by Tulane University. Furthermore, it is quite common to find public health administrators who have a **Doctor of Medicine (MD)** degree coupled with a M.P.H.

DIVERSITY IN THE WORKPLACE

Doctor of Health Administration (D.H.A.): An advanced practice degree in health administration and sometimes health policy for senior executives, clinician leaders, and policymakers in health care.

Doctor of Science (Sc.D.): A research degree most often awarded in epidemiology, biostatistics, or health systems.

Doctor of Medicine (MD): An advanced practice degree in medicine that leads to approval for licensure. An equivalent degree offered by some medical schools is the D.O., Doctor of Osteopathy.

The public health workforce is very diverse. Of the over half-million workers, there is considerable variation in ethnicity, race, age, gender, sexual orientation, socioeconomic background, geography, country of origin, religion, and educational level. In fact, it easily can be claimed that public health is one of the most diverse workforces there is. The United States Coast Guard (USCG) and the Oregon Health Sciences University both use the "diversity wheel" to best capture the full scope of diversity and its various components. This is presented in Figure 11-2 and is useful to public health managers seeking to have a more comprehensive understanding of personal and organizational dimensions of diversity. Most human resource departments have diversity training programs and many have diversity officers. The Office of Personnel Management in the Federal government has advocated for diversity officers in all agencies and many corporations and universities now have Chief Diversity Officers (C.D.O.).

> "The fourfold structure of the human spirit implies four general requirements: be open, be questioning, be honest, and be loving."
> —*Daniel Helminiak, Theologian and Psychology Professor*

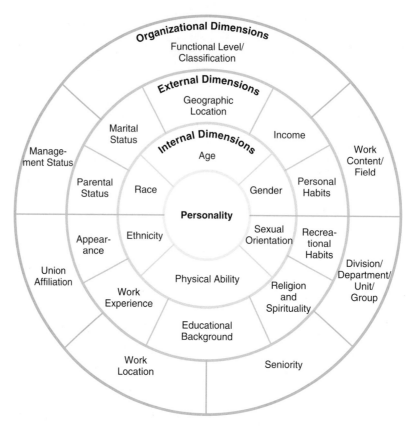

FIGURE 11-2 Diversity Wheel
Source: United State States Coast Guard and U.S. Department of Health and Human Services

Michalle Mor Barak, Ph.D., founder and director of the International Center for the Inclusive Workplace at the University of Southern California, describes the inclusive workplace as a comprehensive way for managing diversity. This workplace is one that:

- values and utilizes individual and intergroup differences within its workplace;

- cooperates with, and contributes to, its surrounding community;

- alleviates the needs of disadvantaged groups in its wider environment; and

- collaborates with individuals, groups, and organizations across local, national, and cultural boundaries.

Her conceptual framework of diversity is very compatible with public health organizations in that the engagement of local communities and the use of prevention/promotion strategies are evident. She also identifies three compelling arguments in favor of diversity management. Some of this is based on a report by the Hudson Institute, *Wokforce 2000*, that predicts the workforce will grow slowly and the proportion of older adults, women, and members of minority groups will continue to increase. These three arguments include the following:

- ***Diversity is a reality that is here to stay.*** The pool of current and future employees is becoming more diverse and organizations have no choice but to adapt to this new reality.

- ***Diversity management is the right thing to do.*** This is the moral and ethical reasoning for diversity management which includes the notion of equal opportunities regardless of individual characteristics such as gender, race, and sexual orientation. This includes providing equal access to jobs and comparable pay for jobs of comparable worth. In many situations, it also includes affirmative action to address past wrongs or imbalances.

- ***Diversity makes good management sense.*** Effective diversity management has been linked to lower absenteeism and turnover, advantages in the competition for talent, reduced risk of discrimination lawsuits, more effective program and service marketing to diverse communities, increased creativity and innovation through diverse work teams, improved agency image.

The primary barriers to inclusion and diversity in the workplace have to do with managers' and employees' attitudes and behavior, specifically, prejudice (biased views) and discrimination (biased behaviors), either overt or covert. These are best addressed through policy, training, and management practices. The U.S. Office of Personnel Management (OPM) provides a useful framework in Exhibit 11-3 for federal-level agencies that is adaptable to public health organizations at the state and local levels as well.

Exhibit 11-3   OPM Framework for Diversity Training

Diversity training, like other federally sponsored training, should adhere to certain principles. It should:

- have clearly stated goals and learning objectives that relate to the mission and needs of the organization;
- use appropriate training approaches, methods, and materials;
- provide advance information to employees on course-content and instruction methods, attendance policy, and alternatives for learning;
- be provided in a supportive and non-coercive environment;
- be conducted only by experienced and fully qualified instructors; and
- be monitored and regularly evaluated.

Goals of Diversity Training

The goals of diversity training are to help Federal employees understand:

- the legal and statutory requirements for Equal Employment Opportunity and Affirmative Action which support diversity in the Federal government and in private industry;
- that diversity is the similarities, as well as the differences, among and between individuals at all levels of the organization, and in society at large; and
- how diversity contributes to a richness in the organization by having a variety of views, approaches, and actions to use in strategic planning, tactical planning, problem solving, and decision-making.

Continues

Diversity training usually focuses on:

- **Interpersonal skills.** Employees need to provide services to, work with, and manage persons and groups with similarities and differences.
- **Behavior.** Employees are expected to exhibit in all workplace contacts—behavior that respects each individual, preserves human dignity, honors personal privacy, and values individual differences as well as common characteristics.
- **The work environment** and its relationship to effectiveness and efficiencies in organizational performance.

Management's goals for diversity training may include:

- increasing employee awareness of equal employment opportunity laws;
- increasing employee understanding of how diverse perspectives can improve organizational performance;
- preventing illegal discrimination or harassment in the workplace;
- improving workplace relations;
- building more effective work teams;
- improving organizational problem-solving; or
- improving service to clients and communities.

Agency goals for diversity training may be achieved through a specific course on diversity, such as "Managing Diversity," or by including diversity content in other agency training programs, such as "Introduction to Supervision," or "Building Effective Work Teams."

Source: U.S. Office of Personnel Management. Retrieved from http://www.opm.gov

WORKPLACE LAWS AND REGULATIONS

discrimination: Occurs when individuals, organizations, or governments (a) treat people differently because of personal characteristics like race, gender, age, religion, disability, national origin, or sexual orientation rather than their ability to perform their jobs and (b) these actions have a negative impact on access to employment, promotions, or compensation.

Discrimination in the workplace occurs when individuals, organizations, or governments (a) treat people differently because of personal characteristics like race, gender, age, religion, disability, national origin, or sexual orientation rather than their ability to perform their jobs and (b) these actions have a negative impact on access to employment, promotions, or compensation. There are many laws and regulations at the local, state, and federal levels of government that prohibit discrimination of this type.

Some of the primary federal laws include the following: The United States Constitution limits the power of the federal and state governments to discriminate. The Fifth Amendment has an explicit requirement that the Federal government not deprive individuals of "life, liberty, or property" without due process of the law. It also contains an implicit guarantee that the Fourteenth Amendment explicitly prohibits states from violating an individual's rights of equal protection and due process. These Constitutional provisions protect employees, former employees, and applicants from unequal treatment based on their affiliation with a group, such as religion, race, or gender. The protection of due process requires that government employees have a fair procedural process before being terminated.

"Discrimination in employment occurs when individuals, institutions, or governments treat people differently because of personal characteristics like race, gender, or sexual orientation rather than their ability to perform their jobs."—*Michalle Mor Barak, Founder of the International Center for the Inclusive Workplace*

The Equal Pay Act prohibits employers from paying different wages based on gender. Employees are not protected from other forms of discrimination in hiring. The Act states that employees should receive equal pay for work that requires "equal skill, effort, and responsibility and performed under similar working conditions." The Civil Rights Act of 1964 covers more areas of discrimination than the Equal Pay Act. The Civil Rights Act protects against discrimination based on race, color, religion, sex, and national origin.

The Pregnancy Discrimination Act of 1978 protects women from employment discrimination based on pregnancy, childbirth, and any medical condition associated with motherhood. It is an extension of other sex discrimination employment laws. The Family Medical Leave Act also prohibits this form of discrimination as well as that related to other family-related medical circumstances.

The Age Discrimination in Employment Act, approved in 1968 and amended in the 1970s and again in the 1980s, prohibits employers from discriminating on the basis of age. An employee over age 40 is protected from employment discrimination under this Act.

The Immigration Reform and Control Act of 1986 protects employees from discrimination based on national origin or citizenship status, provided they are not an unauthorized immigrant.

The Americans with Disabilities Act of 1990 protects individuals with a disability from discrimination. The law prohibits employment discrimination based on physical or mental disability and requires employers to make reasonable accommodations for employees with a disability.

The Genetic Information Nondiscrimination Act of 2008 prohibits employers from using a person's genetic information when making employment decisions.

In federal employment, the Civil Service Reform Act prohibits employment discrimination based on factors that do not affect job performance or actions conducted outside of the workplace. OPM has interpreted this as prohibiting discrimination on the basis of sexual orientation, and in 2009 the interpretation was expanded to include gender identity. The proposed Employment Non-Discrimination Act would specifically target discrimination based on sexual orientation and gender identity.

Aside from federal legislation, state and local laws also offer protection against employment discrimination. Some of these laws expand on existing federal statutes, while some protect against types of discrimination not covered by federal laws, such as discrimination based on political affiliation. Some states extend additional protection to state employees or state contractors. Additionally, most towns, cities, and counties have statutes and codes to provide workplace protection and employment nondiscrimination. Some, as would be expected, are more progressive and broader in scope than others.

HUMAN RESOURCE MANAGEMENT FUNCTIONS

The **human resources department** of a public health organization, sometimes labeled the *personnel department*, has several core functions and numerous management and development responsibilities. The primary functions include planning, recruitment, selection, training, legal compliance, compensation and benefits, career development, performance appraisal, and employee discipline and termination. A simple way of visualizing the core functions can be seen in Figure 11-3.

These functions have many tasks including:

- Workforce Planning
- Job Analysis
- Recruitment
- Training and Development
- Career Development
- Performance Appraisal
- Organizational Development
- Human Resources—Personnel Manual
- Human Resource Information Systems
- Event Management/Celebrations
- Compensation Management

human resources department: Sometimes labeled the *personnel department*, has several core functions and numerous management and development responsibilities. The primary functions include planning, recruitment, selection, training, legal compliance, compensation and benefits, career development, performance appraisal, and employee discipline and termination.

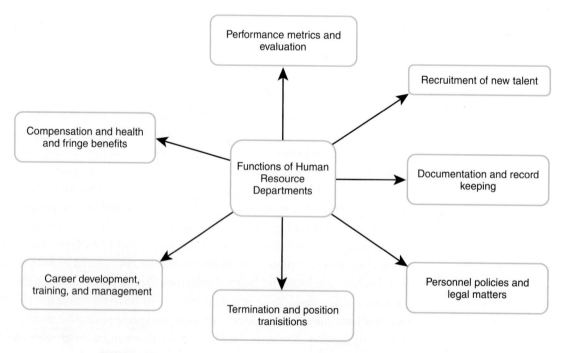

FIGURE 11-3 Core Functions of Human Resources Department
© Cengage Learning 2013

- Sexual Harassment
- Equal Employment and Opportunity
  - Personal Records
  - Statutory Compliance
  - Employee Well-being
  - Employee Communications, Newsletters
  - Relations with Employees Association and Unions
  - Grievance Handling
  - Court Cases and Labor Law Disputes
  - Disciplinary Actions

HUMAN RESOURCE MANAGEMENT PROCESSES

Using a systems approach to human resources, it is best to think of this part of management as a process that involves workforce planning, recruitment, development, retention, and performance management. During the planning phase, the organizational needs are anticipated and the environment is assessed to determine the availability of human resources. This is followed by **recruitment** and **selection** in which positions are created based on organizational needs and policies, and individuals are recruited and selected accordingly. Employees must often be developed through training and other support to be effective in a given position and within the agency they have been hired by. The human resource system also is involved with retention of staff and the processes, measurements, and policies that support performance improvement. This systematic approach can be seen as a cycle, as shown in Figure 11-3.

recruitment: Positions are created based on organizational needs and policies, and individuals are recruited accordingly.

selection: Positions are created based on organizational needs and policies, and individuals are selected accordingly. Employees must often be developed through training and other support to be effective in a given position and within the agency they have been hired by.

"The conventional definition of management is getting work done through people, but real management is developing people through work."—*Agha Hasan Abedi, Philanthropist*

Recruitment and Selection

Due to the complexity and changing environment of the workplace in a dynamic society like the United States, the Federal government publishes guidelines to assist agencies with hiring, retention, promotion, transfers, demotion, and dismissal. The *Uniform Guidelines on Employee Selection Procedures* helps employers comply with federal law. This also helps to delineate the requirements of affirmative action and equal employment opportunity (AA/EEO). The major steps involved in recruitment and selection include:

1. Developing a position (job) description with minimum qualifications
2. Employee recruitment

3. Screening applicants using appropriate forms and/or tests

4. Conducting screening interviews

5. Selecting and notifying the person

6. Notifying other applicants

Steps 1 and 2 are further elaborated upon in Exhibits 11-4 and 11-5 which provide general guidelines to help assure compliance with AA/EEO and what is generally accepted as the desirable standard for human resource-personnel practices.

Performance Measurement and Improvement

performance appraisal:
The formal methods by which an organization documents the work performance of its employees. Performance appraisals are typically designed to change dysfunctional work behavior, communicate perceptions of work quality, assess the future potential of an employee, and to provide a documented record for disciplinary and separation actions.

All public health organizations will have some type of **performance appraisal** process that helps managers know how employees are performing and helps employees know to what extent they are meeting the agency's expectations and requirements. Performance appraisals also are useful in employee development, promotion, and each of the functions identified in Figure 11-3. The best practices in performance appraisal utilize methods that encourage managers and employees to set realistic and measurable goals for job performance. Measurable evaluation criteria are used to motivate, direct, and integrate the employee's learning and development. Furthermore, performance evaluations help managers to distinguish agency-related problems

Exhibit 11-4   Position Description Key Questions

- Does the position description contain clear and specific task statements that describe essential duties and responsibilities?
- Are the knowledge, skills, abilities, educational degrees, and years of experience specified?
- Do the minimum qualifications for the job match the work to be performed?

- Can the agency substantiate the connection between the education and experience required and the tasks of the job?

Source: U.S. Office of Personnel Management. Retrieved from http://www.opm.gov

Exhibit 11-5   Position Announcement Key Elements

- Job title, classification, and salary range (sometimes "open" or "negotiable")
- Location of work, both geographic and organizational
- Description of duties and responsibilities
- Minimum qualifications

- Starting date
- Application process, procedures, deadlines, contact person
- Closing date for applications

Source: U.S. Office of Personnel Management. Retrieved from http://www.opm.gov

---

Exhibit 11-6   Performance Appraisal Interview Key Guidelines

- Set up the interview to allow the employee time to prepare for the discussion.
- Focus on the employee's strengths as well as any performance problems.
- Approach the interview with sincerity and respect for the employee and the process.
- Adopt a coaching model of supervision by using an attitude that provides support and direction in a nonthreatening manner.
- Focus on evaluating without comparison to other employees.
- Focus on performance problems, not individuals.

- Keep the discussion of the performance issues on track.
- Be conscious of word choice, avoiding words such as *always* or *never*.
- Allow and encourage the employee to respond.
- Summarize the review with specific plans for individual goals, improvement, and follow-up directions, expectations, and timelines.

Source: U.S. Office of Personnel Management. Retrieved from http://www.opm.gov

---

that should be corrected through organization-level changes from employee-related performance difficulties that may be corrected in more personalized ways or through training. It is most important that employees are evaluated on at least an annual basis and that this information is utilized in decision making pertaining to pay raises, promotions, future assignments, and the need for discipline. During the performance evaluation interview, the manager might want to consider the guidelines recommended in Exhibit 11-6. These are used by most public health agencies.

Performance improvement is directly related to motivation and abilities. When there are motivational problems there often is a performance deficit that may or may not be directly caused by the employee. The manager must identify performance problems and address them in a systematic way. There are many management tools and solutions that are available.

THE HEALTHY WORKPLACE

Public health organizations, perhaps more than all others, need to attend to the health of their employees. This can easily involve the "3 p's" of public health: protect, prevent, promote.

The U.S. Occupational Safety and Health Administration (OSHA) promotes safe workplaces and healthy work environments. There are both federal and state laws that protect employees from an unsafe and unhealthy workplace. The **Occupational Safety and Health Act of 1970** is the federal law that sets certain safety standards to eliminate threats to workplace safety. OSHA also authorizes states to implement their own safety and health programs. The requirement by

Occupational Safety and Health Act of 1970: The federal law that sets certain safety standards to eliminate threats to workplace safety.

federal and state law is that employers provide a safe and healthy workplace free of recognized hazards. Employers are required to: provide properly maintained tools and equipment; provide a warning system, such as codes or labels, to warn employees of potential hazards or hazardous chemicals; post the OSHA poster in a prominent location; keep records of work related injuries or illnesses; and provide constant examinations of workplace conditions to ensure compliance. The OSHA poster is shown in Figure 11-4.

The World Health Organization (WHO) regards the workplace as a setting for protecting and promoting the health of workers, their families, and the community. The World Health Organization defines a healthy workplace as one in which employees and managers continually work to promote and improve the health, safety, and well-being of all employees. This is accomplished when all workers and managers pay attention to health and safety concerns in the physical workplace, as well as psychological and psychosocial concerns such as organization and workplace culture. Other important aspects of a healthy workplace are access to health resources for employees and employee participation in the improvement of health in the workplace, in their families, and in the community. To broaden awareness of the importance of workplace health, the WHO developed the *Global Plan of Action on Workers Health, 2008–2017* which provides a globally coherent framework for planning, delivery, and evaluation of essential interventions for workplace health protection and promotion.

Following the announcement of the WHO framework, and in support of it in 2009 in Atlanta, GA, the International Association for Workplace Health Promotion adopted a definition of worksite health promotion which states: "Worksite health promotion represents the combined efforts of employees, families, employers, communities, and society to optimize worker health and well-being and overall performance" (The Atlanta Declaration). The American Public Health Association encourages public health organizations to become leaders in promoting health workplaces as an effective way to better achieve overall community health.

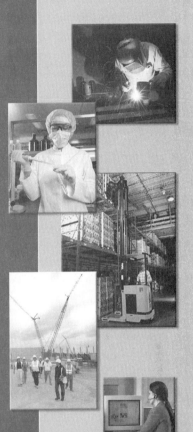

Job Safety and Health

It's the law!

OSHA®
Occupational Safety
and Health Administration
U.S. Department of Labor

EMPLOYEES:

- You have the right to notify your employer or OSHA about workplace hazards. You may ask OSHA to keep your name confidential.

- You have the right to request an OSHA inspection if you believe that there are unsafe and unhealthful conditions in your workplace. You or your representative may participate in that inspection.

- You can file a complaint with OSHA within 30 days of retaliation or discrimination by your employer for making safety and health complaints or for exercising your rights under the *OSH Act*.

- You have the right to see OSHA citations issued to your employer. Your employer must post the citations at or near the place of the alleged violations.

- Your employer must correct workplace hazards by the date indicated on the citation and must certify that these hazards have been reduced or eliminated.

- You have the right to copies of your medical records and records of your exposures to toxic and harmful substances or conditions.

- Your employer must post this notice in your workplace.

- You must comply with all occupational safety and health standards issued under the *OSH Act* that apply to your own actions and conduct on the job.

EMPLOYERS:

- You must furnish your employees a place of employment free from recognized hazards.

- You must comply with the occupational safety and health standards issued under the *OSH Act*.

This free poster available from OSHA –
The Best Resource for Safety and Health

Free assistance in identifying and correcting hazards or complying with standards is available to employers, without citation or penalty, through OSHA-supported consultation programs in each state.

1-800-321-OSHA (6742)
www.osha.gov

OSHA 3165-12-06R

FIGURE 11-4 OSHA Job Safety and Health Poster
Source: Occupational Safety and Health Administration

Summary

The public health workforce is large and diverse. It is comprised of professionals from many different fields and it encompasses a wide range of activities, roles, and responsibilities. There are laws and regulations at the federal and state levels of government that must be adhered to when managing human resources. Additionally, there are processes that help facilitate workforce development and effectiveness. Some of these include: job analysis and design; performance evaluation; selection and placement; training and development; and workplace safety. It is also important for the public health work environment to embrace the concepts and practices of the healthy workplace and health promotion, just as is expected when working with external communities.

The following case studies in Chapter 16, "Cases in Public Health Management," are directly related to concepts and principles presented in this chapter:
- Case 4: A Case of Reverse Discrimination?
- Case 5: Understanding Millennial Employees
- Case 6: Managing Diversity
- Case 7: Sick Building Syndrome
- Case 8: To Hear This Message in Korean, Press '9'
- Case 10: Zero-Tolerance for Smoking
- Case 12: Don't Ask, But Tell
- Case 13: Senior Cyber Café
- Case 16: Healthy Lifestyles Start at Home
- Case 17: Top Ten U.S. Public Health Achievements
- Case 18: Deciding on a Career in Public Health

Public Health Professional Perspective

Victoria Moody, M.S.A., Centers for Disease Control and Prevention, CDC, Atlanta, GA

Interview by Dr. James A. Johnson

Continues

(Q): What is your own working definition of an effective manager?

Ms. Moody: I would define an effective manager as one who consistently uses good people skills to maximize the performance of his or her workers and is one who demonstrates skills and abilities for managing time and resources in order to achieve organizational goals, objectives, and sustainability.

An effective manager communicates performance expectations to workers, identifies and aligns the strengths of workers with positions that enhance worker performance and productivity, provides regular feedback to workers on their performance, and rewards those who make notable contributions to the organization.

(Q): What are the biggest challenges you face on a daily basis?

Ms. Moody: As a program consultant, I serve as a liaison between headquarters and several federally funded public health programs located around the country. It is often challenging to provide technical assistance and guidance to my assigned programs when I am not onsite to observe their daily operations. As a result, I spend a large amount of time on a daily basis communicating with program managers either on the phone, or through e-mail. In addition, my daily activities at headquarters include participation on workgroups, attending meetings, and working on various projects. The coordination and scheduling of these daily activities is often my biggest challenge.

(Q): What skills are most essential for the work you do?

Ms. Moody: I believe the most essential skills needed for being a program consultant include knowledge of epidemiology, surveillance, behavioral science, public health practice, and program management on the local and state levels. In addition, good writing skills are essential in this kind of work because program consultants frequently write reports, including site-visit reports, technical reviews of progress reports that provide feedback to programs, and correspondence to a diverse audience. In addition, good people skills are essential because program consultants frequently work in a variety of settings and with diverse groups of people. And, since public health priorities may rapidly change without much notice, the ability to easily adapt to change is also an essential skill for public health practitioners.

(Q): What is your favorite project or initiative you are currently working on?

Ms. Moody: I am currently working with a colleague to publish an e-mail newsletter that includes articles containing information and updates submitted from state and local health departments. Many of these articles describe prevention efforts and interventions to identify and control communicable diseases. The newsletter is published quarterly and disseminated as an attachment to an e-mail addressed to stakeholders and our public health partners in the field. The format is simple. Contributor submissions are usually only a paragraph, or two, and describe interventions that have resulted in notable outcomes, examples of promising practices, updates to previously published prevention efforts, announcements from public health partners, information about training opportunities, and updates from headquarters. Contributors include contact information following their brief narratives so that readers can contact the authors to get additional information. The newsletter has been published for almost a year now, and the format seems to be popular among our readers.

Continues

(Q): Do you consider yourself a "systems thinker"? If so, how or give an example.

Ms. Moody: Yes, I consider myself a "systems thinker," especially as a public health program consultant. As a "systems thinker" I critically analyze systems that affect program operations and performance before I can identify specific technical assistance needs. I often begin this process by focusing on program evaluation measures. I analyze program processes, or systems of operation, to learn if they are aligned with the program's goals and objectives. I have often found that barriers to achieving successful outcomes are usually the result of inefficient processes or systems. By critically analyzing how program systems operate, I can begin to identify problem areas and to make recommendations for program improvement and, hopefully, sustainability.

(Q): What advice do you have for students who plan a career in public health management?

Ms. Moody: I think it is important for students who want a career in public health management to seek a variety of experiences as a public health practitioner at the operational level. Students should get involved; learn how public health systems impact the health and well-being of diverse communities in a variety of settings. They should get involved in community planning groups that identify target groups within their communities and prioritize public health interventions. In addition, students should learn how stakeholders and partners work in collaboration to coordinate the delivery of public health services to those most in need. These experiences are helpful when managers must make decisions regarding the delivery of public health services, especially when resources are limited.

End

Discussion and Review Questions

1. What is the public health workforce? Describe some of its key characteristics.

2. What are the goals of diversity training, and why is this important in public health organizations?

3. Identify the primary employment laws that a public health manager should be aware of.

4. What are the main human resource processes? Describe at least two of these.

5. Outline the primary steps that need to be taken in a selection process.

6. How would you go about conducting an employment interview? What are the various steps to be taken?

7. Is public health just as concerned about healthy workplaces as it is healthy communities? If so, how and why? Give examples.

Action Learning and Critical Thinking

A. Identify a popular movie that depicts an unhealthy workplace or demonstrates poor human resource practices. Show a clip of the scene or scenes to your classmates and explain how this relates to some of the concepts in this chapter.

B. Conduct a "mock interview" in your class where one person is the employer and the other is an applicant. Frame a set of questions and interview at least three potential candidates. Have the rest of the class critique the interview. Have at least three students take turns in the role of employer so that you can compare styles and effectiveness. Discuss how a "mock interview" can be helpful in management training.

C. Go to the website of the Bureau of Labor Statistics and see what the projected job opportunities are for the coming few years. What opportunities are there for someone with a background in public health and other related health professions? What new opportunities might be emerging in fields such as homeland security, transportation, environmental sciences, agriculture, disaster management, etc., that can be aligned with public health or that might have a public health component to it? Be creative about the future, it's still being developed.

Chapter 12

COMMUNICATION,
INFORMATION SYSTEMS,
AND DECISION MAKING

James A. Johnson, Ph.D., M.P.A.
Bernard Kerr, Ed.D., M.P.H., M.I.M.

Learning Objectives

Upon completion of this chapter, you should be able to:

1. Define communication.
2. Define decision making.
3. Be aware of the barriers to communication.
4. Understand the communication process.
5. Grasp the essentials of decision making.
6. Recognize and understand the purpose of information systems.
7. Be familiar with evidence-based decision making.

Key Terms

communication	information systems	public health
communication process	information	informatics
evidence-based	technology	satisficing
decision making		

Chapter Outline

INTRODUCTION

Public health managers are embedded in an information-rich environment that demands continuous communication. The organizations they work in and the communities being served have a need for a high level of effectiveness when these managers make decisions. This chapter explores the nature of human communication, barriers to effective communication, and skills needed by public health managers. It also looks at information and the rapidly growing field of informatics and its use in public health. Additionally, the chapter addresses the topic of decision making and describes the emerging push toward the use of evidence in this process.

COMMUNICATION

communication: The exchange of information between individuals through a common system of signs, symbols, and behaviors.

In its most simple form, **communication** is the transmission of information from one person to another. This involves a sender and a receiver. The sender is one who initiates the communication by sending some type of message to another person or group of people. This is done through various channels of communication such as language, which can be written, verbal, and nonverbal. Written communication for the public health manager may be in the form of memos, directions, e-mail, and documents. Verbal communication involves speech, and nonverbal messages are often in the form of body language and symbols. In all cases, communication occurs when the message transfers meaning. Central to this process is the receiver being able to decode and interpret the message. In fact, it is so fundamental to the understanding of communication that the very root of the word is derived from the Latin *communis*, which means "common."

Thus communication involves more than simply transmitting information but also the establishment of common meaning. This is especially important for the public health manager who interacts with so many people throughout the day, both within the organization and outside in the community. Every interaction involves some form of communication, either intentional or unintentional. Thus communication is a continuous part of life. In the book *Leadership: A Communications Perspective*, Hackman and Johnson provide five defining characteristics that help our understanding of what communication is. The first of these is that *communication is not a thing, it is a process.* Communication is dynamic and ever changing. Unlike a microbiologist looking at a cell, when studying communications social scientists focus on a continuous, ongoing process without a clearly defined beginning and end. Secondly, *communication is not linear, it is circular.* It has a feedback loop that connects the sender and receiver. The next defining characteristic is *communication is complex.* It involves more than just one person sending a message to another. It involves who you are and who the other person is. It also involves the perceptions of each, such as who you think the other person is and who they think you are. The fourth defining characteristic is *communication is irreversible.* It cannot be taken back. Once the message is sent and received, it will have an impact—either desired or undesired. Finally, *communication involves the total personality.* An individual's communication cannot be viewed separately from the person. It is an integral part of who they are and how they define themselves.

Consistent with the definition of communication as a process that is complex and dynamic, it is important to look further into the communication process and the skills needed to engage in it as a public health manager.

THE COMMUNICATION PROCESS

There are many ways to conceptualize the **communication process**, but one simple way to see it is the public health manager as the sender and the employee as the receiver. Of course, this can and does go in the other direction. All effective communication has feedback that comes to the sender. This might be direct or indirect. Furthermore, all communication channels are subject to distortions that can interfere with the quality of the message received.

In addition to the communication channel and the role of feedback and possible distortions, it is important to consider attributes of the sender and receiver that can affect the message and its interpretation. As described by Kelly in *Nursing Leadership and Management*, the communication process is influenced emotions, needs, perceptions, values, education, culture, goals, literacy, cognitive ability, and the mode of communication (Figure 12-1).

communication process:
A description or explanation of the chain of events involved in communication.

As can be seen from examining the communication process, there are many potential barriers. These are especially evident in the organizational setting.

Barriers in the Communication Process

In their book, *Joining Together*, Johnson and Johnson describe communication problems as coming from the lack of feedback, noise in communication, misuse of language, and listening deficiencies. Some examples would include one-way

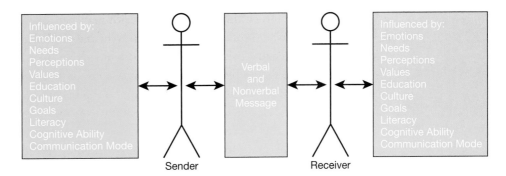

FIGURE 12-1 The Communication Process Influences
© Cengage Learning 2013

communication, in which the receiver provides no return information about whether and with what effect the communication came across. This interferes with the necessary feedback for communication to be effective. Other problems arise when there is interference during the transmission of the message. This could be actual physical noise or distortions and distractions. The misuse of language can also cause difficulty, especially when the language is vague, inaccurate, inflammatory, or overly negative. Other problems arise when the receiver is listening inattentively, passively, or not at all.

Some common barriers to communication faced by the public health manager on a routine basis include filtering, perceptions, time, language, emotions, and nonverbal cues.

- **Filtering:** This occurs when the information is manipulated in some way to make it look more favorable.

- **Perception:** As was shown in Figure 12-1, there are many factors that can alter perceptions. Included would be expectations and past experiences.

- **Time:** Constraints in relation to time can be a barrier by limiting time to gather all the information needed or by creating pressure to interpret the information too quickly.

- **Language:** This can create major barriers especially when there are differences in age, education, and cultural backgrounds. Public health has an abundance of technical words and jargon that can easily contribute to a language barrier.

- **Emotions:** Feelings often enter into the communication process and can result in something being incorrectly heard or expressed. Most emotions, as much as 95 percent, are expressed nonverbally.

- **Nonverbal:** Anytime a nonverbal cue is inconsistent with oral communication, a certain amount of confusion is introduced that can distort the message. It has been shown that as much as 65 percent of meaning comes from nonverbal messages.

"Where observation is concerned, chance favors only the prepared mind."
—*Louis Pasteur, Nineteenth-Century Scientist and Pioneer of the Germ Theory*

There are several things the public health manager can do to offset or overcome these barriers. One of the most powerful is the use of feedback. The manager should have good feedback skills and be comfortable asking questions and seeking clarification. This should be a routine part of communication feedback since it helps to foster clarity and establish the common meaning being sought by the message. Part of the ability to give feedback effectively involves the capacity to engage in active listening. Listening skills are used to gain meaning from the message that can then provide the basis for feedback. Part of active listening includes empathy, in order to relate to the emotional side of the communication.

Communication Skills

Fortunately, the manager has a wide range of skills that can be used and developed to overcome barriers and foster a climate of more effective communication. Examples of some skills commonly used are provided in Table 12-1.

TABLE 12-1 Communication Skills

Skill	Description
Attending	Active listening for what is said and how it is said as well as noting nonverbal cues that support or negate congruence, for example, making eye contact and posturing.
Responding	Verbal and nonverbal acknowledgement of the sender's message, such as "I hear you."
Clarifying	Restating, questioning, and rephrasing to help the message become clear, for example, "I lost you there."
Confronting	Identifying the conflict, for example, "We have a problem here" and then clearly delineating the problem. Confronting uses knowledge and reason to resolve the problem.
Supporting	Siding with another person or backing up another person: "I can see that you would feel that way."
Focusing	Centers on the main point: "So your main concern is …"
Open-ended questioning	Allows for patient-directed responses: "How did that make you feel?"
Providing information	Supplies one with knowledge he or she did not previously have: "It's common for people with pneumonia to be tired."

(Continues)

TABLE 12-1 Communication Skills *(Continued)*	
Using silence	Allows for intrapersonal communication.
Reassuring	Restores confidence or removes fear: "I can assure you that tomorrow …"
Expressing appreciation	Shows gratitude: "Thank you" or "You are so thoughtful."
Using humor	Provides relief and gains perspective; may also cause harm, so use carefully.
Conveying acceptance	Makes known that one is capable or worthy: "It's okay to cry."
Asking related questions	Expands listener's understanding: "How painful was it?"

Since public health managers also communicate outside of their agencies, it is critical that there be an awareness of the intended audience in the community. When developing publication materials, the National Cancer Institute recommends the following five-step process:

1. Define the target audience.
2. Conduct target-audience research.
3. Develop a concept for the program.
4. Develop content and visuals.
5. Pretest and revise draft materials.

Taking this a step further, Ledlow, Johnson, and Hakoyama, in *Social Marketing and Organizational Communication Efficacy*, recommend the following when communicating to populations where a public health intervention will be made: They recommend consistency, having a constant message and purpose and simplicity, to make the communication understandable to all. An example of this is the message of the National Diabetes Trust highlighting the link between obesity and diabetes; the public listens because the message has been consistent and clear.

Communication is such an important part of the function of public organizations generally—and public health agencies especially—that the U.S. Office of Personnel Management offers services to help develop and improve organizational communications, as shown in Exhibit 12-1.

An extension of the communication process and a critical element in communications is the use of information systems. The next section discusses how these systems can be helpful to the public health manager in both the communications and decision-making processes.

Exhibit 12-1   Communication

Continuous communication of agency mission, vision, and direction are keys to success in becoming a high-performing organization. The organization must draw a clear roadmap of agency direction to secure employee commitment. Some technical assistance activities which OPM performs include:

- developing communication plans for agencies that include workforce planning initiatives, desired goals and outcomes, timelines, and executive support;

- identifying appropriate and effective communication vehicles, such as "town hall meetings," intranet, written communication, poster campaigns, etc; and

- developing strategies and processes for line managers to use to analyze communication roadblocks and enhance communication with their own workforce.

Source: U.S. Office of Personnel Management, 2012. Retrieved from http://www.opm.gov

INFORMATION SYSTEMS

Public health organizations and agencies are information intensive. Information is used in decision making, social marketing, organization development, human resource and financial management, communication to communities and constituents, and many more purposes. The information must be managed in a systematic way or there would be overload and inefficiency. This is where information technology and information systems come in. In a 2007 study by the Pew Center on the States, titled the *Government Performance Project*, an assessment of the information systems of 42 states found the following common uses of comprehensive information systems:

1. Development and management of hiring websites for state government employment. This allows prospective applicants to gain information about a public agency and often to apply for a position online. Public health agencies at all levels of government have embraced this use of information technology.

2. Implementation of web portals for employees and consumers to provide information about an agency and its programs. Some are interactive and allow employees to update their human resources records and others are portals open to the public with interactive capability for requesting information.

3. The use of information technology for training and knowledge management. This has helped provide employee-development opportunities and community education.

4. Development of comprehensive state databases on workforce, health, demographics, and other information items that might be useful in organizational strategic planning or program development.

In addition to these macro uses of **information technology** to help improve organizational effectiveness, public health also uses information for health improvement and disease control. At the core of this arena is the Centers for Disease Control and Prevention (CDC) in Atlanta, GA. The CDC works closely with states and local public health agencies to assure quality information sharing and utilization. As was discussed in Part I of this book, there is considerable interdependence between federal, state, and local public health agencies with our federalist system of government. This is especially so with public health **information systems**, also known as *informatics*.

> "Systems of information-feedback control are fundamental to all life and human endeavor, from the slow pace of biological evolution to the launching of the latest space satellite…Everything we do as individuals, as an industry, or as a society is done in the context of an information-feedback system."—*Jay Forrester, Management Professor and Systems Scientist*

information technology:
Technology involving the development, maintenance, and use of computer systems, software, and networking for the processing and distribution of data.

information systems:
Also known as *informatics*; system consisting of the network of all channels of communication within an organization.

Public Health Informatics

A discussion of the **public health informatics** agenda could easily focus on the agenda of The National Center for Public Health Informatics (NCPHI), one of three National Centers within the CDC Coordinating Center for Health Information. The NCPHI mission statement reads: "NCPHI protects the public's health, promotes health equity, and transforms public health practice through the advancement of the science of biomedical informatics in public health practice and through collaborative development of information systems for public health." Certainly this is a worthy mission and agenda. Exploring the public health informatics agenda could also begin at the state level with an entity such as the Colorado Department of Public Health and Environment's Public Health Informatics Unit. The mission of the Unit is "…to improve the performance of public health systems by advancing public health practitioners' ability to strategically manage and apply health information systems." Again, this is a worthy mission and agenda. However, the fundamental merit and value of public health informatics is not found in the mission statements or the agendas of federal or state agencies. The most meaningful opportunities to leverage public health information for the public good are found at the local level and are orchestrated by local public health personnel. These are the frontline informatics warriors in the battle to sustain, improve, and enhance the public's health.

Public health data is collected locally; thus, state and federal databases have local origins. Such databases may have only limited local relevance and value. It is the local data that matters most in forging the core public health informatics agenda. Forging the agenda is not an especially complex task and is depicted in Figure 12-2.

The real complexity is found in the fact that the identification of actionable agenda items involves more than gathering, sorting, and analysis of factual information for use in decision support and action planning. Like it or not, public health decisions

public health informatics:
The systematic application of information, computer science, and technology to public health practice, research, and technology.

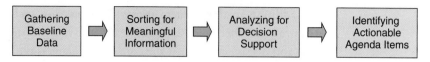

FIGURE 12-2 Health Informatics Agenda
© Cengage Learning 2013

and action plans are born of many variables, among them resources, politics, emotion, and factual information. Therefore, a key responsibility for the public health informatician is to bring factual local information to the forefront while recognizing the role of resources, politics, and emotion in health planning and programming.

The CDC Office of Workforce and Career Development and the University of Washington School of Public Health and Community Medicine's Center for Public Health Informatics partnered to develop a set of Competencies for Public Health Informaticians. The full report with the competencies is available for download at http://www.cdc.gov. The glossary of the report defines a public health informatician (or informaticist) as a "public health professional who works in practice, research, or academia and whose primary work function is to use informatics to improve the health of populations." Since this definition indicates the public health informatician uses *informatics*, a definition of informatics is required. Shortliffe, in the text *Medical Informatics: Computer Applications in Health Care*, defines medical informatics as "…the rapidly advancing scientific field that deals with the storage, retrieval, and optimal use of biomedical information, data, and knowledge for problem solving and decision making." Given these definitions, it is safe to suggest that local public health informaticians should endeavor to use health information for problem solving and decision making in an effort to improve the health of local populations.

This brings us to an examination of the competencies of a public health informatician. Among the 14 competencies outlined in the aforementioned effort, one stands out in terms of the core public health informatics agenda of leveraging health information locally in decision making, problem solving, and program planning: *Ensures that knowledge, information, and data needs of project or program users and stakeholders are met.*

There can be no more significant goal for the public health informatician than to meet the knowledge, information, and data needs of program-users and stakeholders at the local level. While substantial informatics resources are invested at the national, regional, and local levels in terms of technology dollars and human resources, it seems investments in informatics resources are lacking at the local level. Speaking before the Standing Committee on Health, Dr. David Butler-Jones said it best: "Clearly, first of all, public health is a local function. That's where the action happens."

The local level is where public health is delivered and as a result, there is a great opportunity to leverage public health information using the tools and techniques of informatics. A report entitled *Informatics at Local Health Departments: Findings from the 2005 National Profile of Local Health Departments Study* prepared by the National Association of City and County Health Officials stated: "The capacity to use information is fundamental to all public health activities. Consequently, informatics is a key part of the foundation, or infrastructure, on which the public health system is built."

One of the primary uses of information is in the realm of decision making and decision support. This is especially critical for public health agencies. In fact, the Institute of Medicine, in addressing the issue of health safety, identifies decision support as a critical success factor and part of the overall effective use of electronic health information.

DECISION MAKING

Since much of public health practice and management involves decision making, both at the personal and professional levels, it is important to understand the dynamics of decisions. A decision is based on various ways of thinking about a problem and the information attained or assumed about the problem or situation. Some people will rely heavily on intuition to make a decision, others will use data and evidence, while others may be more holistic and involve some mixture of the two. Most individuals will reflect upon a decision to evaluate it against their own perspectives or the perspectives of others. These three approaches are referred to as *intuitive thinking*, *critical thinking*, and *reflective thinking*. An integrative mixture of all three that also takes into consideration the environmental context and systemic impact of the decision is called *systems thinking*. The interaction of these approaches to the way we think and their relation to decision making is depicted in Figure 12-3.

Through this interaction of thought process a decision is usually made. However, in the organizational setting a more structured process is called for. The most commonly used approach involves a six-step process:

Step 1: Identify the need for a decision.

Step 2: Determine the goal or desired outcome.

Step 3: Identify alternatives or actions.

Step 4: Consider the benefits and consequences of each alternative.

Step 5: Decide which action to implement.

Step 6: Evaluate the decision.

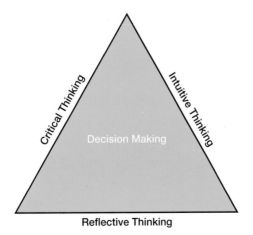

FIGURE 12-3 The Decision-Making Process
© Cengage Learning 2013

While most public health managers will follow this approach or a similar step-by-step process of decision making, there are many instances where decisions are not so rational. Often, due to time pressures, emotional issues, or limited information, the manager will not arrive at an optimal decision but will instead make a satisfactory decision. This is what Noble Prize-winning Herbert Simon referred to as **satisficing**. This occurs when the search for alternative actions in step 3 of the process is limited due to the constraints of a situation.

> "You cannot escape the responsibility of tomorrow by evading it today."
> —*Abraham Lincoln, 16th President of the United States of America*

As an offset to the tendency to satisfice in decision making there has been an increasing trend toward **evidence-based decision making**. This approach involves the use of verifiable data and current information in the decision analysis. Thus every step of the process identified previously would have measurable data elements. As described by Walshe and Rundall in the *Millbank Quarterly*, the rise of evidence-based clinical practice in health care has caused some to start questioning how health managers and policymakers make decisions, and what role evidence plays in the process. Though managers and policymakers have been quick to encourage clinicians to adopt an evidence-based approach, they have been slower to apply the same ideas to their own practice—even in the face of evidence that the same problems of the underuse of effective interventions and the overuse of ineffective ones are widespread. Due to differences between the culture and decision-making processes of clinicians and managers, the ideas of evidence-based practice will need to be adapted for management rather than simply transferred from clinical practice. This is an ongoing process that is still emerging in public health management. The U.S. Department of Veterans Affairs, which manages one of the largest public health care systems in the world, is a major advocate of evidence-based management decision making. Their statement on the subject is presented in Exhibit 12-2.

satisficing: Aiming to achieve only satisfactory results because the satisfactory process is familiar, whereas aiming for the best-achievable results would call for costs, effort, and the incurring of risks. Due to time pressures, emotional issues, or limited information, the manager will not arrive at an optimal decision but will instead make a satisfactory decision.

evidence-based decision making: An approach to decision making that combines expertise, patient or client concerns, and information from scientific literature to derive a decision. The use of verifiable data and current information in the decision analysis.

Exhibit 12-2   A Paradigm Shift Toward Evidence-Based Management in the Department of Veterans Affairs

There are strong arguments for the practice of evidenced-based management. But, currently, most managers do not consistently make decisions on the basis of formal evidence, and, even when they seek it, the availability of systematic evidence is sparse. To remedy this situation—to move toward acceptance and widespread practice of evidenced-based management on a par with evidence-based clinical practice—there must be a paradigm shift in attitude and actions of both managers and researchers.

Managers will need to focus more on using empirical evidence to make decisions rather

Continues

than relying solely on consultants and management gurus without determining if their solutions have been successful in the past. Reviewing empirically based research can provide a reference for what has already been shown to be successful or not. While most healthcare managers do not have a background in research methodology, they need to be more accepting and willing to learn from empirical research.

Researchers need to better focus research questions on the real and immediate needs of organizations. To achieve this goal they must put more effort into establishing closer relationships with management. Researchers' objectives should be to explain and predict the consequences of managerial actions instead of just trying to understand the life of the organization.

Source: U.S. Department of Veterans Affairs, 2012. Retrieved from http://www.colmr.research.va.gov

Summary

Public health managers will continue to face challenges in the management of information and the use of data and evidence in the decision process. However, new technologies and insights into the behavioral and cognitive attributes of decisions will help meet these demands. Furthermore, as public health managers better understand communication processes and barriers to communication, there will be improved effectiveness that benefits the organization and the communities being served. Emerging paradigms such as informatics and evidence-based decision making will continue to evolve and in turn spread throughout public health practice.

The following case studies in Chapter 16, "Cases in Public Health Management," are directly related to concepts and principles presented in this chapter:

- Case 8: To Hear This Message in Korean, Press '9'
- Case 9: A *Giardia* Oubreak?
- Case 13: Senior Cyber Café
- Case 14: Collaborative Approach to Diabetes Prevention and Care
- Case 15: Toy Recall Prompts Attention to Lead Poisoning
- Case 20: Pacific Needle Exchange Program

Public Health Professional Perspective

Josephine M. Bautista, M.S.A., Consumer Safety Officer, U.S. Food and Drug Administration, Washington, D.C.

Interview by Scott D. Musch

(Q): Tell us about your recent positions at the USFDA.

Ms. Bautista: Recently, I transferred to the Center of Biologics in January from the Center for Devices where I worked for 11 years. My current position is as a scientific reviewer and senior advisor. I held several positions during my career at the Center for Devices, most recently as an Associate Director for Compliance and Import Safety, which included corrective actions and removal of devices on the market and ensuring the compliance of devices imported to the United States.

Continues

(Q): What are your main responsibilities?

Ms. Bautista: In my former position, we were responsible for pre-market and post-market review of regulated products. I was a manager within the department. In my new position, I have a similar management role though the regulated product lines are different. These regulated and licensed products are used for donors and donor-patient compatibility testing. Part of my new responsibility includes personalized medicine, which involves devices that are matched with drugs for treating patients, genetic devices, and direct-to-consumer devices.

(Q): You have worked in three sectors—government, private, and military. How would you describe the major differences working in each sector?

Ms. Bautista: In comparing the three sectors, my experiences within the government and military were much more regulated and the requirements were more stringent. The flexibility in your daily responsibilities and work product is not as great as it is in the private sector. In the private sector, the biggest focus is on getting the job done as fast as you can. In the government, the focus is also on getting the job done, but there is a more precise way of doing your job because of regulations. Each sector has its own benefits, and I enjoyed all of my experiences equally. I think there are more opportunities in the government to be exposed to issues in public health, but I have been able to learn equally well from each experience. There are some different skill sets involved in working for the government, particularly learning to deal with a highly regulated environment and the obligation to keep current on all of the regulations. There is not a lot of flexibility when you deal with regulations, so you need the skill set to know [that] if you work for the government there are certain requirements that you will have to meet.

(Q): A distinguishing feature about your career at the FDA is your broad experience in working with teams and committees in decision making. Describe your experiences.

Ms. Bautista: When I was in graduate school and had to work in teams, I really disliked it. I thought it was easier just to do the work myself and not have to deal with the team. However, coming into the government and especially the FDA, nothing is done in a vacuum, everything is done in the open, and 90 percent to 95 percent of the work I do is done with a team. In doing so, I have learned why it's better to do work within a team. You benefit from a group of people making a decision, because there is less room for error. I have changed my opinions on teams quite a bit since school. I have worked on many teams at the FDA that have functioned very well, so I would say that I really enjoy working with teams.

(Q): What communications advice would you have for a professional who is a member of a team and wants to be more effective within the team?

Ms. Bautista: Be a good communicator. Sometimes you work in teams with people who don't want to say anything or who try to control the conversation. A good facilitator is needed in teams, especially when you have a multi-group of people. The facilitator's role is important to get everyone to participate in the group.

Continues

(Q): You have worked at both headquarters and in the field during your career at the FDA. What were some of the major differences in the use of information between the two?

Ms. Bautista: My field roles have primarily involved inspections with field investigators. Working between the two, I haven't really noticed many differences. Professionals in both roles really do their jobs well. I have been really impressed. Sometimes you get the opinion that one is different from the other, but overall the staff between both are equally challenged and prepared with the expertise to do their job. Neither experience is better than the other. You can't do your job in a vacuum on either side. The information flow is similar in either role. The access to information is the same.

(Q): What advice would you give to a student studying public health who wants to enter the field you are in?

Ms. Bautista: Students should gain regulatory education and experience through their course-work and internships at government agencies. Learn how the government works. The FDA has many internship programs to give students training and experience.

End

Public Health Leader Perspective

Beth Taylor, RN, M.B.A., D.H.A., U.S. Department of Veterans Affairs Health System, Milwaukee, Wisconsin

Interview by Dr. James Johnson

(Q): What is your own working definition of an effective manager?

Ms. Taylor: An effective manager is a person who can organize and coordinate the energies of the work unit to collaborate on contributing to the goals and objectives of the organization. It is important to recognize the organic nature of work teams and the energy required to manage these dynamics to collective achievement.

(Q): What are the biggest communications challenges you face on a daily basis?

Ms. Taylor: I think the biggest challenge lies with maintaining focus. Recognizing the interplay of diverse perspectives, personalities, and variables at play in the organization and helping orchestrate the coordination of these while simultaneously keeping the mission at the

Continues

core of each decision is the most difficult aspect of leadership. It is easy to be distracted by a myriad of details and become lost in the weeds. A leader must have the vision to keep moving in a unified direction and not allow the static noise of the work environment to throw them or their team off balance.

(Q): What management and decision skills are most essential for the work you do?

Ms. Taylor: The ability to adapt to continual change is essential for any manager or leader. The health care environment is changing at a rapid pace and requiring us to constantly modify our approach, not only to improve our clinical care but to explore new methods and technologies to improve population health. This requires an open and inquisitive mind of each individual and of the collective culture. It also requires the leader to be somewhat tolerant of failure. Not failure in the sense of incompetence or negligence, but allowing new ideas to be tried understanding that not all will be raving successes. However, sometimes the process of evaluating what did not work will illuminate a new path, and a leader must have the ability to encourage movement forward.

(Q): Are you currently working on any projects that involve evidence-based decision making? Please briefly describe.

Ms. Taylor: I am currently assisting with the development of an Evidence-Based Practice culture in a national health system. It is fascinating to observe the various approaches to implementation and the challenges of supporting a system-wide initiative. It has been estimated that it takes 17 years for clinical research to be implemented at the bedside. With Internet searches becoming easier for all staff, exploring the best evidence for effective treatment of conditions is beginning to shift how clinicians view their work. It is exciting to see migration away from professional practice based in tradition to practice based on the best evidence available to guide care. I believe that better use of evidence in our management and clinical decisions will lead us to more effective organizations as well as improve patient care.

(Q): Do you consider yourself a systems thinker or critical thinker?

Ms. Taylor: I consider myself a student of systems thinking and anticipate remaining in this role throughout my career. A few years ago, I completed a project for a hospital system looking at the referral patterns and movement of patients within their network. It was interesting to see how the various sites were affected by small decisions of others and how these influenced where patients sought health care or where providers referred them. This assignment taught me the importance of looking for answers at the points of intersection within a system and to understand that even the smallest of changes in one facility may have a large, and frequently unintended, consequence in another. This is true when examining micro or macro systems, and underscores the need for communication and collaboration between parts to minimize organizational friction.

(Q): What advice do you have for students who plan a career in public health management?

Ms. Taylor: Health management is a challenging and dynamic profession and provides the opportunity to contribute to healthier lives for individuals as well as populations. What could be a more noble profession than improving the health of fellow human beings? Look for chances to serve at the point of impact, such as direct-patient care in a health facility or field work, as this is the only way you will develop an understanding for how the unique pieces of any health

Continues

system fit together. Understand the core business mission of the organization you work with, and regularly touch bases with your consumers as they can readily tell you what is not working for them. Assertively seek mentors who can help teach you the intricacies of the profession and help open doors to your future. Finally, maintain an open and inquisitive mind as the profession and the world will continue to change rapidly around you.

Note: *The views expressed in this article are those of the participants and do not necessarily reflect the position or policy of the Department of Veterans Affairs.*

End

Discussion and Review Questions

1. Discuss communication and why it is so important to managers.

2. Identify your own barriers to effective communication. Share this with the class.

3. What is the role of informatics? How can it be used in public health?

4. Discuss the step-by-step approach to decision making.

5. What is satisficing? Have you ever done this? Give examples.

6. Why do you think there is a movement toward more evidence-based decision making in public health and management?

7. In the two interviews for this chapter, each person discussed the importance of information, data, or evidence in the work they do for the FDA and the VA. Identify these references and discuss how they relate to topics described in this chapter.

Action Learning and Critical Thinking

A. Verbal Communication Exercise. Emphasis placed on specific words, speed of delivery, volume, and the pitch of one's voice all potentially change the meaning or interpretation of what is being said. To demonstrate this, read this sentence aloud: I can't believe she didn't select that informatician.

Now read and change the emphasis (tone and volume) of the words in bold typeface:

I can't believe she didn't select that informatician.

I **can't** believe she didn't select that informatician.

I can't **believe** she didn't select that informatician.

I can't believe **she** didn't select that informatician.

I can't believe she **didn't** select that informatician.

I can't believe she didn't **select** that informatician.

I can't believe she didn't select **that** informatician.

I can't believe she didn't select that **informatician**.

The instructor might want to have a different student read each sentence. Afterward, discuss the various meanings that were heard as each variation of tone and volume was read.

B. Go to the CDC website mentioned earlier in this chapter, that addresses informatics competencies and compare the competencies identified with those discussed earlier in the book under "Core Competencies for Public Health Professionals" in Chapter 2. Search the Internet and try to identify job opportunities for people seeking positions in public health informatics.

C. Look at the diagram below and identify a decision you could make in each of the domains that would improve your overall health. Did you use an intuitive approach to the decision? A data-based approach? Or some combination of the two? How could evidence-based decision making be used?

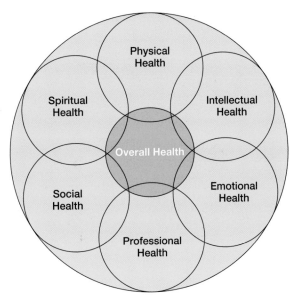

Healthy Decision Making
© Cengage Learning 2013

PART IV

PUBLIC HEALTH MANAGEMENT PERSPECTIVES

This is a set of contributed chapters from practitioners and professors of public health addressing management and practice topics pertaining to working with teams and the community; program planning and development; and future issues for public health leaders. These contributing authors bring extensive public health practice experience to this book and provide perspectives from their own practice backgrounds as well as ongoing research in the field of public health and organizational sciences.

Chapter 13: Groups, Teams, and Working with the Community

Chapter 14: Program Planning, Development, and Evaluation

Chapter 15: Public Health Leadership and the Future

Chapter 13

GROUPS, TEAMS, AND WORKING WITH THE COMMUNITY

Mark J. Minelli, Ph.D., M.P.A.
Donald J. Breckon, Ph.D., M.P.H.

Learning Objectives

Upon completion of this chapter, you should be able to:

1. Understand the roles and functions of teams in public health.
2. Effectively conduct or participate in a meeting.
3. Have a greater understanding of group dynamics in organizations.
4. Establish, meet, and measure group and team goals and objectives.
5. Perform best practices in working with various stakeholders and communities.
6. Understand the central significance of the team and group processes to public health.

Key Terms

agenda	group process	teams
goals	objectives	the SMART rule
group	stages of team	
group decision making	development	

Chapter Outline

INTRODUCTION

Foremost in the field of public health is the health professional's ability to work in and with interagency task forces, committees, teams, groups, and the community at large. Teams or groups will be used interchangeably in this chapter, but in practice may refer to any of the foregoing terms. The synergistic power of working with a diverse group of people to accomplish important goals and objectives should not be underestimated. More insights and resources can be brought to bear on the problems that exist, and importantly, more community and interagency support can be generated by participation that leads to a sense of ownership.

Community agencies and organizations do not stand alone trying to complete tasks the public expects from the services provided. The ability to work in harmony with people from other cultures, settings, and organizations will play a prominent role in the success of any health professional.

This chapter will provide the core foundational skills to effectively engage teams and groups in a public health setting. Information provided will be based on a collection of current literature and reflections of field personnel actively pursuing excellence in their roles as health professionals. The blend of practitioners and scholars will provide a strong theoretical basis on the information to follow in this chapter.

TEAMS AND PUBLIC HEALTH

Teams are often used in the field of public health to examine problems or issues, provide recommendations on matters facing an organization or community, or analyze and investigate the efficacy of a process. Teams need to be empowered to

teams: Often used in the field of public health to examine problems or issues, provide recommendations on matters facing an organization or community, or analyze and investigate the efficacy of a process.

accomplish their tasks and assignments given. This means administrators must trust team members to be free thinkers and provide an open range of discussions and ideas. Although administrators often talk about empowering teams, they must be comfortable in "letting go" over people they may supervise. Even with the chance of turf wars and making mistakes, gains from group participation can outweigh risks. Empowered teams will also become more involved and dedicated if they come up with ideas and are allowed to carry them through (Minelli, 2007).

Teams are frequently short-lived and disband once the objectives or team goals are completed. Members of a work team need to collaborate and feel comfortable with their fellow participants to achieve maximum outcomes. The team members should try to put "politics" aside and not blame or discourage other participants' ideas until they have been fully reviewed. Real synergies of a team can flourish once individual talents are explored and encouraged by other members.

Sharing the workload by using a team approach is another advantage of teams versus individual work. Organizations can maximize their human resources by pooling talent and energizing staff from more than one agency to work collaboratively. This can assist in building ongoing working relationships between individuals and organizations, as people see the potential advantage of team performance. When other issues arise at a later date, individuals may know the talents of others that they can utilize to solve problems. This networking power often enhances an individual's or agency's options in reaching solutions quickly and effectively.

Team Size and Selection

Team size and selection of members may be one of the most important issues in developing a public health work team. Careful thought should be given to the makeup of individuals that will be working together to create a high-performance team. What skills will be needed on the team, such as budget analysis or group skills? Who, if anyone, will be the team leader or facilitator? How will the team members be selected to make up a diverse pool of participants? Who has the background on past initiatives? Who has the needed political or media connections? Who has the trust and respect of the community as well of the ultimate decision makers? These are a few core questions that will need to be addressed on the front end of establishing an effective team.

During the process of team member selection the size of the group must be evaluated. Effective work teams should not be larger than eight as once you get past this number scheduling meetings, obtaining participation by all, and moving the group process along can be slowed. People need to feel actively engaged in the process, and larger groups can distance an individual's feeling of importance and involvement. Remember that successful high-performance teams keep people involved.

Another important factor to consider is the personalities and reputations of the group members. Of course, you may not have control over who represents other agencies, but if you do, avoid members who are known to be overly negative, outspoken, rude, or even overly talkative. Likewise, you may wish to avoid individuals who have a reputation for not maintaining confidence regarding sensitive matters that are discussed, in that matters that arise may have fiscal, political, and staffing implications. A particularly sensitive matter should, as a rule, only have one spokesperson making statements to the media. Of course, these matters should be emphasized early on in the meeting, but may also be issues in selecting members of the group.

TEAM DEVELOPMENT

A classic body of literature on the **stages of team development** was developed by Florida State University professor Bruce Tuckman, Ph.D., in the 1960s. From his intensive study of team development, he found that teams progress through five steps or stages (forming, storming, norming, performing, and adjourning—see Table 13-1).

This section of the chapter has shown the importance and benefits of using teams in a public health setting. In Table 13-2 key concepts in working with teams are summarized.

stages of team development: Consists of five steps or stages: forming, storming, norming, performing, and adjourning.

To bring further realism into the chapter, Jan Hillman (Vice President for Government Relations, Grant Development and Planning at Superior Health Partners and Marquette General Hospital) was interviewed to provide her insight and wisdom for the readers. See the "Public Health Professional Perspective" at the end of the chapter to read her interview.

TABLE 13-1 Tuckman's Stages of Team Development

Forming—This is the first stage of team development as the members are selected, brought together, and identify the objectives to be completed.

Storming—Here the members begin to develop personal relationships, put aside past conflicts, and often select a group leader or facilitator or at least buy into the appointed leadership.

Norming—The members at this step help define the group rules, procedures, etc.

Performing—At this stage the team begins to reach consensus on implementing ideas and suggestions.

Adjourning—As most teams are short-term in nature, the group returns to their individual assignments.

TABLE 13-2 Team Key Concepts

- Teams need to be small in size and members carefully selected.

- Try to maximize synergistic effect on team performance and on agencies that are represented.

- Teams can be used to empower individuals to solve problems and accomplish tasks.

- Administrators must feel comfortable in empowering others for teams to be effective.

- Empowered teams become more dedicated to accomplishing goals for organizations.

- Teams can maximize human resources.

- The more individual team members participate, the more organizational support can be expected.

GROUP DYNAMICS

A major portion of a public health professional's daily and weekly time is devoted to **group process**. The new public health agenda centers on coalition development or, in older terms, "group work." An individual's success or failure may often hinge on their ability to work effectively in groups. Groups may be large or small, formal or informal, short-term or long-term, meet on a regular or infrequent basis, be static or ever-changing as described by Minelli and Brackon in their book *Community Health Education*.

Merriam-Webster's Collegiate Dictionary, 11th ed., defines a **group** as "a number of individuals assembled together or having common interests." One of the first tasks is to decide the goals or objectives to be accomplished, or to fully understand those that have been established as the focus for the group. Once the members have decided on this, emphasis should be given to developing group cohesiveness. Having members introduce themselves and share parts of their background that they bring to the group gives ranking members a chance to build their ego a bit, but it also helps others in the group evaluate the validity of their suggestions. As some ranking members will be modest, the group leader should be prepared to state in generic terms relevant background that the participant did not share. A few group meetings may be required to see who is dedicated to the forthcoming tasks, and some members may drop out. This is a natural process, and while follow-up with the individuals is appropriate (to voice their concerns or just listen), some may feel the group is not something they want to commit to.

To build rapport and cohesiveness it is always appropriate to provide refreshments for the meetings. A cup of coffee or a soft drink help people relax and get comfortable with each other, especially for early arrivers.

Name tags may be helpful in the first few meetings and have members seated so that they can see and hear each other (this may require a circular or semicircular seating arrangement). Sitting around tables is usually helpful, as the need will exist

group process: Working in or with groups. Groups may be large or small, formal or informal, short-term or long-term, meet on a regular or infrequent basis, be static or ever-changing.

group: A number of individuals assembled together or having common interests.

for a place to put materials, coffee, and so on. The group may decide to hold meetings on specified days/times/places, or choose to be more open-ended. Emphasizing that meetings will start on time and end at or before the scheduled time is important in allowing members to schedule the rest of their time effectively.

Meetings usually have an **agenda** sent out in advance so that all members know what is expected to be accomplished. In more formal sessions, approving the agenda may be appropriate, although generally a brief review and asking if there are other things that need to be addressed in this meeting is more common. Handouts should be distributed before the meeting starts so as to avoid wasting meeting time and creating confusion. As groups can be formal or informal, whoever is taking the organizational lead will often coordinate the meetings, at least until another leader is selected.

Group decision making is also an important component of the group process. Reaching consensus can be done through voting or general consensus, depending on whether the group is formal or informal. Frequent review and consensus-checking is always helpful to moving a group along toward its desired outcome. Consensus-checking is typically a function of the group leaders, but can be done by anyone by simply asking "Are we in agreement on …?"

Minutes are often completed to serve as the group history or reports. When new members join they can read through previous minutes and get a good idea of what the group has accomplished and the issues they face. Providing the group members with data on issues prior to or during the meeting can also aid in decision making. A group secretary can be selected, but in smaller groups, the leader often writes up a summary of attendees, areas of agreement, topics for the next meeting, etc.

Cohesiveness is a factor in effective group decision-making process. Factors that come into play are stability, similarity, size, support, and satisfaction. Long-term groups tend to be stable and can attract new members. When group members share common characteristics (e.g., age, ethnic background, education levels, etc.) they tend to be cohesive. As previously mentioned, group size has an impact on performance. Members also know if the group efforts will likely be supported from their superiors in the form of financial commitments, release time, and so forth. Lastly, the social climate of group members with each other will affect their satisfaction levels in being part of a group.

agenda: A list or outline of things to be considered or done.

group decision making: An important component of the group process. Reaching consensus can be done through voting or general consensus, depending on whether the group is formal or informal.

MEETING MANAGEMENT

Meetings can be very effective in group work as trust is built when meetings bring people together to solve real problems. A core concept is meetings need to be productive and efficient, but some fun can also be worked into the setting. Members should be seated so they can see each other and, just like teams, meetings should not be large (8 people for decisions, 18 for brainstorming). Beyond these numbers it can be difficult to reach consensus.

Being sure group members are aware of progress being made is important, as is promoting the likelihood of recommendations being implemented. No one wants to waste their valuable time if there is little likelihood of making a difference. In preparing for meetings, health professionals circulate agendas, provide background

TABLE 13-3 Example Meeting Agenda

1. Call to order

2. Approval of minutes of previous meeting

3. Additions to the agenda

4. Treasurer's report (if needed)

5. Reports of officers (if needed)

6. Committee/subcommittee reports (if needed)

7. Old business (itemized)

8. New business (itemized)

9. Other business (from additions to the agenda)

10. Adjournment

© Cengage Learning 2013

materials, and inform their supervisors. Agendas should always be developed with feedback from the members on any additions or recommendations. This will help make them feel a part of the process and build group morale as a unit working together to accomplish goals. After meetings are completed, minutes should be developed to record the history of the group decisions, actions, and future tasks.

Table 13-3 presents an example of a meeting agenda. As groups tend to be unique, changes can be made to this outline.

Public health professionals need useful strategies for facilitating meetings. Exhibit 13-1 provides some helpful tips provided by the National Center for Chronic Disease Prevention and Health Promotion.

Exhibit 13-1   Facilitating Meetings

- Create an environment conducive to communication. Try seating participants around small tables or in semicircles; move extra chairs out of the way.
- Make participation an expectation. Ask questions frequently and use open-ended questions to encourage thought and participation.

Ask for input from members who have not shared their thinking yet. This may elicit useful information, but it will also help people feel better about participating in the group. Avoid answering your own questions or talking more than participants. Thank participants for comments.

Continues

- Create opportunities for participants to work in teams during the community group meetings. Use some small-group or partner exercise.
- Give small assignments in advance and ask participants to come to meetings prepared to share their work. Preview a question or problem that participants can think about between meetings, or mail out worksheets before meetings.
- Get participants to talk about themselves as a group. Ask them to consider several questions:
  ◦ Are we working together smoothly?
  ◦ Can we improve how we interact?
  ◦ Can we put some more fun into our work?
- Talk with quiet participants during breaks. Help them express their ideas and ask them to share their thoughts with the group.
- Use smart boards, laptops, flip charts, or overhead transparencies to record comments. At intervals throughout the meeting summarize the main points, or ask a group member to paraphrase comments or review the minutes.
- Suggest the next step if the meeting seems to be stagnating.
- Walk around to gain attention, but look directly at participants. Face participants while writing on flip charts or ask someone else to do the writing. Join in. Participants will want to know about you, too, and they should feel that you are part of the group.
- Expect to make some mistakes; acknowledge them, correct them, and move on.

Common Problems

No matter how well planned a meeting is, it may not go smoothly. In fact, a certain amount of discussion and dispute is often necessary

for healthy interaction. However, leaders may lose control of the meeting if certain problems occur. Several common problems are identified below, followed by some suggestions for resolving them.

- No participation. Ask for options, and then remain silent. When participants speak up, compliment them for sharing their views.
- Off the track. Interrupt the discussion and remind participants of the original topic of discussion. Try to select a moment that would not result in anyone being embarrassed. Suggest that the newly introduced issue be discussed at a later time, or refer the issue to a working group.
- Too much talk. Often this can be done informally by summarizing, or suggesting the next step, or calling on those who have been quiet. In more formal or very large settings, it may be appropriate to set a time limit for individual contributions and appoint a timekeeper. Ask the timekeeper to inform participants when they go over the time limit.
- Disputes among participants. Remain neutral and allow the participants to disagree. If the dispute must be resolved, encourage the group to reach a consensus. If more information would help resolve the issue, refer the dispute to a working group for further discussion.
- Unyielding participants. Give the group a chance to bring them around. Often, the majority option will cause participants to reconsider their point of view. Suggest that the participants accept the group's view for now and offer to discuss the issue with them further after the meeting.

Source: Planned Approach to Community Health: Guide for the Local Coordinator, National Center for Chronic Disease Prevention and Health Promotion, Centers for Disease Control and Prevention, USDHHS, 1992.

TABLE 13-4 Group Key Concepts

- A major portion of a typical work day and week is spent in groups.

- Groups may be large or small, formal or informal, short-term or long-term.

- Building rapport and cohesiveness is an important task of all groups.

- Many groups work from meeting agendas and record complete minutes of their business accomplished.

- Facilitating and evaluating meetings are important parts of high-performance groups.

- Developing clear goals and objectives provides guidance and group direction.

© Cengage Learning 2013

Health professions understand the power of working with groups to maximize their efforts and build consensus. Table 13-4 provides key concepts shared in this section.

GROUP GOALS AND OBJECTIVES

Most groups have goals and objectives established to provide guidance and focus. It is important that the group members assist in developing goals and objectives to provide common ground and group cohesiveness. **Goals** tend to be broad statements with **objectives** being more specific and having defined outcomes that can be measured. While groups usually operate with only a few goals, they should align with the objectives and strategic plan of the sponsoring organization. Objectives can be more numerous but caution should be taken not to develop too many, overwhelming the group as outlined by Issel in *Health Program Planning and Evaluation: A Practical and Systematic Approach*.

One method for writing clear objectives is the use of **the SMART rule**. This is S = short, M = measurable, A = action oriented, R = realistic, and T = time-bound. After an objective is written, you should be able to answer "yes" to each part of the SMART rule. If any part is missing, the objective should be rewritten. Developing clear objectives will assist groups in reaching their outcomes and maintain direction.

goals: Broad statements of what needs to be accomplished.

objectives: A short-term goal; something that must be achieved on the way to a larger achievement. More specific than goals and have defined outcomes that can be measured.

the SMART rule: A method used to write clear objectives. S = short, M = measurable, A = action oriented, R = realistic, and T = time-bound.

While it does not fit neatly into the above acronym, it is also important to assign responsibility for action for whatever next steps are needed. As in all accountability measures, having that accountable person report back enhances the likelihood that the appropriate steps will be taken in a timely manner.

Along with setting goals and objectives, groups can be very diverse in their composition. Ms. Jennifer Crawford, who is a prevention coordinator with the Saginaw Chippewa Indian Tribe in the behavioral health area, was interviewed for her knowledge on working with diverse populations. See the "Public Health Professional Perspective" at the end of this chapter to read her interview.

WORKING WITH COMMUNITIES

Often a public health team will work on projects and initiatives out in the community. Many of the same dynamics seen within the organization can become active in community settings. Likewise, the processes of team development and the essentials of team functionality are critical to being able to effectively deliver a program or implement an initiative. As described by the Centers for Disease Control and Prevention (CDC), the relationship the team builds with the community will influence how much community members are willing to trust and thus, ultimately, how they react to public health messages and recommendations. For these reasons, effective community involvement is an important part of the public health process. Community involvement activities should be developed and implemented with the following objectives in mind:

- Earning trust and credibility through open, compassionate, and respectful communications
- Providing opportunities for communities to become involved in public health assessment activities
- Promoting collaboration between the public health agency, communities, and other agencies
- Informing and updating communities about the agency's work through managing and coordinating health communication activities with site communities
- Helping communities understand the possible health impact of not engaging in the desired health behavior

The process used by the CDC and its affiliated agencies is outlined in Figure 13-1.

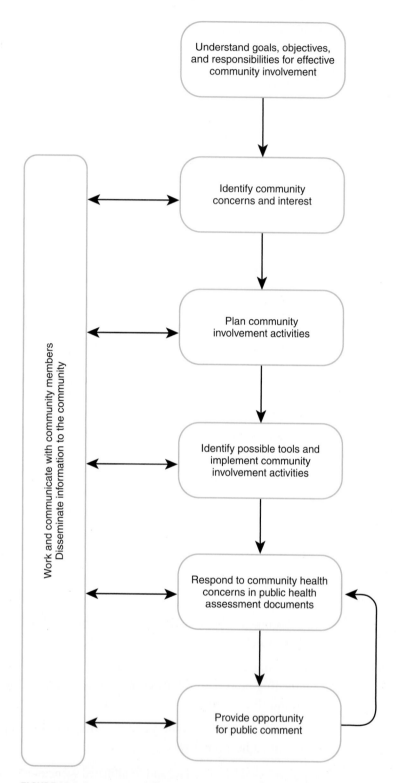

FIGURE 13-1 Components of Effective Community Involvement in Public Health
Source: U.S. Department of Health and Human Services, Agency for Toxic Substances and Disease Registry:
http://www.atsdr.cdc.gov/

Summary

Groups are a useful way to bring disparate entities together and enhance the likelihood of success. The general public likes to see collaboration, because the public assumes that resources are less likely to be wasted. Collaboration brings together many human and fiscal resources. Inasmuch as each group has community constituencies, groups also enhance community support and positive media coverage.

Effective groups do not just happen. They require strong group leadership skills that are applied on an "as needed" basis. The skills do not have to be present in only one person. Shared leadership skills are often more effective.

Interagency taskforces, committees, and groups are an important way to advance community health agendas—and the agendas of interested and sometimes overlapping agencies. Yet these efforts need to be skillfully managed to be effective.

It has been noted for many generations that when health educators are present in a group, things get done. This chapter has presented some of the basic group leadership skills, but the topic is worth studying further, and practicing one or more of these skills in every meeting is usually a worthwhile endeavor.

Often the public health agency and its teams will be working with communities and community groups. It is important to engage these groups in ways that maximize inclusiveness while addressing needs based on assessment. There should always be established objectives and a well-defined process that follows stages designed to meet the goals of the initiative or program.

The following case studies in Chapter 16, "Cases in Public Health Management," are directly related to concepts and principles presented in this chapter:

- Case 3: The Anti-Vaccination Paradigm
- Case 6: Managing Diversity
- Case 7: Sick Building Syndrome
- Case 8: To Hear This Message in Korean, Press '9'
- Case 9: A *Giardia* Outbreak?
- Case 11: Budget Cuts in Home Care Program
- Case 13: Senior Cyber Café
- Case 14: Collaborative Approach to Diabetes Prevention and Care
- Case 16: Healthy Lifestyles Start at Home
- Case 20: Pacific Needle Exchange Program
- Case 21: Community Coalitions and the Built Environment
- Case 22: Neglected Tropical Diseases—A Local NGO's Challenges

Public Health Professional Perspective

Jan Hillman, M.A., Vice President, Chief Integration Officer, Superior Health Partners and Marquette General Hospital, Marquette, Michigan

Interview by Dr. Mark Minelli

(Q): What are some of the most challenging roles in working with teams?

Ms. Hillman:
- Listening, making sure everyone is heard.
- Leading, having the right leader who does the right things at the right time, without being heavy handed.
- Understanding team process. As teams form, they typically go through four phases of forming, storming, norming, and performing. It is challenging to get to high-performing without going through these phases.

Following agreed upon rules is very important. I like Rimmerman's Rules:
(From the patient satisfaction team of the Heart Center at Cleveland Clinic Foundation)
- Leave rank at the door (all team members are created equal).
- No whining.
- At least one bright idea per session.
- No sidebar communications.
- If you have something to say, say it in the room.
- No hostages; leave if you don't want to be here.
- Identify problems but focus on solutions.
- Review the next objectives before leaving—ensure they are realistic in scope.
- Leave with a sense of accomplishment.
- Expect work outside of the meeting—use subgroups and task forces.
- Each meeting is rated by each participant (1 = low and 10 = high).
- Any person ranking the meeting an eight or below gives suggestions for improvement.
- Each participant ranks his or her own participation as well, in the same manner.

(Q): What advice would you give others in working with teams?

Ms. Hillman:
- Be fair and balanced.
- Counter challenges by anticipating solutions.
- Work with a strong agenda and stick to it.
- Develop action plans, review them for status and revise if necessary.

Continues

(Q): What are things to stay away from in working with teams?

Ms. Hillman:
– Rants.
– Overt displays of ego.
– Dominating the conversation/direction of the team.

(Q): Please describe some advantages of working with teams in a community health setting.

Ms. Hillman: Working with a team in a community health setting can bring people from various backgrounds and frames of reference together. Right now we are working in a multi-disciplinary team to develop a community health needs assessment for Marquette County. This team includes nurses, physicians, dieticians, members of the county health department, YMCA leadership, and administrators, among others. Each person brings skills, experience, and a genuine intent for a healthier community. A goal and timeline for the needs assessment have been developed. Problem solving has become a focus. We have just begun, but are off to a very positive start.

End

Public Health Professional Perspective

Jennifer Crawford, MSA, CHES, CPC-M, Prevention Coordinator, Saginaw Chippewa Behavioral Health, Mt. Pleasant, Michigan

Interview by Dr. Mark Minelli

(Q): What are some of the most challenging roles in working with diverse groups?

Ms. Crawford: Whether you are working with individuals who are of different ethnic backgrounds, age, or socioeconomic status, it is imperative to be able to relate to each and every person. So often, curriculums or programs are designed with one type of person in mind. Therefore, it is up to us as the facilitators to peel back the layers or enhance it with information to make it real for our specific audience. We simply cannot rely on "cookie-cutter approaches" if we want the strategies to work with our specific group.

Continues

When working with populations different than ourselves, we need to be sure to take the time to gain as much knowledge as possible about the cultures and traditions within that group. By doing so, we are able to learn about appropriate and inappropriate ways to communicate with the community members in order to establish and maintain respect. It is important to identify key individuals within the group who can help you identify your role within the community, while teaching you at the same time. The process of gaining access and respect from those within a community different from oneself takes time and is never-ending, but is so worth it when achieved.

(Q): What advice would you give others in working with diverse groups?

Ms. Crawford: The advice that I would give someone working with diverse groups is to be respectful at all times, even if a belief of the group contradicts something that you believe in. We can certainly respect and show support for the beliefs of others, while maintaining our own values and traditions. Having a mutual respect and openness allows us to learn so much more about one another and ourselves. We should appreciate, embrace, and celebrate the many unique qualities and traditions of the diverse populations that we live and work with.

(Q): What are things to stay away from in working with diverse groups?

Ms. Crawford: When working with diverse groups, it is imperative to not cast judgment upon others for beliefs, traditions, or customs different from one's own. Doing so would certainly hamper any relationships and ability to effectively work with the members of the community.

Another tip would be to not force oneself upon the community. Identifying and establishing a relationship with a key community leader who could then help introduce you to the community at an appropriate pace would be the most beneficial. By working with a trusted member of the community, one would be more apt to be welcomed and trusted by others.

(Q): Please describe some advantages of working with diverse groups in a community health setting.

Ms. Crawford: There are many advantages to working with diverse groups in a community health setting. First and foremost, having the opportunity to learn about and work with other cultures is amazing and rewarding, and should therefore be regarded as a privilege. There are many health issues that affect different populations in unique ways, so it proposes a challenge to learn new strategies for various target groups, enhancing the skill set of community health workers. Another advantage is the ability to utilize strategies with certain populations that may not be seen as mainstream, depending upon the target audience. For example, utilizing cultural norms and traditions such as language or ceremonies may not be seen as a typical community health strategy. However, when doing so reinforces a tradition that incorporates healthy decision making on many different levels, it is a great supplemental community health tool.

End

Discussion and Review Questions

1. Discuss how teams differ from groups. Give examples.

2. Describe the developmental stages teams go through.

3. What are some characteristics of well-functioning teams? How can they be improved even more?

4. What are the objectives of involving the community in public health programs? Identify the critical components. Give an example of a public health program you are familiar with and determine if it has these in place.

5. Describe the elements of a standard meeting in a professional setting.

Action Learning and Critical Thinking

A. Exercise in Forming a Diverse Team.

A large community grant was just awarded to form a community coalition to fight alcohol and other drug abuse. The participants are in two counties and have unique populations they serve. Both counties have a large African-American population; one county has a Native American Indian Tribe and the other a university campus.

As these are different service populations, describe how you would develop a leadership team to represent each unique group. Build a case for how you would select the leadership team members (i.e., one per group, population-based, and health providers versus community individuals). Your final analysis should present:

• Rationale statement for your team selection

• Number of group members

  ◦ Composition of group members

  ◦ Frequency of meetings and place

  ◦ Starting team goals/objectives

B. Watch the film *Twelve Angry Men* and describe the developmental stages you observe using the Tuckman model discussed in Table 13-1.

C. Identify a community-based public health initiative in your local area and find out through interviews and reading the program's printed material how it went about getting involvement from the community. Share what you found with the class and discuss how you might enrich the initiative or program with your own ideas and suggestions.

Chapter 14

PROGRAM PLANNING, DEVELOPMENT, AND EVALUATION

Carolyn K. Lewis, RN, Ph.D.
Christine Elnitsky, RN, Ph.D.
Joanne Martin, Dr.P.H.

Learning Objectives

Upon completion of this chapter, you should be able to:

1. Describe program development and planning and identify the basic concepts.
2. Analyze the principles of program development in public health.
3. Analyze the various cost analyses in management of health care programs.
4. Critically analyze the components of program evaluation.
5. Compare and contrast theories related to program evaluation.
6. Better understand decision making and its various processes.
7. Be familiar with economic tools used in decision making.

Chapter Outline

Introduction
Planning and Development
Initiating the Planning Process
 Mission Statement Clarification
 Stakeholder Analysis

INTRODUCTION

The landscape of health care is dramatically changing. This transition has evolved from a profitable environment based on cost-plus-payment to a system with capitation and fixed reimbursement. These declining revenue streams demand more comprehensive internal analysis that determines need for new community programs and evaluation of these programs based on a rational decision-making system. Planning for new programs provides a framework and process for attaining goals and gives direction and purpose to the program. No program can be effective without planning. This chapter focuses on the historic development of public health program planning, the framework for planning, the economic analysis for decision making in program planning, and the method of evaluating the impact and effectiveness of the program. More today than ever before, public health managers must be able to identify health problems and plan, design, implement, and evaluate programs that can effect positive changes in the health status of defined clients using population-focused strategies.

PLANNING AND DEVELOPMENT

The history of program planning as a major concept of program development has a different history than that of program evaluation. It is only within the last 10 years that this linkage between planning, development, and evaluation has begun to overlap with synergistic outcomes. Public health historian George Rosen believed that public health planning began approximately 4,000 years ago with the planned cities in the Indus Valley that had covered sewer systems. Planning was related to efforts that were done on behalf of the public well-being and to achieve change. Planning provides a direction and strategies for proceeding with program development. Program development is the strategic alignment of activities undertaken to meet an intended purpose to ensure that an identified problem has the best possible likelihood of success with adequate resources. Planning is the core of program development; it is not a single task and can be time-intensive. It is the planning, more than the plan, that leads to positive outcomes in program development.

Planning is an unconscious act that occurs every day of our life; however, in the context of program development, it becomes a conscious act. In health programs, planning is needed to identify the particular services that will produce the desired results. Planning is an organized, systematic method to conceptualize, detail, implement, and evaluate the effectiveness of a program. Today, there is a need for public health managers to thoroughly understand program planning and development so that the planning process shifts from "What is the problem?" to "What do we need to do about this problem?" and "How do we develop a program that, when executed and evaluated, will provide the desired results or stated goals?" Although there are many models in program planning and development, clinicians most frequently use planning tools that closely parallel the clinical process of assessment, diagnosis, planning, implementation, and evaluation of a program. The major difference is that one set of planning tools are applied to specific populations and the other is applied to individuals, families, or communities. The process, regardless of population, typically follows the flow as demonstrated in Figure 14-1.

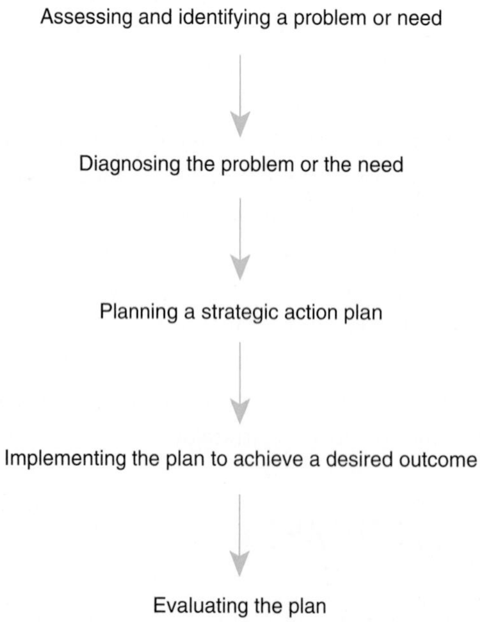

Assessing and identifying a problem or need

↓

Diagnosing the problem or the need

↓

Planning a strategic action plan

↓

Implementing the plan to achieve a desired outcome

↓

Evaluating the plan

FIGURE 14-1 Model of Program Planning
© Cengage Learning 2013

INITIATING THE PLANNING PROCESS

The pre-startup plan includes: (1) mission statement clarification; (2) stakeholder analysis; (3) problem identification; and (4) Strengths, Weaknesses, Opportunities, and Threats (SWOT) analysis. Table 14-1 delineates the critical success factors or core elements of the start-up phase of strategic planning.

This framework is intended only as a starting point in program planning and if implemented should create a flexible planning environment. Management literature emphatically stresses that careful planning at the beginning point in program development will enhance any program.

Mission Statement Clarification

Mission statement clarification requires having a clear sense of direction; this will drive the activities and set the expectations of the program development. No program should occur with an unclear mission or with multiple missions. A well-developed mission statement will clearly state:

- The population served
- What is to be accomplished
- Why the service or program is provided

The mission drives the goals and objectives of the program. The goals set overall direction and are neither concrete nor quantifiable. The objectives are measurable and quantifiable and so can be used to determine whether the goals are met and further used to assess progress and possibly identify other needed programs. A program that does not expand and augment the mission will be unsuccessful.

TABLE 14-1 Concepts for Pre-Startup Planning Framework

Concepts Elements

1. Mission clarification: Statement that drives the program goals and objectives.

2. Stakeholder analysis: Individuals with a vested interest in the program.

3. Problem identification: Identifying the gap of what is needed and what is available.

4. SWOT analysis: Identifying the areas of strengths, weaknesses, opportunities, and threats.

Stakeholder Analysis

Stakeholder analysis involves identifying that group of people who have a vested interest or who may benefit from the program. Successful programs must balance the needs of the stakeholders. When developing a program, carefully consider the potential differences in the stakeholders. If the needs of the stakeholders are not addressed, the program will not be successful or survive. If a public health professional is developing a program on middle school obesity and does not consider the students to be the critical stakeholders, they may feel degraded, intimidated, or embarrassed by the program. Thus, if this step is not completed, it is very unlikely that the identified stakeholders will participate. There typically are four steps in stakeholder analysis:

1. Identify the target group for the program.

2. Determine the criteria the stakeholders will use to assess the effectiveness of the program.

3. Evaluate if the program will meet the stakeholder criteria.

4. Evaluate the importance of each of the criteria.

The stakeholders and their perceptions may be the critical element that will determine the success of a program.

Problem Identification

Problem identification serves as the motivation of any new program. The gap between what is available and what is needed for the stakeholder group becomes apparent to the program planner once the problem is identified. This process may seem simple; however, data to support the identified problem must be collected. A systematic review of evidenced-based research that relates to the program topic and to the effects of an intervention needs to occur. In public health, the best practices must come from evidence that is applicable to communities and populations, and the programs must be based on this evidence and include interventions based on proven theory and research.

Strengths, Weaknesses, Opportunities, and Threats

SWOT are valuable to the development of the program in the pre-startup planning phase. Strengths and weaknesses usually have more of an internal focus, while opportunities and threats have more of an external focus. Strengths are usually easier to identify, but if weaknesses are not identified, they will cause barriers to the success of a program. Strengths and weaknesses are often linked, and in the planning phase a weakness needs to be identified and made into a strength. Opportunities and threats, if recognized, can be used to create new programs.

It is crucial to identify opportunities that may become future threats, and to use creative thinking to plan for these accordingly. These processes become powerful tools in program planning to assist in clarifying the problems and determining the program options.

SYSTEMATIC PLANNING FOR PUBLIC HEALTH

Paul Nutt, in his book *Planning Methods: For Health and Related Organizations*, developed a planning process that has been useful in public health program development to identify steps in planning methodology. His process includes an organized, systematic framework of planning: (1) formulating, (2) conceptualizing, (3) detailing, (4) evaluating, and (5) implementing. Once the public health professional defines the problem, utilizing these five steps will provide tools for successful program planning.

Formulating

This stage in program development is the most crucial; formulating consists of defining the problem based on a needs assessment of the program population. A needs assessment is a systematic set of procedures undertaken for the purpose of setting priorities and making decisions about program or organizational improvement and allocation of resources. The priorities are based on the identified needs. A needs assessment will give information and value perceptions, and can be used as a tool for program planning to identify those needs for a specific population or group of people.

Witkin and Altschuld, in their book *Planning and Conducting Needs Assessments: A Practical Guide*, further delineate a three-phase plan for assessing needs. The first phase is *pre-assessment*, which determines what is already known about needs in the population, decisions on boundaries, sources of data, and how data will be used to determine the need. The second phase is the *main assessment*, or the data gathering. This involves analyzing the data and formulating opinions on the needs and priority setting. The third phase is the *post-assessment* phase and involves using the data to plan for the action. This phase would be the program-planning phase, where the data are collected and analyzed, and the action plans are begun. The information and action plan are then communicated to the stakeholders. The evaluation of the needs assessment is also completed in phase three.

In formulating the plan, the program population must be identified and assessed, the need of this target population must be identified, and the population must be involved in the program planning. The size and geography of the population must be determined and identified if there are other programs addressing the need. The boundaries for the identified population are established by the need and the program goals that are formulated.

Conceptualizing

The second stage of the systematic framework for planning is the conceptualizing phase, that is, the articulation of thoughts and ideas in an objective format. This involves finding solutions to the needs identified in the formulation phase and identifying those risks and potential outcomes.

Detailing

In the third stage, the feasibility of moving forward with the program is assessed in relation to the solutions that have been identified in the conceptualization phase; this is termed *detailing*. Once stakeholders or decision makers are confident about the identified solution, additional planning will follow. Objectives that will meet the program goal(s) are formulated for the identified solution(s). These need to be measured against the activities needed to conduct the alternative solutions. Details of the program plan are outlined for the determined solution as well as any alternative solutions. Goals and objectives derived from learning needs and stakeholders' interests are assumed to have greater value than those goals and objectives derived in other ways. Objectives illuminate and guide all subsequent actions in program design and planning.

Evaluating

In this phase, those alternatives from the previously described detailing phase are evaluated related to costs, economic analysis, benefits, and how the program provider, the population, and the community may react to the alternatives. The feasibility and practicality of conducting the program to meet the desired outcomes are evaluated. Information and data are collected to assist in the evaluative phase, and changes are made based upon the analysis.

Implementing

In the final phase, implementing, the best plan is selected to meet the needs of the target population. The goals and objectives must reflect the solution that has the greatest value in meeting the defined problem/need. The solution chosen must be based on the data collected in the evaluating phase.

If the five planning stages of the systematic planning process are followed, the desired outcomes, which are population focused and consider the well-being of the public, will more likely be achieved. Planned programs bear a distinct advantage over unplanned ones. Planned programs are targeted for a particular population to meet a determined need.

ROLE OF ECONOMIC ANALYSIS IN DECISION MAKING

It is important to recognize the role economic analysis actually plays in decision making. First, it can inform the decision makers, but it is not a major deciding factor. Values such as justice, social welfare, and religious beliefs often trump economic evidence. Policymakers are loath to consider costs when saving lives is at stake. For example, the high-profile debate over end-of-life in Florida eventually reached the floor of the United States Congress in 2005. Economic analysis was not a main criterion for policymakers.

Second, economic analysis does not tell the decision maker if the increased expenditure is worthwhile. When evaluation of a new intervention demonstrates improved outcomes, economic analysis can determine how much more it would cost to achieve better outcomes. The decision makers are better informed, but they still need to judge if the improvement is worth the increased expenditure.

Third, rigorous economic analysis is not always available. It is complex, and doing a proper analysis is not easy. Yet, if not done properly, economic analysis can be misleading. Understandably, policymakers hesitate to base their decisions on results of an analysis they do not understand.

Wise decisions will need to be made about allocating scarce public resources. Policymakers may come to rely more on economic analysis as pressures increase to meet the needs of an aging population. Public health professionals who broaden their expertise to include economic analysis will be prepared to contribute significantly to public policy and decision making. Policymakers can benefit from advice provided by a knowledgeable clinician or public health manager who understands the implications of economic analysis.

TYPES OF ECONOMIC ANALYSIS

A full tutorial on methods and techniques used in performing an economic analysis is beyond the scope of this chapter. The intent of this section is to simply identify the five types of economic analysis and encourage further exploration in subsequent coursework. This is important since we need to move toward improving utilization of economic analysis in public health decision making, program evaluation, and outcomes research.

Cost-Minimization Analysis (CMA)

Cost-minimization analysis (CMA) assumes each approach has equal effects. Therefore, it compares only the costs between alternative approaches. CMA is used to determine which alternative is least costly. CMA is appropriate when alternative approaches truly are equally effective. However, this is rarely the case. Therefore, CMA usually is not an appropriate method of analysis in health care.

Cost-Consequence Analysis (CCA)

Cost-consequence analysis (CCA) measures the consequences as well as the costs. The cost and outcomes for each approach are listed separately so the decision maker can interpret and weigh the findings. For example, a CCA of two home-visiting programs would list the cost for each program and then list the measurable outcomes.

Although CCA can be used in health care, these are examples of questions raised, rather than answered, by the analysis.

Cost-Effectiveness Analysis (CEA)

Cost-effectiveness analysis (CEA) measures outcomes in the same units across alternatives, typically dollars per life-year. This allows the analyst to calculate a cost-effectiveness ratio. It works best when there is a single outcome of interest. The decision maker can learn how much more it would cost to get a defined amount of improved outcome.

Cost-Utility Analysis (CUA)

Cost-utility analysis (CUA) overcomes a disadvantage inherent in CEA: the dollars per life-year gained does not measure the quality of the life-year gained. It does not distinguish between a person who is relatively healthy and functional and a person who has a severe disability. CUA is a variation on CEA because CUA measures both quality and quantity of life. The outcome measure is quality-adjusted life-years or QALYs. This level of analysis is recommended by the U.S. Office of the Assistant Secretary for Health Panel on Cost Effectiveness in Health and Medicine because use of a standardized measure allows comparison across populations and disease states.

Cost-Benefit Analysis (CBA)

Cost-benefit analysis (CBA) measures both costs and outcomes in dollars. This allows the analyst to calculate a single-dollar figure by subtracting benefits from costs. In health care, this can be problematic because it is difficult to assign a dollar figure to life. Even if it were possible to calculate the dollar amount, ethical issues are an important concern; therefore, CBA is not used as much as CEA.

PROGRAM EVALUATION

Program evaluation as described by Rutman and Mowbray, in their book *Understanding Program Evaluation* (SAGE Human Services Guides), is the "use of scientific methods to measure the implementation and outcomes of programs, for decision-making purposes." Evaluation is concerned with the implementation and impact of public health programs. A public health program is defined as an intervention, or set of activities, to meet a social need. The program focus is on implementation and outcomes; understanding how the program activities are delivered informs management decisions about modifications to help achieve program objectives. Evaluation allows assessment of both the quality of administration and the value of the program. Understanding the program processes allows public health professionals to relate the activities to the outcomes.

Program evaluation may be further defined by time elements, methods, and purpose and focus. The evaluation of a public health program may be scheduled as a periodic assessment or as an ongoing monitoring activity. An ongoing measurement system can be incorporated into program delivery and administrative records. Ongoing monitoring allows continued assessment as projects are modified during their life spans and adjustments to program processes as information is provided to decision makers.

Operations, management processes, strategic planning, personnel performance appraisals, and support services, though important to program management, are not the focus in program evaluation.

Program Components, Objectives, Outputs, and Effects

The evaluation focuses on program components, objectives, outputs, and effects. Public health programs are composed of several components. Each component of the program has specific objectives associated with it.

Program objectives are the aims that the public health program is meant to achieve. The program manager directs resources and activities toward the program objectives. Objectives may be immediate, intermediate, or ultimate. Ultimate objectives are long-term benefits to the population.

Program outputs represent the services provided in a public health program. Such services may also be known as the program's activities. The program is accomplished according to these pre-specified activities. Program effects represent the consequences of the program components. Such consequences should include both those that are intended and those that are unintended. To show evidence that the program components resulted in the specific consequences requires linkages between program components, outputs, and objectives. Objectives may include both proximal and distal aims. Public health programs may evaluate knowledge, health and functional status outcomes, as well as cost-effectiveness or cost-utility outcomes.

Program evaluation serves as the mechanism to provide information on the program's interventions and outcomes. The information is used to facilitate management and decision making about the program. The program evaluation may have dual purposes based on the external and internal stakeholder perspectives.

For external sponsors, the program evaluation informs purpose, relevance, and financial priorities. Evaluation is a tool that aids decision making, such as cutting budgets in an environment of economic constraints. External sponsors require evidence that programs have a positive impact, thus evaluation must gather such evidence.

For internal program managers, evaluation has another purpose. In this case, the evaluation facilitates continuous learning about the program, problem solving, program delivery, and program improvement throughout the life span of the program. The program manager uses evaluation as a tool for making decisions about the program. Evaluation results may facilitate program changes and improvements by providing information about:

- Design and delivery of projects

- Type and amount of resources

- Measures of program inputs, processes, outcomes

- Development of indicators and performance metrics

- How programs are being implemented

- Accomplishments, barriers, facilitators, and lessons learned

- Recommendations for program improvement

Phases and Steps in Evaluation Process

Program evaluations consist of five phases: (1) identifying program objectives, (2) selecting or creating measures of impacts, (3) collecting data, (4) interpreting data in terms of the evaluation framework and program context, and (5) disseminating the evaluation information. Steps in the evaluation process vary based on the role of the individual involved. Program evaluations may be conducted internally or externally, that is, the program manager may conduct the evaluation or employ the expertise of an external program evaluator.

Manager Steps

For the program manager, the first step in the evaluation process is to determine the purpose of the evaluation. The second step is to evaluate the pros and cons of internal versus external evaluation and to consider mixed internal and external evaluator roles. Program evaluation purposes include assessment of the impacts and the cost-effectiveness of the program and its interventions.

Evaluator Steps

For the evaluator, the first step is to identify the purpose, objectives, and questions of interest in collaboration with the program manager and base these on an applicable theory. The second step is to design the most rigorous evaluation possible within the practical constraints of the situation. The evaluator considers the level of rigor necessary based on the identified purpose, feasibility, resources, timeline and the availability of data, measurement instruments, and staff.

The evaluator examines the assessment of the program. Using this process, the evaluator will fully understand the program and its true purpose and the environmental context of the evaluation. The process of developing the program theory includes evaluating the assessment of the program. As the theory is developed, the evaluator often discovers that the program is not ready for a formal evaluation. Further program development and refinement of objectives or implementation activities may be indicated. The program design may be altered to be consistent with new information about what is known to work. Program implementation may be improved to increase the likelihood of affecting outcomes.

A formative evaluation may provide a better understanding of the program processes and effects, and may lead to continuous improvement or change in program goals and objectives (Figure 14-2).

The process of developing the program theory often helps the evaluator prioritize evaluation questions and helps the manager decide how to focus the evaluation purpose and allocate evaluation resources. Logical theory or program theory, specific evaluation questions, and practical considerations inform the methodological choices.

The program evaluation will follow a design established by the evaluator to appraise the program's effectiveness, efficiency, and quality objectively and without bias. Evaluation design depends upon the purpose of the evaluation, the objects

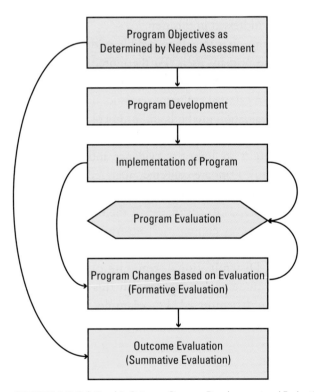

FIGURE 14-2 Relationship Between Program Development and Evaluation
© Cengage Learning 2013

of interest, and the standards of acceptability. Comparisons incorporated into the design may focus on changes over time, between groups, or both. The study design selection aims to omit errors in interpretation of results. Therefore, the evaluation will employ valid and reliable measurement tools and methods in the collection of program information.

The Centers for Disease Control (CDC) "Framework for Planning and Implementing Practical Program Evaluation" is used in public health. The framework is composed of steps in program evaluation practice as well as standards for effective program evaluation. The framework describes six steps taken in any evaluation. The first step is to engage stakeholders in identifying their values and information needs and to help with other steps. Stakeholders include sponsors, collaborators, administrators, staff, clients, families, neighbors, advocacy groups, institutions, organizations, professional associations, and primary users of the evaluation.

The second step describes the public health program, the program mission and objectives, its stage of development, and its relationship with the larger organization and community. It is important to identify expected effects of the program, activities, resources, and setting and environmental context. This step further includes the creation of the program logic model summarizing the planned changes by linking processes to ultimate effects.

In the third step, the focus is on the evaluation design. This requires identifying the evaluation's purpose and the users of evaluation findings as well as specific uses of the evaluation findings. Questions about the various aspects of the program, the scientific research methods used, and the roles and responsibilities of the stakeholders are also addressed in this step.

The fourth step is to gather credible evidence. Credible evidence meets the standards of the primary users. Furthermore, the credibility of evidence depends on the evaluation questions and the planned uses of the findings. It may be necessary to consult an external evaluator on issues of data quality, indicators, sources of evidence, or evaluation methods and protocol.

In the fifth step, the program evaluation conclusions are justified. At this phase, program inputs are linked to evidence and judged in light of agreed-upon values and standards. Data are collected, analyzed, synthesized, and interpreted. Finally, judgments and recommendations are made.

The sixth step is to ensure use of the evaluation and share the lessons learned. This step involves communicating findings with the stakeholders and providing follow-up technical and emotional support for users during and following evaluation. Dissemination or communication of procedures and lessons learned to relevant audiences is included in this step. Lessons learned and evaluation findings are disseminated. For example, findings can be reported to community partners in collaborative meetings. Final reports to the sponsors and those funding the program can provide substantive feedback for future planning by the sponsor.

Summary

The theoretical approaches and frameworks provide models for public health program evaluation design. Program evaluation complements program development by gathering necessary information for documenting program effectiveness. The evaluation results provide information for program changes and improvement. The use of scientific approaches for decision making in public health programs is the basis of evidence-based practice. At the services level in public health, there is concern about how the processes outlined in program development ultimately can affect the quality. Since program planning and economic analysis and evaluation are at the infrastructure level, this will be where the decisions are made on program development.

The following case studies in Chapter 16, "Cases in Public Health Management," are directly related to concepts and principles presented in this chapter:

- Case 3: The Anti-Vaccination Paradigm
- Case 8: To Hear this Message in Korean, Press '9'
- Case 11: Budget Cuts in Home Care Program
- Case 14: Collaborative Approach to Diabetes Prevention and Care
- Case 16: Healthy Lifestyles Start at Home
- Case 17: Top Ten U.S. Public Health Achievements
- Case 19: Smoking Cessation Program Implementation
- Case 20: Pacific Needle Exchange Program
- Case 21: Community Coalitions and the Built Environment

Discussion and Review Questions

1. What type of economic analysis is feasible to use in evaluating public health interventions?

2. What are the greatest barriers to conducting a cost-utility analysis?

3. Consider an existing evidence-based intervention or program. How would you justify continued funding without having some level of economic analysis? Would cost-consequence analysis help or hurt the case for expanding the intervention or program?

4. Suppose you are an external evaluator, employed by the public health department to evaluate the impacts of a childhood immunization program in the county where you live. How would you involve the stakeholders in the evaluation plan? Defend your approach.

5. A school health program is working with middle school students to develop citizenship skills, and the program manager is interested in evaluating the program. Explain how you might proceed.

6. Explain how you would use program evaluation methods and cost-effectiveness analysis to provide evidence of the success of a public health department or program.

Action Learning and Critical Thinking

A. You are a public health professional and attended Parent/Teacher Night at your child's middle school. While attending, you realized that many of these students are overweight. The middle school is in your public health area, and you wish to integrate into the school system an Eat Healthy Program. What information would you need to decide the feasibility of this program and what analysis would you need to conduct before deciding on the program?

B. Read an article in a recent issue of a public health journal in which a program evaluation only reported participants' health or functional impacts. Suggest some possibilities for how collection and analysis of cost-data might have enhanced the analysis and supported the program and its continuation.

C. Watch the film *Rx for Survival* and discuss how you might use program evaluation for each or any of the initiatives presented in the documentary.

Chapter 15

PUBLIC HEALTH LEADERSHIP AND THE FUTURE

F. Douglas Scutchfield, MD
C. William Keck, MD, M.P.H.

Learning Objectives

Upon completion of this chapter, you should be able to:

1. Describe the potential impact of preventive services on health status in the United States.
2. Discuss how changes in the illness care sector can affect public health practice.
3. Describe cultural, professional, and scientific elements that impact public health practice.
4. Describe attributes of local health departments that are key to their effectiveness.
5. Identify and discuss characteristics that will be found in the successful health departments of the future.

Chapter Outline

INTRODUCTION

Significant gains in health status and life expectancy have occurred over the past 200 years in the United States as well as in most other industrialized nations. Many attribute these gains to advances in clinical medicine that tend to be dramatically and impressively chronicled in the electronic and print media. Indeed, our capacity to diagnose and treat illness has advanced rapidly. The reality remains, however, that most of the improvements in quality and length of life have come from measures aimed at protecting populations from environmental hazards and pursuing behaviors and activities that are known to be health-promoting. Health departments and other community agencies are responsible for developing the programs and relationships with individuals and neighborhoods that will continue to improve the health of citizens of this country.

In spite of this fact, the public health system has been largely ignored during the second half of the twentieth century. Resources were focused disproportionately on medical care while the public health system was allowed to atrophy compared to the growing need for its services. The two Institute of Medicine (IOM) reports previously cited in this book, plus the tragedy of 9/11 and the subsequent anthrax episode, provided both a professional and public awakening to the need to reinvest in public health. Despite some positive steps, however, much remains to be done for public health practice to be in the best position to contribute what it can to the

TABLE 15-1 Leading Causes of Death in the United States, 2010

Cause of Death	Number of Deaths
All causes	2,465,932
Diseases of the heart	595,444
Malignant neoplasm	573,855
Chronic lower respiratory diseases	137,789
Accidents (unintentional injuries)	118,043
Alzheimer's disease	82,962
Diabetes mellitus	68,905
Nephritis, nephritic syndrome, and nephrosis	50,472
Influenza and pneumonia	50,003
Intentional self-harm	37,793

Source: Centers for Disease Control and Prevention. Deaths: Preliminary Data for 2010. Retrieved from http://www.cdc.gov/nchs/data/nvsr/nvsr60/nvsr60_04.pdf

effort to improve health status. This chapter reviews the continuing potential for public health contributions to healthfulness, the relationships of public health to the medical care system, challenges facing the changing practice of public health, and likely characteristics of successful health departments of the future. Tables 15-1 and 15-2 show recent data about the leading causes of death in the United States and worldwide, respectively.

PUBLIC HEALTH IN AN EVOLVING MEDICAL CARE SYSTEM

The United States continues to search for the "best" way to finance and deliver illness (medical) care. The nation's citizens are increasingly unhappy because the number of uninsured and underinsured continues to grow despite relative prosperity in the country overall. The insured are asked to carry more of the financial load through increased premiums, deductibles, and co-pays. Rising costs for health coverage are straining the traditional employer-based programs, and United States' businesses

TABLE 15-2 Leading Causes of Death Worldwide

Cause of Death	Deaths in Millions
Ischemic heart disease	7.25
Stroke and other cerebrovascular disease	6.15
Lower respiratory infections	3.46
Chronic obstructive pulmonary disease (COPD)	3.28
Diarrheal diseases	2.46
HIV/AIDS	1.78
Trachea, bronchus, lung cancers	1.39
Tuberculosis	1.34
Diabetes mellitus	1.26
Road traffic accidents	1.21

Source: Data from World Health Organization

offering health insurance are placed at a financial disadvantage in competition with foreign companies in countries that enjoy government-subsidized coverage, or where there is no expectation of coverage. Research continues to demonstrate that the quality of care given to the insured in the United States can often be substandard, and there is no question that the uninsured or underinsured population is less healthy than the population with "good" insurance. Ominously, it is also clear that the nation is increasingly sedentary and overweight, with the result that the prevalence of many associated chronic diseases is on the rise. The question is whether the sum total of these realities has reached sufficient mass to counterbalance well-funded constituencies that oppose change that would diminish their income or influence. Whether the result is continued "tinkering" with the system or a substantial reworking of it, the public health practitioner will be affected. This requires awareness of changes as they occur, at a minimum, or preferably, participation in the policy debates that are sure to continue in this area. The authors believe the United States' medical care system is unsustainable in its current form, and major restructuring is desirable.

The *Affordable Care Act of 2010* moves some elements in the right direction, however in many ways, the debate about health care reform is miscast. For the most part, the wrong question is being addressed. Attempts are made to seek better ways of providing and paying for illness care rather than to determine what should be done to create the healthiest population possible. With the courage and the foresight to frame the debate in these terms, it is readily apparent that improved health status depends on illness care reform *and* on public health reform.

For too long, those professionals who concentrate on the diagnosis and treatment of illness have been separated from those who concentrate on health promotion, disease prevention, and control of the environment. Instead of a seamless web of integrated services and activities focusing first on minimizing risks and then on early diagnosis and treatment of emerging disease, two separate systems have developed and evolved into two distinct cultures that are often at odds with one another. It is the responsibility of public health practitioners to help society understand the value of each approach and the need to integrate them into a quest for improving health status. The major professional organizations representing these two professions, the American Medical Association (AMA) and the American Public Health Association (APHA), have opened a dialogue around this issue and are encouraging discussions designed to bridge the gap between medical care and public health. It is hard to believe that significant progress will be made, however, until health promotion and disease prevention are valued as much as illness diagnosis and therapy.

Obtaining medical care is very important for that segment of the population for whom access is denied or inappropriately restricted, of course. The approximately 10 percent of excess mortality in citizens of the United States that is related to inadequate access to medical care occurs principally in that group for whom access to care is limited by virtue of its cost. No illness is "deserved," and every member of society should have access to those interventions that have been developed to diagnose and treat disease and minimize suffering. It is also worth noting that significant contributions to disease prevention can be made in the context of a single patient's interaction with a physician or other health care provider. The activities described in the *Guide to Clinical Preventive Services* are particularly recommended for their proven capacity to improve health and prevent disease and injury. It is also true that preventive care is underused for the almost 85 percent of the population that has access to primary care. A report released by the Partnership for Prevention notes that the use of key preventive services by Americans remains low despite the evidence of the effectiveness of these services. The report states that increasing the use of just five preventive services (low-dose aspirin for adults, advising smokers to quit, colorectal cancer screening, annual flu immunizations, and breast cancer screening) could save up to 100,000 lives annually. Preventive and population-based services applied in both clinical and public health settings have the greatest potential to contribute to overall gains in health status.

THE CORE FUNCTIONS OF PUBLIC HEALTH

Population-based services are provided from a variety of sources in most communities. These sources include state and local health departments, community health agencies (e.g., family planning agencies, heart associations, kidney associations, cancer societies, mental health agencies, and drug abuse agencies, among others), hospitals, and schools, to name several. However, this chapter focuses on the local health department because it is only the local health department that has statutory responsibility for the health status of its constituent population. It is the health department, in most locations, that is ultimately responsible for the assurance that all citizens have access to the services they need in the community, no matter which groups or organizations ultimately deliver those services. This focus on the health needs of the entire community—by an agency ultimately responsible to that community for its performance—emphasizes the importance of the need for governmental presence at the local level to ensure good health for the citizens of each community.

Institute of Medicine Reports

There exists wide variation in the size, sophistication, capacity, and roles of local health departments in the United States. In its 1988 report, *The Future of Public Health*, the IOM's Committee for the Study of the Future of Public Health described widespread agreement across the country in that "public health does things that benefit everybody," and that "public health prevents illness and educates the population." However, it found little consensus on how those broad statements should be translated into action. Indeed, there is such great variability in resources, available services, and organizational arrangements "that contemporary public health is defined less by what public health professionals know how to do than by what the political system in a given area decides is appropriate or feasible." The committee concluded that "effective public health activities are essential to the health and well-being of the American people, now and in the future," but the variability across the country is so great that this essential system is currently in "disarray."

In an effort to provide a set of directions for the discipline of public health that could attract the support of the whole society, the committee proposed a public health mission statement and a set of core functions. In 2003, the IOM completed a second report focused on the description of a framework for assuring the public's health in the future. The IOM's Committee on Assuring the Health of the Public in the 21st Century looked at health achievements and issues that undercut the potential for improvement in health status, the role of government in protecting and promoting public health, the importance of partnerships between governmental agencies and groups from other sectors of society, and trends that are likely to influence health in the coming decades. The report is highly recommended reading for those engaged in public health leadership and policy-making positions.

Unfortunately the study committee found that the conclusion of the 1988 IOM report, stating that the governmental component of the nation's public health system was in disarray, was still valid 15 years later. To be sure, efforts have been made to improve the circumstances that led to that conclusion, but governmental public health agencies continue to suffer from underfunding, political neglect, and exclusion from forums where their expert advice and leadership are essential for an effective public health system. These agencies continue to be saddled with deficiencies in the tools and other resources necessary to assure population health, and a secure future requires expansion of support for their resource needs and their inclusion in policy-making activities.

In addition, the IOM notes in the most recent report that "the increasingly fragile health care sector threatens efforts to assure the health of the public." Particular problems noted include the growing number of uninsured and underinsured people in this country, the minimal coverage provided for preventive care by the Medicare program, the common lack of treatment options for people with mental health or substance abuse problems, inequality of care provided to racial and ethnic minorities compared to the white population, and the poor distribution of health care resources that limits the ability to address complex medical problems of an aging population or manage a large scale emergency. The IOM committee also noted the importance of broadening the segments of society responsible for, and involved in, activities likely to improve health status. In addition to elements of the public health and health care infrastructure, employers and businesses, the media, academia, and others are important players in a real public health "system" dedicated to creating the conditions necessary to assure the best possible health status.

The committee described six areas of action and change that are central to the desire to create an effective multi-sector health system that can increase levels of health and longevity in the United States in the near future:

1. Adopt a population health approach that builds on evidence of the multiple determinants of health.

2. Strengthen the governmental public health infrastructure—the backbone of any public health system.

3. Create a new generation of partnerships to build consensus on health priorities and support community and individual health actions.

4. Develop appropriate systems of accountability at all levels to ensure that population health goals are met.

5. Assure that action is based on evidence.

6. Acknowledge communication as the key to forging partnerships, assuring accountability, and using evidence for decision making and action.

Public health has been undergoing a philosophic renaissance during the past two decades. Significant problems remain, however, with the structure and funding of local public health services. These problems hinder the capacity of the system to provide the services required for our population to reach the maximum healthfulness our knowledge and technology make possible. The recommendations of the 2003 IOM committee recognize that future progress requires attention and action in the areas listed. Unfortunately, there is little evidence that major policymakers in the Congress or administration at the time of this writing perceive the nature of the problem in any detail, let alone share a commitment to lead the nation in a venture to improve health status. It is not likely that significant progress can be made until the nation commits itself to transforming the current illness care industry into a real health care system and actively engages those with the requisite expertise in such an undertaking.

PUBLIC HEALTH SYSTEM CHANGES

Although the basic organization and structure of local and state health departments has not evolved in a manner that matches the change that has occurred in public health thinking over the past several decades, there have been significant shifts in programmatic emphasis that have affected the public health system and raised questions about future trends. Chief among these, particularly in more recent years, have been the infusion of bioterrorism funds and the push away from the provision of direct medical services to individuals in health department settings.

Bioterrorism Funding

The events of September 11, 2001, the anthrax attacks that came soon thereafter, the SARS epidemic, and growing concern about avian influenza focused attention on the preparedness of the public health system (and others) to respond to natural and man-made events that threatened health on a grand scale. Public health professionals were not surprised by the verdict that readiness was deemed inadequate, at best. It was clear that the diverse practices of more than 3,000 local health departments, each of which had developed and evolved in a unique environment, did not constitute a "system" that could be easily coordinated to meet large national or regional threats. In addition, the public health workforce was small (inadequate) and lacked many of the competencies that an effective response to these emerging threats would require. Technology was limited to the degree that no comprehensive electronic surveillance and information system existed that crossed jurisdictional boundaries.

America responded to these realities with relative speed. The *Public Health Security and Bioterrorism Preparedness and Response Act of 2002* required national initiatives to develop countermeasures to catastrophes, infrastructure to handle mass casualties, and information systems linking relevant agencies, including health departments. The *Homeland Security Act of 2002* was designed to improve the country's ability to prevent and respond to acts of terrorism. President Bush signed an Executive Order in April 2003 designating SARS a communicable disease for purposes of enacting control measures, if necessary. The CDC launched a website to inform the public about avian influenza. In addition, President Bush proposed substantial increases in funding to combat bioterrorism, and new attention was focused on strengthening the nation's public health infrastructure.

These initiatives fostered strong efforts to creatively improve preparedness capacity on the part of all agencies and institutions engaged in the effort, including state and local health departments. These efforts included increasing laboratory capabilities, strengthening disease surveillance and communication mechanisms, performing preparedness training, and conducting drills and exercises. These investments have clearly improved the capacity to deal with communicable disease outbreaks and other threats across the country.

Unfortunately, however, federal funds for other public health programs have been reduced during this period, and most states have experienced revenue shortfalls leading to public health budget reductions. The sum total of these realities is that health departments are faced with supporting ongoing public health service needs and the new preparedness initiatives with little additional funding. The failure to address clearly how national protection activities should be organized and how government public health agencies should be configured to be maximally effective, however, leaves us with a situation where public expectations for the ability to respond almost certainly continue to exceed capacity. The need to reorganize and restructure governmental public health agencies and provide them with the resources necessary for them to meet their obligations is left for the future.

Shift Away from Direct Medical Services

The inadequacies of the medical care system(s) in the United States have driven much of non-environmental public health programming for decades. Health departments are often "courts of last resort" in their communities for populations who are unable to receive clinical preventive services or medical care through other means. Child health clinics, prenatal care services, family planning clinics, and so on, exist in local health departments to fill gaps in medical care. Public health leaders have sometimes bemoaned the fact that their resources would be better spent meeting health promotion and disease prevention objectives, but some have become financially dependent upon third-party payments for clinical services. Nonetheless, there has been a strong push from the federal government to "privatize" Medicaid and move clinical services into the private sector. This transition has largely occurred, and it has moved ahead in the absence of any clear policy initiatives to enhance the ability of health departments to meet national health status goals. As a matter of fact, there has never been a coherent and strong public policy agenda to improve population health in the United States.

An important issue facing leaders in both the medical care and public health sectors is the place of public health in a system when health care access issues are either solved or lessened, or where the provision of medical care services is made difficult for local health departments to accomplish. How does one re-educate the public to embrace and support a new version of public health activities when many continue to view public health's role to primarily be provision of health care to the poor? How does one meld public health with medicine more effectively in a culture that values treatment over prevention? How can one best introduce principles of population medicine into clinical practice?

If we prove unable to provide good answers to these questions in the near future, we are likely to experience a continuation of mission confusion with a poor coherence of approach. That will be characterized by a continuation of disproportionate funding going to medical care and by an expansion of orphan topics that become public health's responsibility alone by default (nutrition, aging, violence, drug abuse, built environment and urban sprawl, exercise, global warming, school health, etc.). We are left, therefore, with the large tasks of developing a national focus on populations as well as individuals and better defining which population-centered programs work and which do not so that appropriate population-based services can be defined and supported. In short, we will be in the business of determining who will fund, direct, control, and evaluate public health services in the future. Local health departments must be prepared to understand and influence medical care policy change because of the impact such change has on public health programs. Questions about how best to organize and deliver health services are once more on the national agenda as we move forward with implementation of the *Affordable Care Act*. It is an opportunity we should not allow to pass without our full engagement.

PUBLIC HEALTH IN RAPID EVOLUTION—NEW CHALLENGES

In addition to the internal and external forces described previously that are impacting the delivery of public health services, other cultural, professional, and scientific elements impacting our society are inevitably affecting the practice of public health.

Information, Informatics, and Communication

We live in a time of incredibly rapid change in our ability to communicate with each other. This age of electronic communication is characterized by continuous enhancement of the speed and sophistication with which large amounts of information can be created, processed, and distributed. The Internet provides a platform for extremely rapid access to huge amounts of information on almost any subject. It can be used for low-cost communication between individuals and groups who share common interests. Every state health department and almost every local health department is now connected to this medium that provides expanding opportunities to communicate with other agencies that have overlapping missions and interests, and to communicate directly with a large portion of the population for whom they have some responsibility. Increasingly sophisticated software allows for the development of electronic medical records, syndromic surveillance systems, new datasets, geographic information systems (GIS), sophisticated imaging and reporting, and on and on. As difficult as it is to keep up with this expansion of hardware and software, the effective public health agency will learn to take advantage of the opportunities that exist in this area to enhance its capacity to develop accurate information about communities, provide effective public health interventions and programs targeted at well-described problems, and evaluate the effectiveness of interventions.

The advent of the electronic medical record provides a growing list of opportunities to use information about individuals from many sources to enhance the understanding of populations. There is a paradox inherent in this situation, however, because the potential for inappropriate use of information about individuals and their health problems has delayed the use of information that might impact individual privacy rights. Significant future energy will be spent on analyzing these competing interests and designing surveillance systems that can both inform public health practice and protect individuals.

Socioeconomic Determinants of Health

In an ideal world, the public health system would be able to turn most of its attention to amelioration of those factors (income, race, family structure, community resources, etc.) that can impact the social fabric in ways that are detrimental to health. In the less than ideal world in which we work, we have the challenge of moving in that direction in the absence of clear policy and funding prerogatives to do so.

To begin, public health will have to find its way to decision-making tables where it has been infrequently represented before. It can be argued that public health should be present whenever public policy decisions are made to assess the likely impact on population health, both positive and negative, of policy decisions. For example, the structure of the so-called "built environment" impacts health, so public health should be represented at forums where construction of housing, factories, parks, and roads is discussed. Programs that engage, or propose to engage, existing social networks should seek assistance in understanding the public health role in building human and social capital, and so on. The effective public health practitioner of the future will need to acquire knowledge and skills that will allow impact in these areas.

Building the Public Health Research Base

Given the lack of a real population focus in health policy and planning in the United States, it is not surprising that the bulk of health research dollars are spent in the area of disease diagnosis and treatment. This bias in investigative scholarship has left the field of public health lagging in understanding the structure, operation, and impact of public health programs and delivery systems. This, in turn, leaves public health policymakers and administrators with a thin portfolio for guidance in the establishment of effective public health interventions. Fortunately, concerted efforts are underway to systematically address public health research needs. The Community Preventive Services Guidelines process identifies community interventions where evidence related to their effectiveness is incomplete or absent, the Council on Linkages Between Academia and Public Health Practice has compiled a list of detailed public health systems research needs, the CDC's Office of Public Health Practice has developed a national agenda for public health systems research, and many of the profession's leading researchers, thinkers, and professional organizations are focusing new attention on improving the science base for public health practice. Academy Health, with funding from the Robert Wood Johnson Foundation, is engaged in a process with major public health research stakeholders of further refining and prioritizing a research agenda in preparation for a strong effort to attract new funding to this field.

Perhaps the best summary of the challenge that lies ahead was penned by Glen P. Mays, Ph.D., M.P.H., in the Conclusion section of his white paper, "Understanding the Dimensions of Public Health Delivery Systems: Theory, Evidence, and Unanswered Questions," prepared for Academy Health in June, 2007:

> Addressing current and future research needs in public health will require more than a few rigorous and timely studies conducted on high priority topics. A successful research enterprise on public health systems will require sustained commitments to building robust data resources that reflect the organizational, financial, and workforce characteristics of public health delivery systems at local, state, and national levels. Data elements that historically have been collected from multiple, episodic surveys of state and local public health agencies need to be standardized and routinely collected to support expanded research on systems. Additionally, public health agencies, professionals, and others involved in the delivery of public health services need to be engaged more directly in the conceptualization, design, and conduct of public health systems research studies. Such engagement will ensure that studies are asking the right questions, using the best data and measures, and capitalizing on opportunities for studying natural experiments that result from organizational and policy changes. Additionally, practitioner engagement—such as through practice-based research networks and participatory research designs—promises to reduce the cycle time required for disseminating and integrating new evidence into practice. If successful, expanded research on public health systems will strengthen the ability of governmental public health agencies and their private-sector partners to deliver services that protect and promote health. The result will be a continuously improving public health system that assures the conditions necessary for all Americans to enjoy healthier lives.

Assuring the involvement of practitioners is an important factor if research is to be useful. Since the 1988 IOM report lament about the major decoupling they found between academia and public health practice, much has been done to expand the connections between town and gown. Much remains to be done, however, and expanding and strengthening the linkages between them will be a required prerequisite for effectively completing public health services research and translating the results into effective patterns of practice. Both academic and practice settings will need to find or create expanded opportunities to develop working relationships that will facilitate the movement of students into practice settings for relevant learning experiences and will establish partnerships for service research. As suggested by Keck in the *Journal of Public Health Management*, the academic health department is one approach to linking health departments and academic institutions that is gaining some traction. One of the most attractive elements of this model is the involvement of practitioners in academic settings and vice versa, and the opportunities presented for training public health professionals in combined academic/practice venues. Practitioners and academics who link now will be in good position to take advantage of funding for service-related research likely to become available during the next decade.

Accreditation of Local Health Departments

The credentialing of the public health workforce has already begun with the development of The National Board of Public Health Examiners and the administration of the first board examination for Master of Public Health (MPH) graduates in 2008. The recent progress in the description of essential services a community must have in place to reach high levels of healthfulness coupled with the development of performance standards for public health services at the national level and in many states, and the development by the National Association of County and City Health Officials (NACCHO) of an "Operational Definition of a Functional Local Health Department" in 2005, have set the stage for a process to measure agency capacity. A report commissioned by the Robert Wood Johnson Foundation in late 2004 noted that there was no real momentum for state health agency certification, but that there are many examples of innovative programming related to agency accreditation at the local level. The importance of making local health departments accountable for their work across the country led to the establishment in October, 2006, of a national Public Health Accreditation Board (see http://www.exploringaccreditation.org). The board has implemented a voluntary national accreditation program. This is an example of "lap over" from the medical care system where concern about quality of service delivery has led to quality improvement activities, pay-for-performance, and so on, and effective health departments should begin to prepare themselves for new levels of accountability.

Population Shifts and Diversity

Health disparities among subpopulation groups in the United States have been well documented and have proved very difficult to resolve. To be sure, if access to care for all can be achieved, it will have some positive impact, but that alone will not cause health disparities to disappear. Writing for the *New England Journal of Medicine*, Marmot points out the evidence is growing that many of the roots of health disparities lie in the areas of social policy, economics, environment, and in our personal perceptions and prejudices, and these are compounded by a constant influx of immigrants from around the world who bring with them their own unique cultural attributes, many of which affect their smooth integration into American society. This is further discussed by Miringoff in the book, *The Social Health of the Nation*. The social environment, or our social health, should be as carefully monitored as the more traditional indicators of community health status. The major difficulty in all of this is deciding the appropriate role for local health departments. Influencing social and economic policymaking and confronting the realities of racism, sexism, and ageism are not simple tasks. They require broadly based partnerships at least, and at most a new paradigm of public health service delivery. It will be important for the public health community to become familiar with this new public health agenda item, to monitor the impact of new models of public health activity developing in some communities, and to determine how best to influence social health in their own constituencies.

This suggests that there may well be a new set of skills that the public health practitioner will need. Practitioners might want to attend a planning and zoning committee meeting to provide input and suggestions for arranging the community to assure opportunities for exercise by providing parks and bike trails, for example. Additionally, one might ask whether the community offers enough opportunities for recreation and interaction of community members, and whether there are community centers where clubs and organizations can meet, parks where families and other groups can gather, bandstands, and so on.

Globalization

International health issues will become increasingly important for local public health. The most obvious issue is the repeated demonstration that many infectious diseases are not constrained by geopolitical boundaries. The reality that relatively large numbers of people travel to almost anywhere else in the world within the 24 hours of any given day creates the potential for any new or re-emerging infection to become a major public health problem in the United States at any time. This risk is compounded by the present-day reality that both domestic and foreign enemies of the United States can choose to attack populations in this country through acts of violence against property (Federal Building bombing in Oklahoma and the World Trade Center and Pentagon on 9/11) or against people through the use of toxic or infectious agents (anthrax) in an effort to create large numbers of casualties and population panic. As described previously, these activities have brought new awareness to the important role of public health in dealing with biological and chemical disasters, and resources directed to public health in recent years have improved response capacity for future disasters but also for more "routine" disease surveillance and outbreak control measures. Maintaining and improving preparedness will be a major public health practice issue for the foreseeable future.

The continuing degradation of the global physical environment has substantial implications for human health in all parts of the world, including the United States. Rainforest loss and desertification, species extinction, populations driven by poverty and hunger massing in so-called mega cities, global warming, and so on, will influence disease patterns around the globe. Persons anxious to escape poverty and conflict are migrating in large numbers to the so-called "developed" countries. In the United States, this results in a growing number and size of minority populations with a tendency to exacerbate the already unacceptable health disparities that exist between majority and minority groups in this country, despite special attention paid to this issue over the past decade or so. The need for cultural awareness and increased cross-cultural competency on the part of public health workers is both obvious and problematic. Bringing minority representatives into the public health workforce and minority students and faculty into academic institutions that train public health workers remains a priority that attains increasing urgency with the growing diversity of the United States' population. The minimal success accomplished to date will need to be significantly enhanced if public health is to remain relevant to the needs of its constituents in the future.

The Human Genome

The deciphering of the human genome has been a remarkable scientific achievement. We now possess the master code for increased understanding of humans. The biologic and medical implications of this feat are increasingly apparent, and there is growing awareness of the ethical challenges inherent in that understanding. Little attention, so far, has been directed at the public health implications of being able to characterize human beings and their risk for disease in this manner, except for the wide practice of newborn genetic screening. Nevertheless, it is likely that human genomic understanding will produce new tools for the practice of public health, as well as significant challenges to the appropriateness of their use. The competencies that will be required of public health practitioners in this area have already been delineated, but few training programs and institutions have developed curriculum intended to assure that future public health graduates have a broad understanding of genomics and future use of the discipline in public health practice.

CAPACITY OF HEALTH DEPARTMENTS TO FULFILL CORE AND OTHER FUNCTIONS

The growing unity of thought about public health's core functions and essential services begs the question of whether or not local and state health departments actually have the capacity to fulfill the core functions and the other tasks that may be required of them by their own communities. Indeed, available evidence suggests that there is great variability in capacity among the diverse agencies found at local and state levels.

Organizational Diversity

Chapter 7, "State and Local Public Health Agencies," in this text reviews the structure and capacities of local health departments. The diversity that characterizes health departments is perhaps an indication of just how problematic it can be to provide public-sector services in a democracy. Competition for attention and resources among many interests in a system with multiple decision makers and policymakers makes it difficult to attain and sustain coherence and consistency of function. In addition to the organizational variability of local public health agencies, there is also a great deal of programmatic variability that results from the deliberate delegation out of public health departments of a number of responsibilities previously considered to be in the purview of public health.

The IOM report noted that the coherence of public health activities is damaged by the administration of environmental health, mental health, and indigent care programs by separate agencies. This separation of responsibilities encourages the development of separate programs and fragmented data systems that impede integrated problem analysis and risk assessment. The result is diminished coherency in the efforts of government to provide service and a division of constituencies that might otherwise coalesce around a broad vision of the mission of public health.

Funding

In addition to the problems noted in the previous section, most local health departments must cope with inconsistent funding sources. Some local departments are comparatively well funded, but many face severe financial constraints and must rely heavily on sources of revenue that may very well result in inadequate and unstable funding. It has been clearly demonstrated by Mays, McHugh, and Shim in the *Journal of Public Health Management Practice* that the performance of essential public health services in local health departments is directly associated with public health spending levels, even after controlling for system and community characteristics. Where to find the needed resources will be a continuing challenge. The realization that the public health system is an integral part of preparedness has resulted in increased funding for that purpose with some positive spillover into more routine public health activities. At the same time, however, the period during which preparedness funding accelerated also saw declines in federal support for other public health functions. Health departments need to be creative to find resources that can be applied to material needs (i.e., housing and equipment) and the solution of population health problems. Possible sources include private foundations, fees-for-service, hospital and other partnerships, research grants, and so on. With a wide diversity of funding sources, public health financial managers need to be more publicly accountable and develop management skills more akin to those found in the private sector.

Public Health Training in the Workforce

Most public health workers, including some public health leaders, have not had formal training in public health. The IOM report noted the need for well-trained public health professionals with "appropriate technical expertise, management and political skills, and a firm grounding in the commitment to the public good and social justice that gives public health its coherence as a professional calling." The report further noted that public health leadership requires an appreciation of the role and nature of government. It also requires the capacity to continue to learn to stay current with the evolution of the discipline. Health status in the future is dependent to a significant degree on the thoughtful deployment and nurturing of an evolving public health workforce.

An important component of public health training is the integration of learning with practical experience. It is critical that public health students and workers receive training linked to practice by requiring practicum experiences in local health agencies for students; improving communication and collaboration among agencies and schools through such efforts as joint programs, research, and technical assistance, among others; making education and training programs more relevant to practice; and increasing the resources devoted to linking academia with practice.

Until consistent, high-quality, easily accessible workforce development is available, on-the-job training will continue to be the major mechanism for integrating professionals into the public health workplace.

Staff Size

An important indicator of the capacity of an agency's staff to fulfill the core functions of public health is the size of its staff. The vast majority of health departments are small. NACCHO's *National Profile of Local Health Departments* reveals that 26 percent of local health departments in the United States at that time had four or fewer employees, and an additional 20 percent had between five and nine employees. Although local health departments, on average, employ 67 full-time staff, the median is 13. Recent information from NACCHO indicates that small local health departments serving small populations usually employ just a few occupations: typically these are a director, nurses, environmental health specialists, and clerical staff. The larger departments, in contrast, are most likely to have significant numbers of staff with public health or related training and the resultant capacity to pursue assessment, policy development, and assurance functions as refined in the 10 essential services.

Technical Capacity

Technical capacity is closely linked to the issue of staffing, although it also includes the availability of equipment that might be required to provide for preventive health services, analysis of environmental health problems, laboratory services, and health education activities, among others. Little data exists regarding the distribution of equipment and facilities, but it is probably reasonable to assume that it follows the same distribution characteristics as the staff required to use it.

Accomplishment of the core functions and essential services relies heavily on the capacity of local health departments to collect, analyze, and use information. Nearly all local health departments are now connected with the Internet, a clear improvement over the situation just five years ago. The current perception of public health leaders is that the larger, more sophisticated agencies are part of the "information superhighway," that the smallest agencies tend not to be involved with much data processing or information sharing, and that medium-sized agencies are improving their capacity to process information.

Leadership

The importance of leadership in public health and its characteristics are described in Chapter 1, "Public Health Mission and Core Functions," and Chapter 9, "Management, Leadership, Strategy, and Systems Thinking." There is no objective scale by which leadership can be measured, although most people seem to have a good notion of whether it is present or absent. Certainly, there are no formal efforts to measure the effectiveness of leadership in the public health world. There have been discussions of the nature of that leadership, however, with some praise mixed in with an apparent consensus that public health leadership is generally lacking. That consensus has fueled efforts to provide leadership-training opportunities at the national, state, and local levels.

Although leadership is difficult to measure objectively, there are several questions to ask to assess whether a local health department is well led. For example, is the department respected in its community by both community leaders and citizens? Is the opinion of department leaders actively sought when the community faces public health problems? Does the department seek and maintain collaborative working arrangements with other community groups and agencies in such a manner that services to the public are provided efficiently and effectively? Is the department successful working within the political system? Are interactions with the medical community (physicians and hospitals) strong and productive? Is the department considered a source of innovative problem solving? Does the department exhibit a history of adequate and stable funding? Is the department involved in teaching and research? There are many other questions that could be listed here as well. The sum total of impressions garnered from pursuing questions such as these leads to a judgment of the quality of leadership present in a particular local health department.

The quality and nature of public health leadership will be increasingly critical as practitioners struggle to bring some focus to the activities of all the disciplines and professions that impact the public's health. Health is the arena where social forces come together, and the growing awareness of the interrelationship of factors that influence health will continue to expand areas of involvement for health departments. Flexible and innovative public health leadership is essential for society to make decisions in all areas of human endeavor that are health-promoting rather than health-destroying.

THE EFFECTIVE HEALTH DEPARTMENT OF THE FUTURE

The public health system in the United States is in a state of significant flux. Some of the characteristics of this evolving system include shifts toward the provision of services based on demonstrated need and potential impact, modeled after the *Healthy People 2010* objectives for the nation; multidisciplinary team-based approaches to problem solving; growing community involvement; closer linkages between prevention and treatment services; and closer linkages between practice and academia.

To be effective, public health agencies of the future must be aware of these continuing waves of change and exhibit the understanding and flexibility required to adapt activities to their environment so that public health services will be appropriately designed and effectively delivered. Also, to be effective, public health departments must be positioned as the health intelligence centers of their respective communities; that is, they must be the source of epidemiologically based thinking and analysis of their community's approach to dealing with health matters. They must be facilitators of strong and meaningful community participation in the assessment and prioritization of community health problems and issues. They must be major participants in public-policy decision making, and they must both deliver and broker the delivery of services needed by their constituent populations. Finally, they must be focused on health outcomes as measures of the impact of interventions.

Accomplishing these tasks will require that health departments work from the strongest organizational base possible, and that they hone and expand the capacities that are necessary to accomplish the core functions of public health and the other services assigned to them by their respective communities. Many local health departments are too small and too resource-poor even to attempt to play the role now expected of them, let alone to be taken seriously as players by community decision makers. To be effective, health departments must represent a constituency large enough that geographic boundaries of authority make sense to the citizenry, that funding is stable, and that the tax base is adequate to provide the local share of resources needed to ensure that at least the core functions of public health are accomplished.

Effective health departments require a governance structure that clearly delineates policy and administrative functions between the board of health (or other governing body) and the director of the department. Additionally, the primary concern of governance must be the description and solution of public health problems in the constituent community rather than the political correctness of the department's actions.

Those of today's public health leaders who are reluctant to embrace community participation and adopt new ways of thinking and acting may actually be significant barriers to the change that is required if every citizen is to be served by a strong and effective public health agency. Effective health departments will have leaders who exhibit commitment, charisma, and drive while embracing collective action, community empowerment, consumer advocacy, and egalitarianism. This was described by John Lloyd in the *Journal of Health Administration Education*.

New technology is moving the nation into an information-rich future. Dealing appropriately with this reality requires computer equipment and analytical skills that provide access to the information available and allow for the correct interpretation of its meaning. Health departments must be able to analyze information about the world they find themselves in and determine the appropriate response to it. This means they must be connected to the information superhighway and be capable of recognizing information and trends that are relevant to the health of their constituents. Every department should have a high-speed connection to the Internet with e-mail capability. Departments must be able to collect and analyze information from their own communities, as well. They should be tracking the demographics of their communities and be thinking imaginatively about the potential use of home computers and interactive television in assessing community perceptions of health needs and priorities. These capacities are basic to future policy and program development and evaluation.

The effective health department will enable individual citizens to take responsibility for decision making related to the community's health as well as their own. Citizens will be involved both in setting the community's priorities for public health issue study and action and in assessing the impact of programs and services designed to improve community health. Effective citizen involvement will require a new level of cultural sensitivity and awareness, and a growing representation of minority groups among the public health workforce.

It is doubtful that any health department has the necessary resources available to carry out the community's full public health agenda. Thus, ensuring that all citizens receive the services they require for good health will require that public health departments build strong collaborative and cooperative linkages with other community health agencies and with the illness care system in the community. These collaborative arrangements will be with other health departments, other departments of local government, community health centers, school systems, and community agencies such as Planned Parenthood, the American Lung Association, the American Cancer Society, neighborhood block clubs, and environmental groups, to name just a few. Such collaboration is necessary for effective health promotion and disease prevention efforts to occur. Joint programming and service and referral arrangements with hospitals, managed care companies, group medical practices, individual physicians, and other providers of illness services are necessary to ensure that each citizen has access to a seamless web of services that promote health, prevent illness, diagnose disease early, and provide disease treatment that is efficient and effective.

Health departments should take the lead in assessing their community's capacity to deliver the 10 essential services by coordinating the use of the national performance standards. The partnerships inherent in such activities can, additionally, provide the base for responding to the threat of terrorism, adjusting the local health care delivery system so that universal access to care can be realized, and ensuring social health can be monitored and deficiencies addressed.

Improvements in those activities and services intended to advance the public's health are strongly dependent upon increasing knowledge of the effectiveness of current or planned actions. They also depend upon the ability to bring well-trained professionals into the field of public health. The practice of public health and the academic base for it have been allowed to become relatively isolated from one another. This reality has been recognized, and work is underway to link the two settings in a manner that will improve the level of training of local public health workers and increasingly focus research efforts on public health administration and service delivery concerns. If at all possible, the effective local health department will welcome students and faculty from academic settings who have the potential to contribute to the understanding of local public health issues and strengthen the capacities of the local public health workforce. The health department should also be supportive of its current employees who want to pursue additional public health training and become adjunct or part-time faculty members. In addition, public health workers should be encouraged to join appropriate professional associations at the state and federal level. These groups can be very helpful in creating networking opportunities, keeping their members up-to-date on technical and organizational advancements, and representing member opinion in public-policy setting processes.

Summary

This is an extraordinary time, and change is in the air. It is a time when no one is clearly in charge of the public health world. Consequently, there are remarkable opportunities for entrepreneurial efforts to reshape the public health system. It is a time for public health leaders to take responsibility for shaping the profession's collective destiny. If that leadership can be exerted so that the public health system can break out of old molds that are no longer functional, there is every reason to believe that public health workers will provide a valuable service to their communities and that it will be recognized as such. The most important element of that recognition, of course, will be steady, measurable gains in community health status.

The following case studies in Chapter 16, "Cases in Public Health Management," are directly related to concepts and principles presented in this chapter:
- Case 5: Understanding Millennial Employees
- Case 8: To Hear this Message in Korean, Press '9'
- Case 11: Budget Cuts in Home Care Program
- Case 14: Collaborative Approach to Diabetes Prevention and Care
- Case 16: Healthy Lifestyles Start at Home
- Case 17: Top 10 U.S. Public Health Achievements
- Case 18: Deciding on a Career in Public Health

Discussion and Review Questions

1. What potential exists for public health to continue to contribute to gains in health status in the United States?

2. What recommendations were made by the Institute of Medicine (IOM) to increase levels of health and longevity in the United States in the near future?

3. List some of the new challenges confronting public health leaders.

4. List some of the traditional challenges faced by public health departments that will continue to be relevant in the future.

5. What are some of the key characteristics you think effective health departments of the future will illustrate?

Action Learning and Critical Thinking

A. Research past issues of the *American Journal of Public Health* and the journal *Health Affairs* and summarize five articles on changes in public health that might shape the future. Share this with your class.

B. Go to the website homepage of the Human Genome Project (http://www.genomics.energy.gov) and read about its development and plans for the future. Discuss in class the social and public health implications and promising possibilities. Also discuss any ethical concerns.

PART V

PUBLIC HEALTH MANAGEMENT IN PRACTICE

This section of the book is provided to help students connect principles and concepts from the book to real-world situations and scenarios. The case approach is used to accomplish this and serves to facilitate understanding within the context of public health agencies and organizations. The student is able to see the many challenges faced by public health managers on a daily basis. This section also includes a chapter that provides common terms used by public health managers. This helps the student expand their professional vocabulary, while also providing a learning resource for this book and future studies in public health and management.

Chapter 16: Cases in Public Health Management   Chapter 17: Terms for Public Health Managers

Chapter 16

CASES IN PUBLIC HEALTH MANAGEMENT

Scott D. Musch, D.H.A., M.B.A.

Learning Objectives

Upon completion of this chapter, you should be able to:

1. Apply management and leadership principles to case situations reflecting real-world scenarios in public health.

2. Think critically about how to approach challenging situations, analyze issues and assumptions, consider stakeholder concerns, and make fair and comprehensive recommendations.

3. Gain an understanding of the nuances of management in public health across various organizations and agencies.

4. Define a problem precisely and recognize the essential information necessary to reach a management solution.

5. Appreciate the roles and responsibilities of public health professionals and managers as they assume leadership roles in the industry.

Chapter Outline

Introduction
Case-Study Approach
Structure
Summary of Common Themes

INTRODUCTION

The case-study method brings interesting, real-world experiences into the classroom. Case scenarios expose students to management roles and responsibilities. They provide students with the opportunity to assume varying roles within case situations and reflect on the different perspectives of the characters involved. One benefit of the case-study method is students learn to understand in professional and managerial situations that there are no clear-cut right and wrong decisions. Students often need and want guidance to find the "right decision." In management, however, many times no right decision exists, but rather decisions that may be better than others given a particular set of circumstances. Oftentimes, decisions are dictated by policies or codes, such as legal, ethical, or organizational regulations. Decisions which have a clear outcome on the basis of these policies are often rare in practice. More often, professionals must balance competing stakeholder interests which offer no clear-cut resolutions. Within these types of predicaments lies the real challenge for managers. Experience, reflection, and consultation of others are the necessary guides for reaching effective outcomes. As students work through these case scenarios, they will gain an understanding of such competencies for making quality decisions. They will develop the ability to think through how to approach challenging situations, analyze the issues and assumptions involved, consider stakeholder concerns, and make comprehensive and fair recommendations.

The case scenarios presented in this chapter provide a foundation for analyzing critical issues facing the public health professional and highlight important concepts discussed in the preceding chapters. They reflect the myriad of realities facing public health professionals. In writing cases, an author is faced with the challenge of narrowing down the universe of possible management scenarios into a collection that is both comprehensive and manageable. The cases in this chapter aim to capture "real-life" scenarios in real or fictional public health settings. They were written to reinforce the understanding of and to stimulate creative thinking about the many nuances of management in public health. Their scope involves professionals at varying levels of authority in a wide range of organizations both inside and outside the public health sector. The case scenarios are intended for teaching and discussion purposes only. Each case is based on a fictionalized scenario from a real or fictional public health setting. Unless specifically referenced, the characters and events are fictional.

CASE-STUDY APPROACH

Students will find many sources available on how to analyze a case scenario and the elements to include in a written or oral report. The purpose here is to highlight a few features to enhance the case-study approach.

Case scenarios often leave out complete information. This is a deliberate strategy by the author. Managers often have to make decisions in a context of incomplete information. This is decision making in a real-world environment. Students should learn to seek out additional information efficiently and effectively. This involves learning both what pertinent questions to ask to collect the right information and how to gather such information. Time-constraints in the decision-making process require managers to learn to define a problem precisely and recognize the essential information necessary to reach a solution. Students should understand the importance of making reasonable assumptions in the case scenario and being flexible to modify those assumptions to different iterations of character and event interactions. Moreover, students should recognize that their analytical method in reaching a decision is often just as important in the case-study method as the actual solution. No prescribed solutions are offered in the cases. This enables instructors to guide students toward a particular lesson or objective.

At the end of each case scenario are discussion questions specific to that case to consider. In addition, the student may benefit by reflecting on the broader issues inherent within the case and how such issues may affect decision making. Some larger considerations might include:

- What factors—history, culture, politics, environment, organizational structure, communication, and character attributes—contributed to the problem or success of the situation?

- Identify all the stakeholders affected by the current scenario. Identify additional stakeholders who may become involved after implementation of the decision.

- Is there more than one issue involved in the case? Do the issues require different and potentially contradictory decisions?

- How does the context of the scenario facilitate or inhibit decision making?

- What are the likely short-term and long-term consequences of the decision?

- Evaluate the temperature level of the decision response. Is it appropriate for the current situation or might it raise the temperature, i.e., is the professional under-reacting or over-reacting?

- Does the professional have support of key stakeholders for the decision or will it involve building allies?

- What is the appropriate timeliness of the decision response? When is the best time to pull the trigger? Does the situation require immediate action or is there time for reflection and consultation?

- What is the professional's level of authority? Does the decision require prior approval of senior management or does the professional have the necessary authority to execute the decision on their own?

As students work through these case scenarios, they should try to resolve the immediate management situation, but also should aim to serve a greater role and responsibility. Public health professionals should strive for leadership. In doing so, students should reflect on the different roles implicit in any given situation as they develop recommendations for the cases:

- **Professional:** Works within the boundaries of their job description and responsibilities; successfully executes their duties.

- **Manager:** Supervises professionals in carrying out their job responsibilities to ensure successful and timely completion to accomplish an organization's goals; focuses on efficient and effective execution; works within boundaries established by role.

- **Leader:** Assumes role beyond immediate management goals and questions effectiveness of existing roles and responsibilities to achieve a strategic goal or objective; thinks "outside the box" to develop solutions; moves beyond existing boundaries to ensure goals and strategy are aligned properly to succeed in a dynamic environment.

The case scenarios in this chapter will assist students to think through important management concepts and help augment their skills to fulfill effectively their responsibilities as public health professionals, managers, and as students striving for leadership roles in the industry.

STRUCTURE

The case scenarios in this chapter are all related to key topics presented in this textbook. Table 16-1 categorizes the cases according to the main topics covered in the chapters. Table 16-2 categorizes the cases according to the public health organizations involved in the scenarios. These matrices should help guide instructors and students in integrating the cases into their coursework.

TABLE 16-1 Relationship Between Cases and Chapter Topics

	Ch. 2	Ch. 3	Ch. 4	Ch. 8	Ch. 9	Ch. 10	Ch. 11	Ch. 12	Ch. 13	Ch. 14	Ch. 15
Case 1: A Friend's Dilemma	●						○	○			
Case 2: Stolen Briefcase	●	○						○	○		
Case 3: The Anti-Vaccination Paradigm		●	●	○	●	●		●	●	●	
Case 4: A Case of Reverse Discrimination?	○					○	●	○			
Case 5: Understanding Millennial Employees					○	○	●	○			●
Case 6: Managing Diversity	○					○	●	○	●		○
Case 7: Sick Building Syndrome	○	●			●	●	●	●		○	
Case 8: To Hear This Message in Korean, Press '9'	○				●	○	●	●	●	●	●
Case 9: A Giardia Outbreak?	○				●						
Case 10: Zero-Tolerance for Smoking	○	○		○	●	●	●	○			
Case 11: Budget Cuts in Home Care Program	○	●			●	●		○	●	●	●
Case 12: Don't Ask, But Tell	○	●			●	●	●	●	○		
Case 13: Senior Cyber Café	○					●	●	●	●	○	○
Case 14: Collaborative Approach to Diabetes Prevention and Care		●	●		●	○		●	●	●	●

	Ch. 2	Ch. 3	Ch. 4	Ch. 8	Ch. 9	Ch. 10	Ch. 11	Ch. 12	Ch. 13	Ch. 14	Ch. 15
Case 15: Toy Recall Prompts Attention to Lead Poisoning	o	●			●	●		●	o		o
Case 16: Healthy Lifestyles Start at Home		o	●				●	●	●	●	●
Case 17: Top Ten U.S. Public Health Achievements		●	●				●	o	●	●	●
Case 18: Deciding on a Career in Public Health							●				●
Case 19: Smoking Cessation Program Implementation			●	o		o			o	●	
Case 20: Pacific Needle Exchange Program								●	●	●	
Case 21: Community Coalitions and the Built Environment			●					o	●	●	
Case 22: Neglected Tropical Diseases—A Local NGO's Challenges	●	●		●		●		o	●		

Legend: ● = directly related o = indirectly related

TABLE 16-2 Relationship Between Cases and Public Health Organization Sector	Ch. 6 Federal	Ch. 7 State	Ch. 7 Local	Ch. 8 NGOs	Ch. 8 Global
Case 1: A Friend's Dilemma		○	●		
Case 2: Stolen Briefcase		●	○		
Case 3: The Anti-Vaccination Paradigm		○	●		○
Case 4: A Case of Reverse Discrimination?			●		
Case 5: Understanding Millennial Employees			●		
Case 6: Managing Diversity			●		○
Case 7: Sick Building Syndrome	●		○		
Case 8: To Hear This Message in Korean, Press '9'	○	○	●		○
Case 9: A *Giardia* Outbreak?		●	○		
Case 10: Zero-Tolerance for Smoking			●		○
Case 11: Budget Cuts in Home Care Program		●	●	○	
Case 12: Don't Ask, But Tell	●				
Case 13: Senior Cyber Café		●	○	●	
Case 14: Collaborative Approach to Diabetes Prevention and Care	○	○	○	●	
Case 15: Toy Recall Prompts Attention to Lead Poisoning				●	○
Case 16: Healthy Lifestyles Start at Home				●	
Case 17: Top Ten U.S. Public Health Achievements	●	●			
Case 18: Deciding on a Career in Public Health	○	○	●	○	○

(Continues)

TABLE 16-2 Relationship Between Cases and Public Health Organization Sector *(Continued)*	Ch. 6 Federal	Ch. 7 State	Ch. 7 Local	Ch. 8 NGOs	Ch. 8 Global
Case 19: Smoking Cessation Program Implementation	o	●	●	o	o
Case 20: Pacific Needle Exchange Program		●	●		
Case 21: Community Coalitions and the Built Environment		●	●		
Case 22: Neglected Tropical Diseases—A Local NGO's Challenges				●	●

Legend: ● = directly related   o = indirectly related

SUMMARY OF COMMON THEMES

Across the case scenarios, regardless of responsibility level or organization type, common themes appear that are instructive "take aways" for professionals in public health.

1. *Engage stakeholders in the decision-making process.* At the beginning of a problem or opportunity, the health care professional should identify all stakeholders affected and take the time to understand their primary concerns. Managers need to involve key stakeholders during the process. Managers can learn from the diverse perspectives of stakeholders and at the same time ensure their concerns are being addressed. By including stakeholders at the appropriate time and level in the decision-making process, a manager can gain their support in implementing and accepting a tough decision.

2. *Learn to effectively work in and manage teams.* Teamwork is a critical component within public health work. The workforce in public health is highly educated and eager to participate in the decision-making process that affects them and the long-term interests of the organization they serve. The benefits of a team approach are too numerous to list, but they primarily involve integrating the diversity of experiences, skills, and perspectives of team members to reach an optimal work product. The development and operation of productive teams require a skill set gained through education and experience. Important considerations include team member selection, size, diversity, type, and structure.

3. *Be in front of a problem or opportunity.* Managers need to ensure that the appropriate organizational structures are in place to assist professionals and staff

to make sound decisions in the first place. It takes less time, energy, and cost to prevent a problem from emerging than it does to fix a problem once it occurs. Likewise, having structures in place will enable an organization to seize on an opportunity, exemplifying the old adage "prepare for an opportunity, rather than wait for an opportunity to prepare."

4. *Learn to communicate effectively.* Aside from having proficient communication skills, managers need to recognize when to communicate. There are several stages to apply effective communication in a decision-making process. At the beginning of any process, the manager should make sure everyone has a clear understanding of roles, responsibilities, and expectations, and that they are openly receptive to questions and concerns. During the process, the manager should offer guidance and seek feedback along the way to avoid any surprises at the end. Finally, at the end of the process, the manager should take the time to seek constructive feedback and share lessons learned. Every scenario presents an excellent learning opportunity.

5. *Embrace systems thinking.* Systems thinking has become a necessary competency for public health professionals. We live and operate within systems. Interconnections, relationships, and interdependencies affect public health behaviors and the performance of policies and programs aimed at addressing key concerns. Leaders in public health have embraced systems thinking and have learned to realize the many complexities inherent in a systems-wide approach.

6. *Recognize and embrace diverse backgrounds.* The scope of the public health field is vast, encompassing a wide range of specialist and generalist areas and drawing on a large diversity of professional backgrounds and talents. Managers need to value this diversity. They should incorporate the wealth of experiences and perspectives within their programs and organizations.

7. *Remember public health is a service industry.* At the core of all service industries are people. In all professions dedicated to serving people, managers will encounter human fallacies. It is to be expected, but it should not deter managers as it can also be a great source of inspiration and creativity. Public health professionals need to recognize that human behavior cannot be modeled or anticipated. They cannot plan for every contingency. They need to be prepared to encounter and embrace this human dimension of public health.

8. *Embrace your role as a professional.* It should be the role of each individual employee to take responsibility to uphold an organization's mission and standards. It does not serve anyone in the long run to defer this responsibility to someone else, to another manager, or otherwise. Professionalism requires resisting the temptation to just "get the job done" or to fall back on the old adage "well, it's not my responsibility." Professionals should not let opportunities slip away. Take the time to communicate, motivate, evaluate, coordinate, educate, and most importantly, lead.

9. *Sustain the mission of public health.* The case scenarios presented in this chapter illustrate the far-reaching aspects of public health and its primary mission to promote the health and safety of all citizens. Public health touches so many dimensions of our daily lives. In fulfilling their job responsibilities, public health professionals serve not only the immediate purposes of their organizations,

but the greater overall mission of public health. They embrace the opportunities to have a significant effect on people's lives and make a difference in the future health and well-being of our global community.

CASE 1: A FRIEND'S DILEMMA

Situation

Stacy is an administrative assistant at the Los Angeles-Downtown Wellness Center, an HIV testing site funded by the California Department of Public Health (CDPH). In addition to HIV testing, the Wellness Center provides HIV prevention education services, HIV/AIDS medical treatment, and HIV support services such as case management and counseling. Stacy's job primarily involves data entry and processing. Her main responsibility is to assist in filling out the HIV/AIDS case report forms required by the CDPH for confirmed HIV tests.

Although she has worked at the Wellness Center for only eight months, she enjoys the work and recognizes the highly sensitive nature of her job. In the course of her work, she handles patient medical record files and sees the names of patients who have tested positive for HIV. Given the routine of her work, she typically processes the information without much thought to patient names, until this afternoon. In the patient file she is holding, she recognizes the name—Eric—her best friend's boyfriend. He tested positive for HIV and gonorrhea. Linda, her best friend, has been dating Eric exclusively for the last year, and she knows that Linda has not had sexual relations with anyone else during that time.

Background

The Wellness Center is administered by a county health department and operates pursuant to the California Health and Safety Code. The Health and Safety Code (Section 121022[a]) requires health care providers and clinical laboratories to report HIV infection by patient name to the local health officer and mandates local health officers to report HIV cases by patient name to the CDPH. The report consists of a completed copy of a HIV/AIDS case report form which is coordinated with the CDPH, Office of AIDS, HIV/AIDS Case Registry. Prior to 2007, patient names were not reported. In 2007, the California Department of Health repealed non-name code and partial non-name code used for HIV reporting and required health care providers, laboratories, and local health officers to use patient names when reporting cases of HIV infection.[1] This change decreased the reporting burden for reporting entities and the name-based HIV reporting system ensured that California remained eligible for federal funding.

All local health department employees and contractors with access to confidential HIV-related information are required to sign a confidentiality agreement form, which informs staff of the penalties associated with a breach of confidentiality as well as the procedures for reporting a breach. As an employee of the Wellness

Center, Stacy signed a confidentiality agreement form prior to being allowed to handle confidential HIV-related health records. In addition, Stacy attended a mandatory Data and Security Training session offered to new staff who will handle patient-data entry. The training program outlined the policies and procedures of maintaining confidentiality. During the training, Stacy learned that any person who willfully, maliciously, or negligently discloses the content of any confidential public health record to a third party, except in accordance to a written authorization or as authorized by law, can be subject to a civil and criminal penalties, including imprisonment.

Next Steps

After entering Eric's information into the case report form, Stacy reaches for the telephone to call Linda but then stops to think. Stacy knows that Eric isn't the type of person who will tell Linda and admit his infidelity. If Stacy tells Linda, she will be upset and will confront Eric. Eric will try to figure out how Linda found out about his test and will likely inquire at the Wellness Center, which might lead back to Stacy. If the Wellness Center's administrator finds out, Stacy will be terminated and could face additional penalties. But is her job worth the risk of potentially putting her friend's health in jeopardy?

Discussion Questions

1. What should Stacy do in her situation?

2. Does the confidentiality protection facilitate or inhibit those interests of public health when involving infectious diseases?

3. How will Stacy's supervisor handle a breach of confidentiality?

4. If you were Stacy's supervisor and she asked for your advice, what would you recommend?

Reference

[1] California Department of Public Health. (n.d.). R-06-014E-Reporting HIV infection by name. Retrieved from http://www.cdph.ca.gov/services/DPOPP/reg/Pages/R-06-0141E—ReportingHIVinfectionbyName.aspx

CASE 2: STOLEN BRIEFCASE

Situation

After two years as a Disease Intervention Specialist for the Texas Department of State Health Services—Infectious Disease Control Unit, Carlos was aware of the many challenges associated with his job. Although the title doesn't sound dangerous, the job can be at times. His responsibilities include not only informing people who test positive for sexually transmitted diseases (STD), including HIV, but also tracking down their sex partners. These situations can become confrontational, particularly when working with marginal information and dealing with irate people who don't want to face the news. Today, however, didn't involve any confrontations, but rather something more serious. After finishing a field visit in an economically depressed inner-city neighborhood, Carlos returned to his car to find the passenger door window broken, door ajar, and his briefcase containing case interview files missing.

Background

A disease intervention specialist (DIS) is a trained public health professional who is responsible for finding and counseling patients, sex partners, and others suspected of having an STD or other communicable disease. The main objective of this front-line public health work is to prevent and control disease transmission by ensuring that all people who have been diagnosed or exposed to a communicable disease are promptly examined and adequately treated. Among his or her many duties, the DIS conducts field visits to locate, motivate, and refer communicable disease patients and their partners/contacts for medical evaluation and treatment at public or private health care providers. Given the sensitive and personal nature of STD information, the DIS must follow a strict protocol to maintain confidentiality.

The DIS has the responsibility to ensure that persons who are infected with a STD, or who are at risk of acquiring a STD, receive appropriate medical care at the earliest possible time. Although reaching a person by the telephone for initial follow-up activities is permitted, it is not the preferred method for in-depth investigation and dealing with highly sensitive issues such as HIV or HIV-partner notification. A field call is the most effective follow-up method and frequently the most efficient. The Texas Department of State Health Services has an established set of operating procedures and standards (HIV/STD Public Health Follow-Up Confidential Information Security Procedures) for all HIV/STD field and support staff involving the handling of confidential information.[1] The Department's local responsible party (LRP) implements and enforces these policies and procedures which are designed in part to ensure that the DIS observes certain safeguards to protect the nature of his or her professional capacity and the privacy of individuals in the course of disease intervention activities. The LRP also has the responsibility of reporting and assisting in investigating breaches. Some of the standard procedures for field visits include:

- Field visits need to be conducted in unmarked vehicles to ensure client confidentiality.

- Field records containing confidential information are not to be left unattended outside the office.

- Documents used in the field should contain the minimum amount of confidential information necessary to conduct the field investigation.

- Contents of field records should not be divulged to any unauthorized persons.

- Field records should be properly coded, and code sheets should not be kept in the same container as the field records.

Next Steps

Carlos planned multiple calls today to make the most efficient use of his field time. His briefcase contained a number of files that contained information to identify the addresses and names of people in the neighborhood who he planned to visit. Although the field records were coded, there were other papers in his briefcase that would make it obvious in what capacity he was working. Carlos had locked the files in his briefcase after reviewing them, placed the briefcase under the passenger seat, and locked the car before heading off to his first client's apartment. Although he knew this neighborhood had a high crime rate, he thought his car would be safe parked on the street. After all, his briefcase wasn't even visible.

Discussion Questions

1. How should Carlos handle this situation?

2. Did Carlos violate any operating procedures?

3. What should the LRP do in this situation?

Reference

[1] Texas Department of State Health Services. (2010, September 28). HIV/STD security policies and procedures. Retrieved from http://www.dshs.state.tx.us/hivstd/policy/security.shtm

CASE 3: THE ANTI-VACCINATION PARADIGM

"Free your mind…from the vaccine paradigm."
Vaccination Liberation home page (http://www.vaclib.org)

Situation

Dr. Anne London, Chief of Immunization at the Franklin County Health Agency, reviewed the reports on her desk on the progress of the immunization program in her county. She was particularly concerned as she studied the reports: the overall rate of vaccine refusal remained low at 2.7% but has continued to climb over the last five years. She wondered if Franklin County was setting itself up for a potential public health issue. Outbreaks were no longer unheard of in the United States, especially when considering the measles outbreak in San Diego in 2008, the *pertussis* (whooping cough) outbreak in California in 2010, and even more troubling, the measles epidemic in Great Britain over the last decade.

Dr. London has seen the websites, blogs, and homemade videos—Mom's Against Vaccine Enforcement, among others—claiming a link between vaccines, particularly MMR (measles, mumps, and rubella) and autism. In implementing the immunization program, Dr. London made sure to emphasize education to dispel such beliefs. She recognized that most parents who refuse vaccines for their children are concerned about possible adverse effects and are skeptical of the government, pharmaceutical industry, and medical community. She could empathize to a degree with these parents, as they are probably acting in good faith and love for their children. After all, she seriously weighs every decision she has to make that may affect her daughter's health. However, don't these parents realize that by failing to immunize their children they place not only their children at a greater risk of disease, but also the community as a whole?

Background

Vaccines have been successful and with that success a new generation of parents in the United States has emerged who have not experienced the terrible effects of polio, measles, whooping cough, and smallpox. Measles outbreaks started to recur in the United States nearly eight years after the virus was declared dead in the United States, largely attributed to a successful vaccination program that began in the 1960s. In 2008, the United States experienced its largest outbreak of measles in more than 10 years, affecting 15 states.[1] In 2010, California experienced an outbreak of *pertussis* with more than 4,000 reported cases and nine infant deaths linked to the outbreak.[2] These outbreaks have ignited concern over community clusters in which a growing number of parents are intentionally refusing to vaccinate their children. Parents are permitted to do so by signing a personal-beliefs exemption. In the United States, all states require children under law to be properly immunized before attending school. However, exemptions are permitted. In addition to medical exemptions offered in each state, 48 states allow for religious exemptions and 20 states allow personal-belief exemptions for day-care and school.[3] Fears that vaccines cause autism, attention deficit hyperactivity disorder (ADHD/ADD), asthma, and allergies are continually fed through viral marketing—websites and blogs purporting vaccination conspiracies—despite the many studies and expert commentary that dispel any scientific link.

The potential seriousness of vaccination noncompliance can be witnessed by looking at the measles epidemic that reemerged in Great Britain over the last decade. After a British medical journal published a study in 1998 in which British researcher Andrew Wakefield suggested that the MMR vaccine triggered autism, vaccination rates in parts of Great Britain fell precipitously, from a national average of 92% in the mid-1990s to 88.4% in 2000, to a low of 75% in some areas of London and Wales.[4] The World Health Organization states that a community needs a vaccination rate of 95% to ensure the herd immunity threshold.[5] Cases of measles have grown annually in Great Britain and Wales as a result of children not getting immunized. (Notably, not only was the Wakefield study retracted in 2010, another British medical journal, *BMJ*, published an analysis in 2011 that found Wakefield's research to be fraudulent.[6])

Despite the public health consequences, anti-vaccination campaigns still continue in communities within Great Britain and the United States.

Next Steps

Later in the week, Dr. London has a meeting scheduled with her team to review the new immunization-program data. After seeing the continuing rise in the rate of vaccine refusals, she plans to ask her team to suggest changes to the immunization program campaign to increase vaccination compliance rates. As Chief of Immunization at the Franklin County Health Agency, Dr. London wants to be proactive. We need to remain vigilant, Dr. London reflects, and we need to use multiple angles—education, access, and outreach.

Discussion Questions

1. What strategies should the team recommend to Dr. London?

2. How do you deal with parents who refuse to vaccinate their children?

3. As a public health official, should you promote vaccination compliance as a civic responsibility?

4. How do you manage a conflict among individual behavior, organizational behavior, and public health goals?

References

[1] Dunham, W. (2008, July 9). Measles outbreak hits 127 people in 15 states. *Reuters.* Retrieved from http://www.reuters.com/article/2008/07/09/us-measles-usa-idUSN0943743120080709

[2] Mitchell, D. (2010, September 27). Most toddler vaccination rates near national goals but outbreaks show need for docs to continue educating parents. *AAFP News Now.* Retrieved from http://www.aafp.org/online/en/home/publications/news/news-now/clinical-care-research/20100927toddlervaccs.html

[3] Institute for Vaccine Safety, John Hopkins Bloomberg School of Public Health. (2011, January 6). *Vaccine exemptions.* http://www.aafp.org/online/en/home/publications/news/news-now/clinical-care-research/20100927toddlervaccs.html

[4] Laurance, J. (2000, August 8). UK measles outbreak feared after Dublin deaths. *The Independent.* Retrieved from http://www.aafp.org/online/en/home/publications/news/news-now/clinical-care-research/20100927toddlervaccs.html

[5] Georgette, N. (2007). The quantification of the effects of changes in population parameters on the herd immunity threshold. *The Internet Journal of Epidemiology,* 5(1). Retrieved from http://www.ispub.com/ostia/index.php?xmlFilePath=jounrals/ije/vol5n1/population.xml

[6] Deer, B. (2011, January 8). Secrets of the MMR scare: How the case against the MMR vaccine was fixed. *BMJ, 342*(7788), 77–83. doi: 10.1136/bmj.c5347

CASE 4: A CASE OF REVERSE DISCRIMINATION?

Situation

NPMC Care Clinic (NPMC) provides community-based primary care to adults requiring specialized health care and social services in North Philadelphia. The clinic operates under the guidance of St. Joseph's Hospital in North Philadelphia and offers medical services, support services, and medical case management. Brad, a recent graduate from the Boston University School of Social Work, joined NPMC six months ago as a case manager in the HIV/AIDS Services Program. Brad earned his Masters in Social Work and wants to become certified as a Licensed Clinical Social Worker (LCSW). He enjoys performing HIV/AIDs social work as he finds it extremely rewarding. Most individuals with AIDS are poor and must rely on the limited benefits of public health insurance and usually cannot afford to purchase additional services when they are needed. Case managers help people living with HIV/AIDS get primary medical care and medications, adhere to treatment plans, and access supportive services such as housing, transportation, food, and mental health counseling. As a LCSW, Brad would develop comprehensive, individualized care plans for clients and work closely with other team members in the clinic to ensure his client's medical, mental health, and social services are being addressed. As part of the licensure requirements in Pennsylvania, Brad needs to complete three years or 3,000 hours of supervised work experience in a clinical setting. Brad was excited to join NPMC as it had an active patient case load and his supervisor seemed eager to help him work towards his licensure requirements.

In the HIV Services Program at NPMC, Brad works closely with two other case managers, Tim and Michael, who have been with the clinic for approximately two years. His working relationship with his colleagues was at first very amicable. He seemed to be accepted by them, and at times they joked with him for being the "straight advocate" or "token" in their group. Tim and Michael are gay, as is the supervisor of the program, while Brad is heterosexual. Tim and Michael are open about their sexual orientation and Brad doesn't feel uncomfortable, though at times he does not always understand their humor. Tim and Michael often share their dating adventures of their previous night's encounters in the office, and Brad would look forward to hearing their humorous stories. Brad enjoyed conversing with colleagues. He also had a good initial relationship with his boss. His supervisor was well respected in the department and he offered Brad much encouragement. Gradually, Brad noticed that his supervisor seemed more inclined toward Tim and Michael, but he didn't make much out of it as he figured it was probably due to their being able to relate better, given their shared culture.

After five months, however, the general atmosphere at work changed. Brad felt increasingly like an outsider. While the case load at NPMC was fairly distributed, Brad's cases seemed to get less attention from his supervisor than Tim's and Michael's cases. The majority of Brad's patients were heterosexual and he sensed reluctance on the part of his supervisor to assign him more cases involving gay patients. From Brad's perspective, Tim and Michael seemed busier and their cases tended to receive more exposure throughout the clinic. Brad tried to defuse his impression of the situation by approaching his supervisor to volunteer to handle a greater "variety" of cases. However, while his supervisor acknowledged his interest, he told Brad that Tim and Michael had a more appropriate background to handle these types of cases. Brad tried to dismiss his concerns over the apparent favoritism in the office and focused on doing his work. Adding to his suspicions of favoritism, Brad often found Tim and Michael in his supervisor's office in what appeared to be formal meetings. On occasion, Brad tried to join these meetings by hanging outside his supervisor's office door to give the impression of wanting to be involved. His supervisor would call him in and generally did not seem to mind; however, he never directly addressed Brad's lack of invitation. Gradually, Brad stopped making the extra effort to be involved and just concentrated on his case load at his desk.

Brad's relations with his colleagues Tim and Michael grew increasingly strained. What was once a collegial atmosphere in the office was now tense. Tim and Michael no longer included him in their "water-cooler" talk and even if he tried to join in, they seemed to tense up and shortly end their lively discussions. On several occasions, Brad thought he heard Tim and Michael making off-handed comments about him, referring to him as the "breeder" in the office. In addition, they seemed particularly extra-sensitive to any comments Brad might make that appeared critical of their behavior, including comments on risky sexual behaviors that he may have relayed from a patient case. Brad felt increasingly isolated in the office. He tried to dismiss his concerns as just "being in his head" as he really needed the hours at the clinic to meet his goal of obtaining his license.

Background

Federal laws prohibit discrimination based on race, color, sex, religion, national origin, age, and disability for private employers. Sex discrimination claims by workers are most often filed under Title VII of the *Civil Rights Act of 1964* (Pub. L. 88-352). Sexual discrimination prohibited under Title VII includes discrimination based on pregnancy, sex stereotyping, and sexual harassment. Title VII does not prohibit discrimination based on sexual orientation though some state discrimination laws do. Almost half of the U.S. states, including the District of Columbia, have active laws that prohibit sexual orientation discrimination in both private and public workplaces. A few states prohibit sexual orientation discrimination in only public workplaces, such as for state employees, as is the case with Pennsylvania (as of 2010). Sexual orientation discrimination involves a situation when someone is treated differently solely because of his or her sexual orientation: gay or lesbian (homosexual), bisexual, or straight (heterosexual). This type of discrimination may also occur on the basis of a perception of someone's orientation, whether that perception is correct or not. The *Employment Non-Discrimination Act* (ENDA) is proposed federal legislation that would add sexual orientation as a protected class against discrimination. While ENDA has been proposed in the United States

Congress numerous times, it has failed to pass. Sexual harassment is a form of sex discrimination that is prohibited by federal law and the law of most states, regardless of whether the state also has a law making discrimination on the basis of sexual orientation illegal. The victim as well as the harasser may be a woman or a man, and the victim does not have to be of the opposite sex to be able to bring a legal claim for sexual harassment.

Next Steps

Brad once looked forward to getting up in the morning and going to work. He really had a passion for helping his clients. However, increasingly he had to drag himself out of bed. He felt isolated and dreaded having to face his colleagues in the office. He knew he had to address the situation as he didn't want it to start to affect his love for social work. He considered meeting with NPMC's human resources director. What would he say? There was not any direct evidence to identify to build a case for discrimination. Who would believe that a heterosexual male among gay workers could be the object of discrimination? Brad believed the human resources director was also gay, so he was not confident he would get a fair hearing. His perceptions would probably just be dismissed as paranoid. In addition, if his supervisor found out about his meeting with human resources, the situation would only become worse. Brad thought that it might be time to seriously look for another job.

Discussion Questions

1. What should Brad do?

2. If you were the HR director, what issues would you address?

3. Is Brad a victim of reverse discrimination?

4. How might Brad's supervisor make for a more inclusive work environment?

CASE 5: UNDERSTANDING MILLENNIAL EMPLOYEES

Situation

"Stephen just quit," Betty interjected as Katherine walked by the desk. "Apparently, he felt frustrated in his job. He found an opportunity with more responsibility at Riverside Health Clinic." Katherine, the Human Resources Director for the State Department of Health and Environmental Control (DHEC), paused and absorbed the news. "Stephen is the third employee to leave the Program Department in the last 12 months," Katherine replied. "Why can't Bill hold on to his younger employees?" She thought there must be more behind the departures than simply better opportunities.

Stephen had worked in the central office of the Public Health Programs department under the supervision of Bill, a 30-year veteran with the DHEC. The department oversaw and coordinated program initiatives for three branches: Health Services, Health Regulations, and Environmental Control. Bill supervised approximately 25 employees in various capacities, including three managers with responsibility for programs in each of the three branches. Bill had worked his way up through the organization, starting his career at a local health department within the state and eventually earning his current position. Bill was a seasoned professional within the DHEC, with a wide breadth of experience, and he had a strict, almost authoritative, management style. The three other managers were also long-term employees with an average tenure of 20 years. On the other hand, Stephen was a recent undergraduate recruit from a well-respected school of public health. The other two employees who resigned were also relatively young employees, having worked in the department for less than two years.

Katherine had spoken with Bill after the other two employees departed. Katherine felt that Bill needed to re-evaluate his management style and recognize how his workforce was changing, particularly with the millennial generation, adults who were born after 1982 and are just now starting to enter the workforce in greater numbers (see Table 16-3). However, Bill was resistant. He echoed a comment that she often heard from other managers in the office: "Why do we need to change our culture for these new employees?"

Background

In its report, *Confronting the Public Health Workforce Crisis*, the Association of Schools of Public Health (ASPH) estimated that 250,000 additional public health workers will be needed by 2020, largely attributed to the current workforce slowly diminishing as approximately 23% will be eligible to retire by 2012.[1] For some state health agencies, this percentage is more drastic, reaching over 50% as reported in the Association of State and Territorial Health Officials' *2007 State Public Health Workforce Shortage Report*. To replenish the workforce and avert a crisis, the ASPH estimates that schools of public health will need to train three times the current number of graduates over the next 11 years.[2] While there are many implications from these statistics, one is clear: the public health workforce will gradually be younger and employees from the millennial generation will become a larger part of the workforce.

The multigenerational workforce in public health, as with all industries, presents numerous challenges. While casting stereotypes within any demographic group can lead to simplistic conclusions, each generation has a slightly different paradigm for

TABLE 16-3 Generations

Generation	Veterans	Baby Boomers	Generation X	Millennial
Years born	1925–1942	1943–1964	1965–1981*	1982*–2002
Ages in 2011	69–86	47–68	30–46	9–29

* Sources differ on ending and beginning dates.

the role of work in life and the standards for that work. Employers who understand how each generation's values, ethics, and expectations affect the workplace may be able to better optimize employee productivity, retention, and success. Incorporating this understanding into management practices may reduce generational conflict and miscommunication. Much has been written on the subject of the millennial generation, including recommended techniques for recruiting, managing, motivating, and retaining these employees. Among the research, some general characteristics are apparent. Desirable attributes in a job for millennials include a preference for an inclusive work environment, team collaboration, challenges and opportunities to learn new skills, flexibility, and life-work balance. Employers tend to go wrong with millennials when they do not provide clear growth opportunities, discount their ideas for lack of experience, and feel threatened by their technical knowledge.

Next Steps

Sitting in her office, Katherine reflects on the loss of another employee in Bill's department. As a human resources professional, Katherine has come across many articles and presentations on the topic of the millennial workforce and related challenges of a multigenerational workforce. With all the challenges of recruiting and retaining employees in public health, Katherine reasons that being sensitive to this new generation should be an easier one to tackle. Katherine considers taking a proactive approach by implementing a training program for Bill and his managers to discuss the issue. A training program might give managers, of all generations, the tools to successfully adapt their culture and better incorporate the values of different generations rather than just dismissing them.

Discussion Questions

1. What should be the main objectives of the training program?
2. What would you include in the training curriculum?
3. What multigenerational management challenges are facing the public health sector?
4. Will a training program help address these challenges?
5. How should Katherine implement this training program for managers? How should she deal with resistance?

References

[1] Association of Schools of Public Health. (2008, February). *Confronting the public health workforce crisis: ASPH statement on the public health workforce.* Retrieved from http://www.asph.org/UserFiles/PHWFShortage0208.pdf

[2] Association of State and Territorial Health Officials. (2008). *2007 State public health workforce survey results.* Retrieved from http://www.astho.org/Display/AssetDisplay.aspx?id=500

CASE 6: MANAGING DIVERSITY

Situation

Jennifer, a supervisor for the food safety division within the Health Department of a major metropolitan area, wanted to throw her hands up and shout at the next employee who walked through her office door to complain. She had reached her limit in hearing complaints from her staff members over other coworkers in the department. It seemed like every other day a staff member would come into her office and tell her about a coworker making an insensitive comment or not doing their work the way they "should." Although Jennifer was sensitive to reports of any activity contributing to a hostile work environment, she started to think that her employees were being too sensitive and intentionally looking out for comments to support their cases. When her employees joined the department, they participated in diversity training as part of their orientation session, but the lessons they learned seemed to have dissipated.

Supervising a diverse team of employees has its rewards and challenges. Jennifer appreciated the wide range of perspectives and views on public health concerns. The overall staff at the health department was, what Jennifer liked to call, "truly cosmopolitan." The staff was reflective of the diversity of the metropolitan area. In Jennifer's department, the cultural diversity was even more pronounced. Jennifer supervised the program responsible for monitoring food service workers and inspecting community restaurants for food safety and health violations. The diversity of her workforce was absolutely necessary to interact successfully with the multicultural restaurant workers within the city. Her employees' diversity contributed greatly to the success of the food safety division.

Jennifer had recently selected a group of her employees to work on a team to evaluate new policies and procedures for restaurant and food safety inspection. She felt the policies-and-procedures team would give coworkers a better opportunity to get to know each other and improve their working relationships. The objective of the team was to standardize a set of restaurant policies among different counties within the greater metropolitan area. The team needed to discuss what policies worked and which didn't, and then agree on a set of recommendations. The work would require team members to share their cultural perspectives of the food and restaurant practices within the city. Selecting the team was a challenge, as Jennifer wanted to make sure members represented the city's diverse ethnic communities. The final team included Meihui, a Chinese woman; Manual, a Catholic Hispanic Latino; Susan, a Caucasian lesbian; Knitasha, an African-American, who was a recent hire from a public health school graduate program; Tom, an Indian, who was a veteran with the department and near retirement; and Alima, a female Sunni Muslim. Since inception, the team has been dysfunctional. Certain team members refuse to speak directly to other members. Members make insensitive comments to others, leading to arguments and members storming out of meetings. Other members are completely silent and don't participate during meetings.

The animosity between team members has bled over into the general atmosphere of the department, contributing to the increased frequency of complaints arriving at Jennifer's office door.

Background

Many managers feel unprepared to lead departments and project teams comprised of diverse individuals of different cultures, ethnic backgrounds, educational levels, ages, genders, sexual orientations, religions, and other heterogeneous mixes. This discomfort can manifest in a lack of understanding and recognition of the competencies necessary to manage a diverse workforce and project teams. The result can be a dysfunctional work environment, with workers becoming less productive, motivated, and easily offended. Low-satisfaction levels can increase employee turnover and lead to formal complaints against coworkers, contributing to hostility and suspicion. Managers need to proactively refine and improve their techniques to recognize diversity and improve the overall climate and encourage cooperation. Enhanced skills are required not only to manage a diverse workforce, but to lead productive teams comprised of diverse members.

Effective teamwork offers obvious benefits to team members, including a chance to be creative and share ideas, an opportunity to build stronger working relationships with colleagues, an opportunity to learn new skills or enhance existing ones, among many others. The satisfaction gained from working in teams and creating a collective work product can be very rewarding. Facilitating and managing a team, however, requires education and experience. Most teams go through four development stages before they become productive, as identified by Bruce W. Tuckman: forming, storming, norming, and performing.[1] The stages can be cyclical, and individual team members may be at different stages with other team members. The project manager needs to lead the group through these four stages and keep the members focused on their objective. Incorporating additional levels of diversity into the mix of a team places greater responsibility on the project manager to effectively facilitate the team and root out underlying hostility and insensitivity.

Next Steps

Jennifer is growing increasingly concerned that the team will not succeed in meeting its objectives. Moreover, she is upset that many of her employees seem to be contributing, directly or indirectly, to the heightened level of animosity towards each other in the department. Her department and the policies-and-procedures team have become dysfunctional. If this continues, her boss and other supervisors at the health department are going to think she is not capable of managing and she may lose her job.

Discussion Questions

1. How would you handle this situation?

2. How could Jennifer manage diversity more effectively in the department?

3. What steps should be taken to reduce the animosity within the department?

4. How would you facilitate the policies-and-procedures team and get it back on track?

5. Create a cross-cultural sensitivity training program, using the current team members as the audience, to serve as a tool for career development.

Reference

1 Tuckman, B.W. (1965). Developmental sequence in small groups. *Psychological Bulletin, 63,* 384–399.

CASE 7: SICK BUILDING SYNDROME

Situation

Mary hung up the phone and sighed. Larry, the building supervisor, was furious and he vented his emotions to Mary. Larry had just spoken with a project officer from the National Institute for Occupational Safety and Health (NIOSH). The project officer reported that a Health Hazard Evaluation (HHE) request was made by an employee of one of his corporate tenants, and the officer wanted to arrange a site visit. NIOSH, a part of the Centers for Disease Control and Prevention (CDC) in the Department of Health and Human Services, is responsible for assuring safe and healthy working conditions. Larry wanted to know which one of Mary's employees had contacted NIOSH and why. He was upset that he was not informed about this ahead of time. His company had completed the renovation of the building and there should not be any health hazards. In addition, if word leaked out about an inspection, he might have trouble leasing the other vacant floors, not to mention the reputational damage with current tenants. Who would want to lease office space in a building being investigated by NIOSH? Mary had listened patiently while Larry vented. She didn't know who contacted NIOSH, and even if she did, she definitely wouldn't share it with Larry.

Mary was the human resources director of Triade Billing Services, a medical billing and claims processing company. Triade was a rapidly growing company with an expanding workforce. The company was headquartered in a large office building in downtown Atlanta and had occupied the building for five years. The office building was constructed in the mid-1990s, but the floors were recently renovated within the last year. The renovation went well and the employees seemed happy with the updated accommodations. Given the nature of the business, the floor layout consisted of closely arranged desk cubicles with computer terminals and other electronic equipment. The office was not unlike most business offices in downtown Atlanta. Mary thought the office space was suitable for employees though employees occasionally complained of headaches and dry eyes. Everyone blamed the bad air and lighting. Given the nature of their work—long hours in front of computer terminals—Mary felt the problem was most likely due to the glare on their computer screens. However, as the complaints persisted, she contacted Larry to evaluate the fluorescent lights on the floor. After some evaluation, Larry reluctantly agreed to change the power of the lights and within days, the headaches disappeared.

Mary thought this might be the end of the complaints and for most part, it was. However, a few employees continued to express concerns over the quality of the air in the office. Mary noted that absenteeism due to sick days had gradually trended up over the last year for several employees. One employee in particular concerned her. Doug had recently come down with a chronic breathing problem. He had seen a doctor who thought it might be the onset of asthma, but was unable to determine a direct cause. Doug was convinced that it was building-related asthma, and he was not shy sharing his concerns to his fellow workers. Mary, on the other hand, was skeptical. However, she witnessed Doug growing increasingly frustrated at work due to his illness and discomfort. He started to call in sick more often, which had been unlike him in the past. There were other employees who reported similar problems but none to the extent of Doug's.

Background

Sick Building Syndrome (SBS) is a situation in which building occupants experience health symptoms as a result of time spent in a specific building and the illness cannot be traced to a specific cause. Another condition, building-related illness (BRI), is a situation in which the symptoms of an illness can be identified and directly attributed to building contaminants. For instance, BRIs have traceable causes, such as the spread of a virus throughout an office, allergies or asthma due to dust or mold in the workplace, or cancer caused by asbestos or other chemicals. Experts differ in their opinions on the causes of SBS, as to whether it is due to poor indoor air quality from inadequate ventilation, other pollutants, or even work-related stress. Complaints of SBS appear more often in newer, energy-efficient buildings where windows are sealed shut and there is limited circulation of outside air. Although experts differ on the causes, they recognize SBS as a serious problem for employees who are suffering with real symptoms and employers who are losing billions of dollars each year in lost productivity.

Next Steps

Mary realized that Doug was likely the employee who contacted NIOSH, probably out of frustration. She wished Doug would have approached her first, but would she have recognized that the work environment may be to blame? She might have tried to convince Larry to run some tests, but given Larry's negative reaction to changing the fluorescent lights, she knew how he would have reacted. The NIOSH project officer is scheduled to visit the building next week to begin the HHE. The evaluation could take several months to a year. In the meantime, Mary, Larry, and Doug will just have to wait.

Discussion Questions

1. How should the NIOSH project officer interact with a skeptical Mary, a disgruntled Larry, and a sick Doug?

2. Did Doug do anything wrong in contacting NIOSH to request an HHE?

3. Can Mary reprimand Doug for contacting NIOSH?

4. What should Mary have done once employees complained of SBS at their workplace?

CASE 8: TO HEAR THIS MESSAGE IN KOREAN, PRESS '9'

Situation

Angela, the Program Coordinator for a federally qualified health center (FQHC) in Queens, New York, was concerned that the language and cultural capabilities of the staff at the health center were not keeping pace with the diverse community. The FQHC, one of several in the Queens Borough, is located in a designated Medically Underserved Area (MUA) neighborhood and assists underserved populations, homeless people, and migrant workers. MUAs are areas designated by the federal government as having too few primary care providers, high infant mortality, high poverty, and/or high elderly population. Most of the health center patients are at incomes below the poverty level and nearly two-thirds are racial or ethnic minorities. The mission of the health center is to be community-based and patient-focused, which can be a challenge given the cross-cultural and language differences.

Immigrant populations have swelled around the health center over the last decade. The clinic's staff is increasingly confronting language and cultural challenges. Almost daily, Angela shares in the frustrations of practitioners trying to best serve their patients in spite of these barriers. Most immigrants can speak enough English to get around in their daily activities, but that skill level is usually insufficient in the doctor's office when discussing medical terms. Miscommunication or lack of communication due to cultural sensitivities can lead to ineffective patient care, including errors in diagnoses, mistranslations, and misunderstandings in treatment instructions. These language and cultural challenges may even discourage people from seeking health care at the center. Angela recognizes that the center may not be fully realizing its mission to serve the community.

Much of the staff at the center is bilingual, but they predominantly speak only Spanish and English. This has served the clinic generally well as the largest demographic group aside from Whites is Hispanic or Latino minorities (see Table 16-4).

TABLE 16-4 Selected Demographics: Queens County, New York	
Race	**Percentage of Population**
White (alone)	30.2%
Hispanic or Latino (of any race)	26.9%
Puerto Rican	5.3%
Mexican	3.6%
Other	18.0%
Asian (alone)	21.9%
Chinese	8.5%
Asian Indian	6.0%
Korean	2.6%
Filipino	2.0%
Japanese	0.2%
Other	2.6%
Black or African American (alone)	17.6%
American Indian and Alaska Native (alone)	0.3%
Other race (alone)	1.6%
Two or more races	1.5%

Source: Queens County, New York, ACS Demographic and Housing Estimates: 2009, American Community Survey, U.S. Census Bureau.[1]

However, as the community has become more diverse, there is a need for other languages and cultural skills, particularly to serve Asian communities. The existing interpretation services at the health center are largely insufficient to deal with this evolving problem. The majority of residents in the community speak a language other than English at home (see Table 16-5). However, the health center is inadequately prepared to handle multiple languages. The operator service on the phone, for instance, provides language services only in English or Spanish. Angela wonders how

TABLE 16-5 Selected Demographics: Queens County, New York

Language Spoken at Home (Population 5 years old and over)	Percentage of Population
English only	44.2%
Language other than English	55.8%
Speak English less than "very well"	28.5%
Spanish	23.8%
Speak English less than "very well"	12.6%
Other Indo-European languages	16.8%
Speak English less than "very well"	7.2%
Asian and Pacific Islander languages	13.5%
Speak English less than "very well"	8.1%
Other languages	1.7%

Source: Queens County, New York, Selected Social Characteristics in the United States: 2009, American Community Survey, U.S. Census Bureau.[2]

many potential patients hang up when trying to schedule an appointment at the center due to frustration of not being able to understand enough to get through the menus. The management team recognizes the increasing need to recruit more multilingual staff and hire interpreters. The health center has hired interpreter services, but they can cost up to $190 an hour, which can be very expensive for a not-for-profit organization.

Background

The demographics of the United States population over the next 40 years will experience significant changes. The Pew Research Center estimates that 82% of the increase in the United States population (117 million) will be attributed to new immigrants (67 million) arriving from 2005 to 2050 and their United States-born descendents (50 million).[3] The report states that by 2050 nearly one in five Americans (19%) will be an immigrant. According to the U.S. Census Bureau's American Community Survey, the percent of people who are foreign born in New York State is 21.3%, which is above the national average of 12.4%, and within Queens County in New York, the percent is more than double at 46.6%.[4]

The demographic trends in the United States population highlight the need for more diversity among health care professions. Greater diversity will lead to improved public health by providing patients with increased opportunities to see practitioners who share their common race, language, ethnicity, and culture. In its study, "The Rationale for Diversity in the Health Professions: A Review of the Evidence," the Health Resources and Services Administration found compelling evidence to support a diverse health professions workforce:

> "Minority patients tend to receive better interpersonal care from practitioners of their own race or ethnicity, particularly in primary care and mental health settings; Non-English speaking patients experience better interpersonal care, greater medical comprehension, and greater likelihood of keeping follow-up appointments when they see a language-concordant practitioner, particularly in mental health care."[5]

Next Steps

Angela recognizes that there are tremendous needs in the immigrant communities in Queens County that are not being met. While the health center provides quality care, there needs to be a mechanism in place to deal with language and cultural barriers to improve interactions between patients and health professionals.

Discussion Questions

1. How should Angela and the management team address this challenge?

2. Do patients have a fundamental right to an interpreter?

3. Should the staff of a community health center and FQHC reflect the diversity of the population they serve?

4. If so, what are some of the challenges an organization will face trying to realize that objective?

References

[1] U.S. Census Bureau. (n.d.). Queens County, New York, ACS Demographic and Housing Estimates: 2009, American Community Survey. Retrieved from http://factfinder.census.gov/servlet/ADPTable?_bm=y&-geo_id=05000US36081&qr_name=ACS_2009_1YR_G00_DP5&-context=adp&-ds_name=&-tree_id=309&_lang=en&-redoLog=false&-format=

[2] U.S. Census Bureau. (n.d.). Queens County, New York, Selected Social Characteristics in the United States: 2009, American Community Survey. Retrieved from http://factfinder.census.gov/servlet/ADPTable?_bm=y&-geo_id=05000US36081&-qr_name=ACS_2009_1YR_G00_DP2&-context=adp&-ds_name=&-tree_id=309&-_lang=en&-redoLog=false&-format=

[3] Passel, J.S., & Cohn, D. (2008, February 11). *U.S. population projections 2005-2050.* Pew Research Center Report. Retrieved from http://pewhispanic.org/files/reports/85.pdf

[4] U.S. Census Buearu. (n.d.). 2005-2009 American Community Survey 5-Year Estimates. Retrievedfromhttp://factfinder.census.gov/servlet/GCTTable?_bm=y&geo_id=01000US&-_box_head_nbr=GCT0501&-ds_name=ACS_2009_5YR_G00_&-_lang=en&-mt_name=ACS_2008_5YR_G00_GCT0501_US9F&-format=US-9F

[5] U.S. Department of Health and Human Services, Health Resources and Services Administration, Bureau of Health Professions. (2006, October). The rationale for diversity in the health professions: A review of the evidence. Retrieved from ftp://ftp.hrsa.gov/bhpr/workforce/diversity.pdf

CASE 9: A *GIARDIA* OUTBREAK?

Situation

"This is the tenth confirmed case of giardiasis we received this week," relayed Eric, to one of the department's environmental engineers. Eric works as an environmental health specialist in the Northwest Region office of the Pennsylvania Department of Environmental Protection (DEP), Bureau of Water Standards and Facility Regulation. Several physicians in the Local Township called his office this week to report positive laboratory tests of *Giardia* cysts in their patients, who were experiencing flu-like illnesses with symptoms of persistent diarrhea, nausea, and abdominal cramps. The physicians were growing concerned of a potential outbreak of a waterborne contaminant in the community's water supply, yet they hadn't seen any public announcements from the DEP. Officials from the local health department had also called earlier in the day to ask if any "boil water advisories" should be in effect.

One of Eric's essential duties in his job as an environmental health specialist was to respond to and investigate complaints and violations of Pennsylvania's water supply and wastewater treatment facilities. His department develops surveillance strategies that direct field inspector activities at water supply and wastewater treatment facilities. In addition, he works closely with the Bureau of Watershed Management which is responsible for planning and managing the water resources in Pennsylvania, including monitoring and regulating water sources to ensure safe drinking water, as required by the *Safe Drinking Water Act* (SDWA).

The Local Township is a small city in rural Pennsylvania, with a population of less than 8,000, located near the Allegheny National Forest. Eric knows that many rural cities in the mountainous areas of Pennsylvania are particularly susceptible to waterborne contaminants since their water supplies from lakes, ponds, or streams can become contaminated with animal droppings or human sewage discharge. Although water treatment plants have been constructed in many communities, some of the more remote areas still did not have completely effective water systems that were fully risk-compliant. Eric remembered studying the *Giardia* outbreak that occurred in 1979 in Bradford City, a community not too dissimilar to the Local Township.

Background

Giardia and *Cryptosporidium* are the most common etiologic agents causing water-borne outbreaks in the United States. *Giardia* and *Cryptosporidium* are protozoan intestinal parasites that cause diarrheal illnesses in people. The parasites are found in every region of the United States and throughout the world. The cysts of the organisms are commonly transmitted from the environment to humans through contaminated water or food. The illnesses associated with the parasites, giardiasis and cryptosporidiosis, are usually acute and can become chronic and last up to one or two months. From 1965 to 1996, there were 118 outbreaks of giardiasis in the United States with 26,305 reported cases of illness, mainly attributed to the consumption of contaminated drinking water from public and individual water systems with the majority of cases occurring due to inadequately treated surface water systems.[1]

The state of Pennsylvania was once among the leaders nationally in the number of recorded waterborne disease outbreaks.[2] The *Giardia* outbreak in Bradford City in 1979 is an informative reference case. Bradford's water system is supplied from three upland reservoirs. A reservoir is an artificial lake created in a river valley by a dam or built by excavation to store water. Prior to the outbreak, the water from the reservoirs was delivered directly to consumers without any filtration or other barriers. Treatment relied exclusively on chlorination. The water passed out of the reservoirs into the transmission mains. During September to December 1979, 3,500 cases of giardiasis occurred in Bradford.[3] A number of events lead to this outbreak. First, even though chlorination treatment was provided, it was interrupted and deficient at times. Second, heavy rains caused runoff in the watershed leading to high turbidity. Turbidity is a key test of water quality and represents the cloudiness in water caused by suspended particles. Incidentally, Bradford had applied for and was granted a waiver from the U.S. Environmental Protection Agency of its obligation to notify the public of the high-turbidity measures in the water supply. Although chlorinated, the water was unfiltered prior to passing through the transmission mains. Third, beavers in the watershed were infected with *Giardia* cysts contributing to the infection of the water supply. In order to ensure that no future outbreaks of the disease occurred, Bradford City constructed a water treatment plant to treat all water delivered to the city. The facility was capable of removing all microorganisms from the water through chemical treatment and filtration.

Next Steps

Eric's department had been in the process of evaluating local monitoring and sampling equipment in the area, so the field inspection surveys for the Local Township might have been delayed. If this turned out to be the beginning of an outbreak, his department could be in store for some harsh criticism. The environmental engineers were in the process of coordinating with local inspectors to collect more data, and Eric thought that this may be the best course of action before alerting the public of a waterborne disease outbreak. Eric sat down and reflected on the best course of action to take. He considered calling the local health officials to update them on the situation. Eric thought it might be prudent to ask the local media to alert residents to boil water before consumption. However, his department still needed to determine the cause, and he didn't want to risk alarming the public unnecessarily. He knew he should coordinate any external communication activity first with his supervisor, even if it delayed getting the message out to the public. He picked up the phone to call his supervisor and ask for recommendations.

Discussion Questions

1. What course of action should Eric follow if inspection tests confirm the Local Township's water supply is contaminated by *Giardia*?

2. What parties should Eric involve in the process of determining an appropriate response by the department?

3. Should Eric release an official "boil water notice" to inform the public as a precaution?

References

[1] United States Environmental Protection Agency, Office of Water. (1998, August). Giardia: Human health criteria document (EPA No. 823R002). Retrieved from http://water.epa.gov/action/advisories/drinking/upload/2009_02_03_criteria_humanhealth_microbial_giardia.pdf

[2] Pennsylvania Department of Environmental Protection, Bureau of Water Standards and Facility Regulation. (2009, November). Cryptosporidium and Giardia… Are they in YOUR drinking water? (3800-BK-DEP0524). Retrieved from http://www.elibrary.dep.state.pa.us/dsweb/Get/Document-77461/3800-BK-DEP0524.pdf

[3] Karanis, P., Kourenti, C., & Smith, H. (2007). Waterborne transmission of protozoan parasites: A worldwide review of outbreaks and lessons learnt. Journal of Water and Health, 5(1), 1–38. doi: 10.2166/wh.2006.002

CASE 10: ZERO-TOLERANCE FOR SMOKING

Situation

Theresa arrived early in the office. As supervisor of a Mandover Health Clinic, a large community health center (CHC) in a suburb of Chicago, she had a full agenda planned for the day. However, she couldn't stop thinking about what she witnessed the previous evening. After work, she had taken her family to the Olive Garden restaurant for dinner. As she was walking into the restaurant, she noticed out of the corner of her eye one of her employees, Hanna, smoking in the parking lot. Theresa was dismayed—what a surprising and disappointing sight. She didn't expect to see any of her employees smoking, not to mention one of her most senior ones. Hanna was well liked by the staff at Mandover. She performed her duties well at the clinic, and the rest of the staff often sought her out for advice; however, by smoking Hanna was setting a poor example for the organization and even more so as a seasoned health professional.

The Mandover Health Clinic is a smoke-free workplace as required by the *Smoke Free Illinois Act* that went into effect in 2008. The Act prohibits smoking in a public place or place of employment. Employees who smoke at a workplace can be fired for violating the law. Theresa has not seen any employees smoking outside the building so she assumed, incorrectly of course, that none of her employees smoked. Moreover, she expected that as public health workers they would know the dangers of smoking and would naturally choose not to smoke. The more Theresa thought about the situation, the more upset she became. Mandover offers a smoking cessation program to new employees and she thought the program was successful. Theresa wondered how many other employees might be smoking off-duty. Theresa felt somewhat embarrassed thinking about her public health employees smoking behind her back. Don't they realize that smoking increases our health care insurance premiums, not to mention it reflects badly on the image of Mandover as a community health clinic?

Background

More companies are adopting zero-tolerance smoking policies that prohibit employees from smoking in their private lives. Employers are firing employees who fail to quit smoking after a period of time and are even banning the hiring of people who smoke. The adoption of zero-tolerance policies has accompanied the enactment of smoke-free work and public places laws by states, municipalities, and companies. Twenty-four states and commonwealths in the United States now have 100% smoke-free laws that prohibit smoking in all workplaces, restaurants, and bars.[1]

Employers support these policies as a means to curb rising health care costs. However, there may be a more idealistic objective. Health care companies, including public health agencies, may well consider the example they are setting by accepting employees who smoke despite the knowledge of the inherent health risks of such behavior. The thinking goes that if an employee of a health care company who should know the health consequences can't be responsible enough not to smoke, then who can be? The World Health Organization (WHO) has set an illustrative policy. According to the WHO's Smoking and Tobacco Use Policy, the organization will not recruit smokers or other tobacco users. The policy states that "In the case of tobacco, the importance for WHO not to be seen as 'normalizing' tobacco use also warrants consideration in the Organization's recruitment policy" and "The Organization has a responsibility to ensure that this is reflected in all its work, including in its recruitment practices and in the image projected by the Organization and its staff members."[2]

Next Steps

Theresa debated whether to set a strict example of Hanna by showing that smoking would not be tolerated by any employee at Mandover. She had a range of options from asking employees to sign a pledge not to smoke as a condition of employment to mandating random testing. If an employee chose not to take a test or the test came back positive, then their employment would be terminated. She wondered whether there would be much resistance in implementing such programs, particularly considering they worked for a health clinic. However, first she needed to decide what action to take with Hanna. She could ask Hanna to participate in the clinic's anti-smoking program, but if she refused, Theresa may have to let her go.

Discussion Questions

1. What would you do if you were the supervisor faced with this situation?

2. Should an employer fire an employee who refuses to stop smoking?

3. What human resources policies are available to encourage employees to quit smoking?

4. What do you think of the WHO's Smoking and Tobacco Use Policy? Should a public health organization, in its role as an employer, observe a higher standard with respect to specific health behaviors that are deemed unacceptable for its employees?

References

[1] American Nonsmokers' Rights Foundation. (2011, January 2). U.S. 100% Smokefree laws in workplaces and restaurants and bars. Retrieved from http://www.nosmoke.org/pdf/WRBLawsMap.pdf

[2] World Health Organization. (2008, September). WHO policy on non-recruitment of smokers or other tobacco users: Frequently asked questions. Retrieved from the World Health Organization's website: http://www.who.int/employment/FAQs_smoking_English.pdf

CASE 11: BUDGET CUTS IN HOME CARE PROGRAM

Situation

Pauline, a Director of the California Department of Social Services (CDSS) for San Martin County, returned to her office after a meeting with the County Board of Supervisors. The Board of Supervisors was considering drastic reductions in the proposed funding for the County's In-Home Supportive Services (IHSS) program. Similar to most municipalities in California, San Martin County faced a substantial budget deficit in the upcoming fiscal year. The economic downturn coupled with the state's budget problems had a lingering effect on the County's revenues.

The County relied on matching state funds to support the IHSS program. Given the state's fiscal woes, the governor was likely to propose significant cuts in all social programs, including IHSS, to try to stop some of the fiscal bleeding. In fact, the previous governor, in his last year of office, had proposed cutting roughly half the funding for the IHSS program. Therefore, it was unlikely that the County would escape funding cuts from the state, and it had to make some drastic decisions.

The Board of Supervisors tasked Pauline with working with San Martin County's IHSS Public Authority Governing Board to come up with some budget recommendations. Primary among those recommendations will be significant cuts in the wages and benefits of the home care workers for the IHSS program. Pauline knows that entertaining such discussions will ignite a backlash from the Service Employees International Union—United Healthcare Workers West (SEIU), which represents the County's home care workers. The County's collective bargaining contract with the Local SEIU expires in two months and the Board of Supervisors wants to begin negotiations. Despite the valuable services these home care workers provide, they will likely suffer some form of wage and benefit cuts. Pauline realizes that those reductions in turn could have a debilitating effect on the County's senior and disabled citizens who might not receive the level of care they require.

The Board of Supervisors and members of the Governing Board want to take a hard negotiating position with the union and ask for a cut of $2.00 in the hourly wage rate of $11.50 and require workers to pay for a greater percentage of their health insurance benefits. A few Supervisors think workers should cover their own health benefits given the current fiscal crisis for the County. Pauline believes this aggressive position will antagonize the president of the Local SEIU, although she thinks he must realize that the County is hurting for money and the state funding reductions are imminent. Pauline recognizes that these wage cuts might force home care workers to leave the profession to look for jobs with better wages and benefits, leaving many clients without care. As a result, these clients might end up in nursing or long-term care facilities to get the care they need, costing the County more money in the long run. The Board of Supervisors and Local SEIU are headed for a heated, public debate over the next few months, and Pauline will likely be in the middle of it.

Background

In-Home Supportive Services is a division within the California Department of Social Services of the Health and Human Services Agency. The CDSS provides services to needy children and adults through 51 offices throughout California, 58 county welfare departments, and a number of community-based organizations.[1] The IHSS Program provides personal care and domestic services to persons who are elderly, disabled, or blind and who live in their own homes. These services can include household chores, food shopping, non-medical personal care services, assistance with medications and prosthesis care, accompaniment to medical appointments, and protective supervision. The IHSS program is provided as an alternative to placement in nursing homes and long-term care facilities. As of December 2010, more than 442,000 individuals received services under the program at a monthly cost of over $400 million.[2]

IHSS is offered in every county in the State of California. Each county has an IHSS Public Authority which is a public agency established by each respective County Board of Supervisors. The IHSS Public Authority serves low-income elderly and disabled citizens who require home care services in order to remain in their homes. The Public Authority Governing Board is advised in its recommendations by an advisory committee composed of appointed citizen members who are consumers or providers of in-home supportive services, consumer advocates, or advocates for related interested community organizations.

Next Steps

Pauline has an upcoming meeting scheduled with the executive director of the Public Authority Governing Board to discuss the proposed budget cuts. She needs to develop a social services programs funding recommendation to present to the County Board of Supervisors at its next meeting. The Board of Supervisors will use the recommendation as their first proposal to the SEIU to begin contract negotiations.

Discussion Questions

1. If you represented the Local SEIU, what would be your position and how would you defend it?

2. If you represented the County Board of Supervisors, what would be your position and how would you defend it?

3. Do you think the County Board of Supervisors and SEIU can reach an agreement?

4. What will be the likely public health implications of drastic budget cuts in the IHSS program?

References

[1] California Department of Social Services. (n.d.). About CDSS. Retrieved from CA.gov website: http://www.dss.cahwnet.gov/cdssweb/PG190.htm

[2] California Department of Social Services. (2011, January 10). In-Home Supportive Services Management Statistics Summary Report – December. Retrieved from http://www.cdss.ca.gov/agedblinddisabled/res/pdf/2010DecMgmtStats.pdf

CASE 12: DON'T ASK, BUT TELL

Situation

The Company Commander, Captain Ronald, listened to the report from the emergency room (ER) physician on the phone. One of his unit members, Army Specialist (SPC) Garrett, was in observation at the Military Treatment Facility (MTF) on the Main Operating Base (MOB) station for severe injuries. The physician relayed the specific details of the situation. After completing the day's pre-mobilization training and having dinner, SPC Garrett reported to his barracks around 2000 hours (8 p.m.). At 2200 hours (10 p.m.), he came to the MTF dazed and bleeding and was immediately assessed by a medical technician. The medical evaluation intake showed that SPC Garrett suffered contusions, lacerations, and abrasions to his head and torso. In explaining the cause of his injuries, the patient stated that he "fell down" in the barracks. However, his injuries were inconsistent with a fall, and the medic suspected that he had been beaten, and possibly kicked. The medic reported the incident to the ER physician on call, who further evaluated the patient. Given the seriousness of the injuries, the physician recommended that SPC Garrett remain under observation for several days as he suspected possible mTBI (mild traumatic brain injury), due to blows to SPC Garrett's head.

Captain (CPT) Ronald absorbed the report. While at first he was shocked by the news, he later realized there had been early signs of escalating aggression. There had been an increasing level of animosity directed toward SPC Garrett by several of his fellow unit members throughout that week's training sessions. SPC Garrett was a good soldier. He was disciplined, physically fit, and technically competent. However, he was more reserved than the other men and as a result seemed to be a bit of an outsider. Some of the other unit members fed on this, and regularly taunted him, including making off-handed remarks about him being gay or "having sugar in the blood." The taunting escalated after news of the repeal of the Don't Ask, Don't Tell (DADT) policy. While CPT Ronald was aware of the remarks, he generally dismissed them as they didn't rise to the level that warranted any action. He realized now that a few of his men in Charlie Company resented the repeal of DADT, and they might have acted out. The company was preparing for an extended mobilization in the AOR (Area of Responsibility), and CPT Ronald knew he had several decisions to make regarding this potential violation of Uniform Code of Military Justice (UCMJ) against SPC Garrett.

Background

The ban on gay service members dates back to 1950 when the United States Congress passed the UCMJ which included the basic policies, discharge procedures, and appeal channels for the disposition of homosexual service members. In January 1981, President Reagan issued Defense Directive 1332.14, which directed the Department of Defense to discharge any gay, lesbian, or bisexual service members pursuant to the UCMJ, declaring homosexuality incompatible with military service. In 1993, in his first year in office, President Clinton called for legislation to end the ban and allow all citizens to serve in the military regardless of sexual orientation. In response, Congress inserted text into the *Defense Authorization Act for Fiscal Year 1994*, passed in December 1993, requiring the military to abide by regulations essentially identical to the 1982 absolute ban policy (10 U.S.C. § 654). In response, President Clinton issued Defense Directive 1304.26 as an enforcement guideline for the law, which became known as "Don't Ask, Don't Tell." The Defense

Directive served as an enforcement policy mandating that military officials not ask about or require members to reveal their sexual orientation, that members may be discharged for claiming to be homosexual or having an intent to engage in homosexual activities, and that military officials are not to pursue rumors about the sexual orientation of the service members or condone harassment or violence against service members for any reason.

In December 2010, the United States Congress passed the *Don't Ask, Don't Tell Repeal Act of 2010* ending the ban on gay service members. Prior to the repeal taking effect, the President, Secretary of Defense, and Chairman of the Joint Chiefs of Staff have to certify to Congress that the Department of Defense is prepared to implement the repeal and that in doing so there will be no harm to military readiness, military effectiveness, unit cohesion, and recruiting and retention of the Armed Forces. The repeal will take effect 60 days after Congress receives the certification. Upon passage of the new law, Robert M. Gates, Secretary of Defense, noted that "successful implementation will depend upon strong leadership, a clear message and proactive education throughout the force."[1]

Next Steps

CPT Ronald planned to visit SPC Garrett in the MTF the next day and press him for the names of the men he suspected were involved in the incident. Once he got their names he would arrange through the Security Forces to handle the interrogation. While an established military justice protocol was in place to deal with this type of situation, CPT Ronald was more concerned about how to defuse any potential for further violence within his unit. He couldn't have more of his unit members heading to the MTF with injuries from altercations or mental health issues. The repeal of DADT was a sensitive topic for some members, and the incident with SPC Garrett may affect unit cohesion. He could not risk any division on the battlefield. Above the individual health and safety concerns of his unit members, he was concerned that the policy might impact the Battle Buddy system that has been an essential part of the military in a deployed environment. CPT Ronald recognized that he needed to send a clear message to his company to defuse any conflict and strengthen the cohesion of his unit.

Discussion Questions

1. What message should CPT Ronald deliver to his unit in response to the incident with SPC Garrett?

2. How did the military's policy on homosexuality imperil the health of service members, the military, and the country (consider undiagnosed STDs, medical history intake, mental health)?

3. What implications will the repeal of DADT have on the health of armed service members and the community at large?

Reference

[1] Wong, S. (2010, December 18). "Don't ask" repeal wins final passage. *Politico.* Retrieved from http://www.politico.com/news/stories/1210/46576.html

CASE 13: SENIOR CYBER CAFÉ

Situation

Linda, President of the Mid Florida Area Agency on Aging in Gainesville, was concerned about complaints she had received from several seniors at the local Senior Center. The complaints involved two of her volunteers, Kim and Mark, college students from a local technical school. Kim and Mark were new volunteers at the agency and given their computer proficiency, they were greatly needed. They had explained to Linda that they were volunteering in order to "give back to the community," but probably also to augment their resumes. Linda put their computer skills to great use and asked them to teach computer-training classes two times a week at the local Senior Center as part of a Senior Cyber Café program. The program was a new initiative for the agency and Linda had great expectations. The program consisted of a 10-week computer-training class that provided instruction on basic computer use including how to access the Internet and use e-mail. Linda had heard of similar programs that offered many benefits to seniors aside from just learning how to use the computer, including increased connectivity to family and friends, increased empowerment and autonomy, and access to information about health and activities. She saw the Senior Cyber Café initiative as a vital component of the socialization programs offered by the agency in its partnership with senior centers.

Linda reviewed her notes on the complaints. She was sensitive to the seniors' concerns as she recognized that many of them were adapting to "aging," as she had learned in her gerontology training. Some of the class participants might even feel embarrassed over their sense of helplessness with computers and the Internet. In terms of the complaints, apparently during the classes Kim and Mark came across as condescending to the seniors. For instance, one senior complained that Kim had a patronizing attitude when she answered their questions and tended to dismiss their concerns, often replying "Why?" Another senior said that Mark sometimes acted like they were mentally impaired, over-compensating when he spoke to them and showed them how to use the applications. These behaviors were interfering with the seniors' enjoyment and their patience in the learning process. Enthusiasm for the classes was high—there was already a waiting list for the next class session when the current one ended in eight weeks—and Linda didn't want anything to jeopardize it.

Background

The Mid Florida Area Agency on Aging office in Gainesville is one of 11 Area Agencies on Aging (AAA) in Florida. The AAAs are private not-for-profit entities that plan, coordinate, and fund support services for seniors in their respective services areas. They are an integral component of the elder-services network of the Florida Department of Elder Affairs, the designated State Unit on Aging which was created by the *Older Americans Act of 1965*. Through partnerships with local agencies, faith-based and nonprofit community organizations, and local governments, the AAAs deliver an array of services to residents age 60 and older to continue to live active, healthy lives in their senior years.

One of the most important partnerships for the AAAs is with Florida's senior centers. The senior centers are community facilities that provide a broad range of educational, recreational, and wellness services to independent seniors. They provide seniors with the opportunity to join together to visit with friends and participate in community-based activities. The majority of senior centers are located in freestanding buildings, within community or recreation centers, or in local government buildings. The senior centers use their own funds to operate and as a result must rely heavily on volunteers. Florida, with one of the largest concentrations of residents age 60 and older, has approximately 260 senior centers which draw approximately 380,000 visitors per year and more than 18,500 visitors per day.[1]

Next Steps

Linda evaluated her alternatives. She recognized that with budget constraints, public organizations like her agency and the senior centers needed the time and skills of volunteers. The success of the Senior Cyber Café program was important to her agency and she needed to ensure she had volunteers with the necessary computer skills to teach the classes. However, she also recognized that many of these volunteers, including Kim and Mark, did not have any formal training or experience in teaching, especially to senior citizens.

Given the existing complaints, Linda realized that she may need to replace Kim and Mark as instructors. This action might set a good example to other volunteers that they need to be more sensitive in how they interact with seniors. However, this action will be difficult to implement as she doesn't have many other volunteers with that level of computer proficiency and she doesn't want to interrupt the class sessions. Moreover, it might backfire on the agency by giving a negative impression for other volunteers, especially if Kim and Mark react poorly to the decision. Kim and Mark may be well-intentioned and simply not be aware of their offensive communication behaviors. Linda recognized that intergenerational communication was often based on stereotypical expectations. She didn't want to overreact, and replacing them might send the wrong signal. Linda wanted to create an enjoyable experience for volunteers so that they would continue to come back as well as encourage others to volunteer through positive word of mouth.

Another alternative might be to move Kim and Mark into another role that did not require teaching or direct interaction with the seniors in the class. Again, this might be difficult as she did not have many other volunteers with the same computer skills. She could not afford to hire professional computer trainers to teach the Senior

Cyber Café project given budget constraints. In addition, it would be hard to find an alternate role in the agency that did not involve direct interaction with seniors at least on some level. Another option might be to pair a staff member or a more senior volunteer with Kim and Mark in the classroom to offer some mentoring. Linda even considered a more far-reaching solution—offer an age-sensitive communication training program for all volunteers. Linda weighed her alternatives. She needed to make a decision before next week's class at the senior center.

Discussion Questions

1. How would you respond to the complaints?

2. Would you replace Kim and Mark as instructors for the classes?

3. Explain what intergenerational communication issues may be present. How would you manage them?

4. Describe the challenges of managing and motivating volunteers within the public health workforce.

Reference

[1] Florida Department of Elder Affairs. (2010, November 20). Florida's Senior Centers. Retrieved from http://elderaffairs.state.fl.us/english/seniorcenter.php

CASE 14: COLLABORATIVE APPROACH TO DIABETES PREVENTION AND CARE

Situation

In 2010, United Health Group (UHG), a leading health benefits and managed care company (http://www.unitedhealthgroup.com), announced an innovative new model, the Diabetes Prevention and Control Alliance (Alliance), to help prevent and control diabetes, prediabetes, and obesity.[1] The Alliance is anchored by two integrated programs: the Diabetes Prevention Program (DPP) and the Diabetes Control Program (DCP). The DPP is a partnership between the YMCA of the USA (YMCA) and UHG that offers, through local community YMCAs, a group-based lifestyle intervention for people at high risk of developing diabetes. The YMCA provides lifestyle coaches to help participants learn to eat healthier and increase their physical activity through a 16-session program, with monthly support thereafter to maintain their progress. The YMCA's DPP is based on the Diabetes Prevention Program funded by the National Institutes of Health (NIH) and the CDC.[2] UHG will reimburse YMCAs offering the DPP. The DCP is a partnership between UHG and Walgreens that provides diabetics with access to community-based pharmacists who will provide education and behavioral intervention in the convenient setting of a local pharmacy. Health plan participants whose employers offer the programs and who are identified with diabetes or prediabetes through UHG's screening model are invited to participate voluntarily in the programs at no cost.

Karen, the Director of Government Funding in the office of Accountability and Funding at the YMCA, recognizes that the Alliance has the potential to have meaningful system-wide effects on the diabetes epidemic. In particular, the program extends service delivery beyond the traditional physician office setting. The YMCA and Walgreens have considerable reach and scale, and they increase access to a much larger group of people in the community at high risk for diabetes. For instance, 57% of United States households are located within three miles of a YMCA.[3] Reception from local communities in the pilot cities has been generally positive, but there will need to be an education campaign to fully inform qualifying candidates to optimize participation. Karen has been working with the program coordinators within the YMCA and UHG to develop informational campaigns. The YMCA trainers and the community-based pharmacists represent significant access points to increase responsiveness and equity in the system. The YMCA is making the DPP available to everyone who meets the criteria regardless of their health insurance coverage.

Background

The diabetes epidemic in the United States is accelerating at an alarming rate. According to the Centers for Disease Control and Prevention (CDC), approximately 24 million people or 7.8% of the United States' population had diabetes in 2007 and another 57 million had prediabetes.[4] By 2020, an estimated 52% of the adult population will have diabetes or prediabetes and more than 90% of those with prediabetes will be unaware of their condition.[4] Private spending, largely borne by employers and employees, is currently estimated at $57 billion a year and is projected to reach nearly $1 trillion in total between 2011 and 2020.[5] The epidemic will have major implications for people's health and health care costs, placing a financial strain on families, employers, insurers, states, and the federal government.

Progression to diabetes among those with prediabetes and to complications among those with diabetes is not inevitable. Research from the CDC indicates that two-thirds of all diabetics do not follow their physicians' advice or treatment guidelines on how to manage their disease.[6] People struggle to maintain a healthy lifestyle and often lack knowledge about diabetes and prediabetes conditions. There is substantial evidence that interventions ranging from lifestyle changes to early support for diabetic-related complications can make a meaningful difference in reducing the health and financial toll of diabetes. For instance, research shows that a typical prediabetic person who reduces body weight by 7% through a combination of exercise and caloric restriction can reduce the risk of becoming diabetic by 58%.[7]

Successful interventions will require new approaches outside of medical management of the complications of diabetes, which has been the traditional focus of treatment for the disease. Not only will this require engagement of patients and health care providers, but also health insurers if a real meaningful impact is to be made on the epidemic. Employers are increasingly looking to insurers to do more to manage health care costs than just collecting premiums and paying providers.[8] With enactment of the new federal health care law, insurers will be required to cover people regardless of their medical condition, so the financial implications are clear. Despite the benefits of early intervention, until recently no insurance company has paid for evidence-based diabetes prevention and control programs.

The initiative by UHG represents a new paradigm in health care focused on prevention. As indicated in a statement by the Chairman of UHG's Center for Health Reform & Modernization, Simon Stevens, there is recognition of the new role health insurers must play in the system: "It will mean a focus not only on the 'flow' of health care consumption, but on managing the 'stock' of population health risk."[9] UHG is using its broad assets in technology, health data, evidence-based medical decision making, and disease management to ensure the dissemination and use of reliable and timely information to use in the program. UHG, as one of the nation's largest health insurers, is providing the primary source of financing. UHG will cover the services at no charge to plan participants enrolled in employer-provided health insurance plans. The Alliance represents the first time in the United States that a health plan will pay for evidence-based diabetes prevention and control programs.[9] To fortify these efforts, UHG has committed $2.25 million to support the YMCA's healthy-living and obesity prevention initiatives.

Next Steps

Karen is impressed with how the Alliance brings together partners from the private, public, and nonprofit sectors to provide leadership and governance to successfully implement the programs. The YMCA and UHG are slowly rolling out the programs nationally, starting with seven markets in four states: Cincinnati, Columbus, and Dayton, Ohio; Indianapolis, Indiana; Minneapolis and St. Paul, Minnesota; and Phoenix, Arizona. This coordinated approach recognizes that the programs will evolve as they are implemented in different markets. Prevention and control of diabetes in the health care system are tightly linked. UHG and employers understand that by engaging individuals to take preventative steps they can decrease the odds of employees moving into higher-cost treatment categories. Participants who regularly follow the programs will receive financial incentives, positive encouragement, and motivation through improved health.

As the benefits become tangible, more employers, employees, and insurers will likely offer similar programs. Reimbursing a community-based organization for delivering prevention and control programs may seem counter-intuitive for a profit-oriented company. However, UHG may protect itself in the long run as diabetic patients who do not control their disease could become future liabilities if they change jobs and join employers who are fully insured by UHG. All insurers benefit from healthier members. It is cheaper to give up co-payments and premiums rather than pay for full-blown diabetic disease conditions later. Ultimately, interventions to a system that rely on behavioral modifications are likely to face resistance to change. Although the benefits of prevention and control appear obvious, participation is not assured and insurance coverage for these programs and the financial incentives offered are crucial steps to get more people engaged. Karen recognizes that as a relatively new intervention program, both at the YMCA and UHG, the Alliance will face future challenges.

Discussion Questions

1. Discuss how the initiative by the YMCA and UHG represents a new paradigm in health care focused on prevention.

2. What are some of the challenges of bringing together partners from the private, public, and nonprofit sectors to successfully implement programs, such as the Alliance?

3. How should each organization measure the success of the programs?

4. How are public health program initiatives enhanced by private- and public-sector partnerships?

5. Do you think a profit-oriented company working with a community-based, nonprofit organization to deliver a public health program is counter-intuitive?

6. What issues do you think the partners will face as they slowly roll out the Alliance on a nationwide basis?

References

[1] UnitedHealth Group. (2010, April 14). UnitedHealth Group launches innovative alliance providing free access to programs that help prevent and control diabetes and obesity [Press release]. Retrieved from http://www.unitedhealthgroup.com/newsroom/news.aspx?id=199e50a5-557b-4353-b96d-ff060fba10fc

[2] YMCA of the USA. (2010, April 14). YMCA of the USA, UnitedHealth Group collaboration offers new model for chronic disease prevention [Press release]. Retrieved from http://www.ymca.net/news-releases/20100414-ymca-unitedhealth.html

[3] Vaughan, L. (2010, July 10). The YMCA's Diabetes Prevention Program. Presentation at the Alliance for Health Reform Briefing Co-Sponsored by UnitedHealth Foundation.

[4] U.S. Department of Health and Human Services, Centers for Disease Control and Prevention. (2008). National diabetes fact sheet: general information and national estimates on diabetes in the United States, 2007. Retrieved from http://www.cdc.gov/diabetes/pubs/pdf/ndfs_2007.pdf

[5] UnitedHealth Group. (2010, November). *The United States of Diabetes: Challenges and opportunities in the decade ahead* (UnitedHealth Center for Health Reform & Modernization Working Paper 5). Retrieved from http://www.unitedhealthgroup.com/hrm/UNH_WorkingPaper5.pdf

[6] UnitedHealthcare. (2009, January 15). UnitedHealthcare launches first diabetes plan with incentives for preventive care [Press release]. Retrieved from http://www.uhc.com/

news_room/2009_news_release_archive/unitedhealthcare_launches_diabetes_plan_with_incentives_for_preventive_care.htm

7 UnitedHealthcare. (2009, January). Diabetes Health Plan: Fact Sheet January 2009. Retrieved from http://www.uhc.com/live/uhc_com/Assets/Documents/DiabetesHealthPlan.pdf

8 Abelson, R. (2010, April 13). An insurer's new approach to diabetes. *The New York Times*. Retrieved from http://www.nytimes.com/2010/04/14/health/14diabetes.html?_r=1

9 UnitedHealth Group. (2010, October 4). UnitedHealth Group pledges $2.25 million to fortify the Y's efforts to prevent obesity and related chronic diseases [Press release]. Retrieved from http://www.unitedhealthgroup.com/newsroom/news.aspx?id=d0be9be3-b4ef-46ae-bfe3-e2f5c10ac959

CASE 15: TOY RECALL PROMPTS ATTENTION TO LEAD POISONING

Situation

Ryan, the Chief of the state's Bureau of Lead Poisoning Prevention, has received numerous calls, e-mails, and letters from concerned parents of young children after the recent recall of toys found to contain lead-based paint. The toys were imported by a well-known United States company from its contract manufacturer in China. The company, in coordination with the U.S. Consumer Product Safety Commission, announced the recall last month. The toys represented a very small fraction of the company's overall business and product line, so there seemed to be a perception of the lack of urgency in dealing with the recall. Parents have been outraged, not just about the possibility of lead poisoning, but frustrated over how the company is dealing with the problem. The company has refused all interview requests and has issued one brief statement saying an investigation is underway and "We are implementing a corrective action plan." No other details have been offered. Parents are angry as they feel the company is keeping them in the dark as the recall only applied to one of its many toy product lines that are popular with young children. Parents want to know what the corrective action plan reveals. In addition, how safe are the company's other products? Is a recall coming? Ryan is concerned by the company's insufficient communication strategy both with his agency and the general public. His calls to the company's executive office have been returned with simple, prepared statements that offer no additional insight. He did manage to connect with an employee within the company through an old networking contact. The employee revealed that he hasn't seen any internal communications via e-mail or memo on the issue. The employee really didn't know what was going on with the company's management team and why they have been so silent. Ryan joined the parents' frustration. His primary concern is to protect the well-being and safety of the state's children. Without the company's cooperation, however, he cannot perform his job.

Background

Lead exposure in American children has fallen significantly in the last several decades after concerted efforts by public health officials to reduce lead exposure among children from lead-based paint and lead-contaminated dust in deteriorating buildings. Despite this progress, a renewed concern has emerged from exposure to products containing lead that have been imported from developing countries, namely China. Lead poisoning in children causes learning disabilities, kidney failure, anemia, and irreversible brain damage. The U.S. Consumer Product Safety Commission (CPSC) has announced the recall of numerous children's products containing hazardous amounts of lead imported from China over the last several years, including metal jewelry, toys, gloves, and chalk.

The CPSC is an Independent Federal Regulatory Agency created in 1972 by Congress under the *Consumer Product Safety Act*. The CPSC protects the public from unreasonable risks of injury or death from consumer products that pose a fire, electrical, chemical, or mechanical hazard or that can injure children. The *Federal Hazardous Substances Act* (FHSA) requires that certain hazardous household products are labeled to alert consumers to potential hazards and to inform them of measures they need to protect themselves from those hazards. The FHSA gives the CPSC the authority to ban any hazardous substance if it determines that the product is so hazardous that the labeling required by the act is inadequate to protect the public. Under the FHSA, any toy or other article that is intended for use by children and that contains a hazardous substance is banned if a child can gain access to the substance.

The American public is growing increasingly concerned over the safety of products imported from China. Recent headline stories of Chinese scandals, involving pet food poisonings, bacterial parasites in contact lens solutions, and deadly toothpaste containing a solvent used in antifreeze, have only contributed to the alarm. Although inspected and banned if necessary, not all products containing hazardous materials are discovered before making it into the American marketplace. The ultimate responsibility for this exposure to hazardous contaminants lies with United States companies purchasing the foreign products.

Next Steps

Ryan weighs his options on how to respond to the company's insufficient communication and at the same time protect the public from any additional exposure to lead poisoning. He needs to coordinate an effective approach by drawing on federal and state agencies, the media, consumer advocates, and even the group of outraged parents.

Discussion Questions

1. What are the most pressing problems for Ryan?

2. What steps could Ryan take to force to the company to communicate with his agency and the public?

3. Aside from the announced recall, does the company have any further obligation or ethical responsibility to provide additional information to the public?

4. The employee within the company revealed that he had not seen any internal communication about the recall and public response. What does this suggest about the company's organizational communication?

5. If you were an executive at the company, how would you deal with this situation?

CASE 16: HEALTHY LIFESTYLES START AT HOME

Situation

Andrew, a lifestyle coach at a community Family YMCA, has started a meeting with a mother and her 10-year-old son to discuss the YMCA's new program, Healthy Family Home. Kristi, the Program Director at the Family YMCA, is also in attendance since Andrew is new with the organization and this is his first time personally consulting with members. After introductions, it is apparent to Andrew that the son is overweight, and may even be obese for his age, but he cannot make that determination definitively without weighing the child. The mother also appears overweight. The mother begins discussing her frustration with her son's weight as she feels helpless over the situation and is concerned that his weight will only get worse. Her son fidgets in his chair as his mother talks. They are obviously sensitive about the issue, and Andrew needs to be cautious with how he discusses the topic of obesity prevention and healthy living. In addition, although Kristi is sitting in the background quietly listening, Andrew knows she is monitoring his personal interactions with the family. Kristi places a high value on members feeling comfortable with her staff so that they would be encouraged to participate in the programs offered by the YMCA. Families such as this one need positive, ongoing support to make healthy living a reality in their lives, and Kristi wants the community YMCA to be a primary resource to them.

Instead of beginning the discussion with a series of questions about the family's eating habits and physical activities at home, which may be perceived as an interrogation, Andrew starts his discussion with the recognition of the many challenges families face. Families are busy and they confront many barriers to healthy lifestyles, including long work hours, overscheduled activities, unsafe neighborhoods, and poor eating choices. Andrew suggests that a solution to overcome these challenges is to make incremental changes toward incorporating healthy activities into family routines. The Healthy Family Home initiative is a program that can help families adopt and maintain healthy behaviors by taking small steps using the tools and resources developed by the YMCA. These tools revolve around The Pillars of a Healthy Family Home:[1]

- Eat Healthy
- Play Every Day
- Get Together
- Go Outside
- Sleep Well

Each Pillar presents examples of objectives for a family to work toward together. They are realistic and achievable goals that recognize that the busiest of families can discover small ways to live healthier. Andrew recommends that the family set goals together each week and keep track of their performance in each of the Pillars.

Background

The YMCA (also referred to as the Y) is a nonprofit community-based, cause-driven organization that promotes programs for youth development, healthy living, and social responsibility. The YMCA's mission "is to put Christian principles into practice through programs that build healthy spirit, mind, and body for all."[2] The YMCA operates on the belief that a strong community can only be achieved by investing in our children, health, and neighbors. In the United States, the Y is comprised of YMCA of the USA, a national resource office, and more than 2,600 YMCAs with approximately 20,000 full-time staff and 500,000 volunteers in 10,000 communities across the country. The Y engages 21 million men, women, and children—regardless of age, income, or background.[2]

During the past four decades, obesity rates have soared among all age groups, increasing more than four-fold among children ages 6 to 11, and today, nearly a third of children and adolescents are overweight or obese, representing more than 23 million kids and teenagers.[3] The prevalence of childhood obesity is a great public health concern as obesity tracks from childhood into adulthood, resulting in significant personal, social, and economic costs. A recent study projected that obesity will account for more than 16% of all healthcare expenditures by 2030.[4]

There are many public health initiatives and programs aimed at addressing this epidemic. The YMCA's Healthy Family Home initiative is centered on the understanding that healthy living begins at home. An objective of the initiative is to support families to sustain healthy lifestyles, as the relationship between a parent and child is a primary source for positive healthy behaviors. It can also serve as a motivator for adult parents to be healthier in their own lives to set an example for their children. Many families, however, need help and direction on how to build health into their lives. Through the program, the YMCA has made an effort to ensure that families are equipped with the tools and knowledge to create healthy environments. The YMCA recognizes that a one-size-fits-all strategy will not work for all families.

Next Steps

After the discussion, Andrew gives the mother and son a Healthy Family Home Starter Kit which explains each of the five pillars and provides family goal examples. The family seems positive about the program and expresses interest in reading the material. Kristi appears happy with their reaction and smiles encouragingly at Andrew as they leave his office. Andrew hopes the family will take an active interest in adopting the self-directed program and will reach out to him for more information, tips, and activities along the way. He plans to recommend some fitness activities at the Y for the son, and perhaps even for the mother, during their next visit. Although Andrew is positive about the meeting, he realizes that the many barriers of everyday living can present formidable obstacles to change. He hopes to have the opportunity to continue his discussions with the son as well as support the family on its continuing journey toward making healthy living a top priority.

Discussion Questions

1. What are the goals of the YMCA's Healthy Family Home initiative? What might be some of the benefits and challenges of this type of public health program that concentrates on the family unit?

2. If you were Andrew, how might you have engaged the family to adopt and maintain healthy habits?

3. As Andrew's supervisor, how would you evaluate his communication approach with the family?

4. Should Andrew have asked if the family had regular primary health care?

5. What actions can public health professionals take to help facilitate changing unhealthy family behaviors?

References

[1] YMCA of the USA. (2010). Build a Healthy Family Home. Retrieved from the YMCA of the USA at http://www.ymca.net/healthy-family-home/

[2] YMCA of the USA. (2010). Facts & Figures. Retrieved from the YMCA of the USA at http://www.ymca.net/organizational-profile/

[3] Robert Wood Johnson Foundation. (2010). Retrieved from http://www.rwjf.org/childhoodobesity/challenge.jsp/"http://www.rwjf.org/childhoodobesity/challenge.jsp

[4] Wang, Y., Beydoun, M.A., Liang, L., Caballero, B., & Kumanyika, S.K. (2008, October). Will all Americans become overweight or obese? Estimating the progression and cost of the US obesity epidemic. *Obesity, 16*(10), 2323–2330.

CASE 17: TOP TEN U.S. PUBLIC HEALTH ACHIEVEMENTS

Situation

Ethan is the Training Coordinator for a large state public health agency in the Northwest. He is in the process of preparing the new-employee orientation program for the agency. The objectives of the program are to provide a general overview of the department, services offered, and administrative policies and procedures to efficiently prepare the employees for their job duties. Among the standard topics included in the orientation session will be the requirements of confidentiality surrounding health services to ensure full compliance with the law as well as other functional responsibilities.

One of the goals of the agency's workforce recruiting program has been to focus on hiring qualified workers for the public health system overall and not just for individual programs and agencies. This recruitment strategy has been successful in attracting professionals from the business field and other areas outside of public health. The pipeline of new recruits will help ensure an adequate supply of professionals for the agency to eliminate the critical public health workforce shortage experienced by many employers within the field.

As many of the agency's new employees will come from positions outside of the field, Ethan believes that the orientation program should contain a session or workshop on the 10 greatest achievements in U.S. Public Health over the last century. He hopes that by including this instruction in the program new employees will develop a base public health competence, enabling them to understand the crucial role public health has played in all aspects of society. The workshop will provide an opportunity for new employees to learn the significance and scope of public health initiatives as well as to broaden their awareness of the needs and challenges within the field.

Background

In 1999, the Centers for Disease Control and Prevention (CDC) prepared a list of the notable public health achievements that occurred during the twentieth century (Table 16-6). The choices were based on the opportunity for prevention and the impact on death, illness, and disability in the United States. The list was not ranked by order of importance.

Next Steps

To develop the workshop, Ethan has arranged for several health analysts in the agency to prepare background research on each of the topics on the list. Ethan wants the session to be highly informative so the new employees will appreciate these contributions of public health and understand their effect on the health of persons in the United States.

Discussion Questions

1. If you were the Training Coordinator, how would you design the workshop to meet the goals of the agency?

2. How will understanding the history help new professionals develop a base competence in public health and help their career development?

3. What other accomplishments could have been selected for the list? Consider international as well as national initiatives.

TABLE 16-6 Ten Great Public Health Achievements in the U.S. (1900–1999)
1. Vaccination
2. Motor-vehicle safety
3. Control of infectious diseases
4. Treasurer's report (if needed)
5. Decline in deaths from coronary heart disease and stroke
6. Safer and healthier foods
7. Healthier mothers and babies
8. Family planning
9. Fluoridation of drinking water
10. Recognition of tobacco use as a health hazard

Source: "Ten Great Public Health Achievements—United States, 1900–1999," Centers for Disease Control and Prevention, *Morbidity and Mortality Weekly Report, 48*(12), 241–243.[1]

Reference

[1] Centers for Disease Control and Prevention. (1999, April 2). Ten Great Public Health Achievements—United States, 1900–1999. *Morbidity and Mortality Weekly Report, 48*(12), 241–243. Retrieved from http://www.cdc.gov/mmwr/preview/mmwrhtml/00056796.htm

CASE 18: DECIDING ON A CAREER IN PUBLIC HEALTH

Situation

Kylie is a summer intern at a large metropolitan community health center in Washington, D.C. She has one week left in her internship program before heading back to college to start her sophomore year. She really enjoyed her work at the clinic and was encouraged by the favorable feedback she received from her supervisor during her performance review last week. Her positive summer experience has inspired her to consider seeking a career in public health. She finds the public health field exciting as it offers exposure to a diverse number of emerging issues including food safety, disease outbreaks (influenza), environment (climate change, safe water, green focus), obesity epidemic, sexual health, genetics, and emergency preparedness, among others. As a public health professional, she would have the opportunity to work at different levels of community involvement, including local, state, national, and international. She feels that a public health career could offer personal fulfillment and satisfaction by working to protect the health of the public. She could really make an impact.

Background

Public health professionals come from varying educational backgrounds and experiences. Kylie realizes that one of her first objectives will be to gain an understanding of what she likes to do best—what is her passion—as well as where her talents lie. Is it crunching numbers, conducting research, writing policy, or working directly with people? There is an abundance of career opportunities available in specialist and generalist public health content areas. Kylie recognizes that she will develop a better understanding of her preferences over time as she gains more education and exposure through internships and informational interviews. However, she does feel pressure to make a general decision now as she has to select her major this year in school.

Through her college's Recruiting and Career Services website, Kylie has discovered that there are anticipated shortages in public health positions for epidemiologists, public health nurses, and public health physicians. In addition, there is projected demand in careers for environmental health specialists, disaster preparedness specialists, public information officers, health policy experts, and health informatics specialists/managers. From preliminary research, Kylie has summarized the possible career paths available for a particular educational focus. Although not an exhaustive analysis, the list does provide her with some general guidance to aid in her decision making.

- **Sciences degrees** (e.g., biology, chemistry, pre-med, mathematics, statistics): Suited for positions in epidemiology, biostatistics, medicine, nursing, environmental health, and health analysis.

- **Social sciences degrees** (e.g., sociology, psychology, education, economics): Suited for positions in behavioral and social medicine, education, health analysis, and program administration.

- **Public health degree**: Suited for positions such as public health official, health administrator, health program director and specialist, and health promotion specialist.

- **Business degrees** (e.g., business administration, management, finance, communications, marketing): Suited for positions in health services administration, finance, business analysis, health insurance, and program coordination.

Next Steps

As a starting point, Kylie decides to review the Association of Schools of Public Health (ASPH) website at http://www.asph.org to learn more about the public health field and career opportunities available. By understanding the educational programs offered, she may be able to select a major now that will serve her well in the long run as she pursues a career in public health. During her last week in the internship program, Kylie has scheduled informal meetings with different professionals within the clinic to learn more about their educational backgrounds and career paths.

Discussion Questions

1. What factors would you consider in deciding a public health career to pursue?

2. Is Kylie being too analytical in her approach? What are some advantages and disadvantages in being regimented in an early career choice?

3. How can Kylie augment her educational experiences to better prepare her to work in public health?

4. How do your interests and talents align in your planned public health career?

5. How can you apply your experiences to an international public health career assignment?

CASE 19: SMOKING CESSATION PROGRAM IMPLEMENTATION

James Allen Johnson, III, M.P.H.

Situation

Dr. Whitten is the director of a community health clinic in Lake Sophia, Florida. Lake Sophia is a small town with approximately 2,000 residents located in a rural area of central Florida. The town of Lake Sophia is located in one of the poorest areas in the state. The health of the population of Lake Sophia reflects its socioeconomic status (SES) in that not only does it have some of the lowest SES indicators (income, education, and occupation) in Florida, but its population has some of the worst health as well.

Dr. Whitten was concerned about a report recently released by the State Department of Health on tobacco use. The report indicated that 32% of the population in Lake Sophia used tobacco. This statistic was not only well above the national average, approximately 20%, but was the highest in the state. In response to this revelation about the significance of the problem of tobacco use in Lake Sophia, Dr. Whitten decided to implement a smoking cessation program at the health clinic.

To develop, implement, and eventually manage the program, Dr. Whitten hired Ali Jones, a recent college graduate who majored in Public Health. Remembering her public health education, Ali concluded that to ensure success she must use an evidence-based approach. She decided to refer to recent literature written about smoking cessation as well as the Centers for Disease Control and Prevention (CDC) and the World Health Organization (WHO) websites.

Background

Ali concluded the consensus was that tobacco dependence showed many features of a chronic disease and that only a minority of tobacco users achieves successful cessation while the majority continue to use tobacco long-term, typically cycling through multiple periods of relapse and remission. Further inquiry revealed that only about 5% of smokers who quit smoking maintained abstinence for 3 to 12 months.[1] It is suggested by the American Cancer Society that one of the reasons for the low success rate may be attributed to the fact that most individuals who try to quit do not use effective treatments.[2] In 2000, the U.S. Public Health Service published and in 2008 updated *Guidelines for Treating Tobacco Use and Dependence* which includes both recommended treatment strategies for clinicians and implementation stages for administrators.

Next Steps

Ali adopted the recommended treatment strategies from the *Guidelines for Treating Tobacco Use and Dependence* and had all the clinicians and practitioners at the health clinic properly trained. The program seemed to be going well, but Ali knew there was room for improvement. She noticed that on breaks some of the employees of the clinic would sit on benches near the front entrance and smoke cigarettes. This was a designated smoking area and next to the benches ashtrays were provided. Ali realized that to further the success of the smoking cessation program she must employ a systemic approach. To help in the formulation of ideas for a systems intervention approach, Ali called a meeting which included clinicians, practitioners, and administrators.

Discussion Questions

1. Discuss some possible opportunities and concerns Ali may want to introduce at the meeting.

2. What are some possible opportunities and concerns the other participants at the meeting (clinicians, practitioners, and administrators) may have?

3. Should Ali address the issue of employees smoking outside in front of the building? Why or why not? If so, what changes should she recommend and how should they be implemented?

References

[1] Centers for Disease Control and Prevention. (2006). *A practical guide to working with health-care systems on tobacco-use treatment.* Retrieved from http://www.cdc.gov/tobacco/quit_smoking/cessation/practical_guide/pdfs/practical_guide.pdf

[2] American Cancer Society. (2003). Cancer Facts and Figures, 2003. Atlanta, GA: American Cancer Society.

CASE 20: PACIFIC NEEDLE EXCHANGE PROGRAM

James Allen Johnson, III, M.P.H.

Situation

Pacific Needle Exchange (PNEX), a one-for-one syringe exchange program funded by the Hawaii Department of Health, is a not-for-profit organization dedicated to the reduction of HIV prevalence amongst injection drug users (IDU) in the state of Hawaii. PNEX provides hypodermic syringes to IDUs through a one-for-one exchange (one new syringe is provided for every used syringe discarded at a designated PNEX exchange location) along with condoms and health education materials relevant to that particular population. PNEX was established in 1989 and has been successful in reducing the prevalence of HIV within Hawaii's IDU population from around 50% in 1989 to around 1.5% where it has persisted since 2001. PNEX is regarded nationally as a success and has served as a model for emerging syringe exchange programs in other states.

Stephen Maturin, M.P.H., the executive director of PNEX, received the annual report on the status of the IDU population it serves. Because of the program's success in reducing the spread of HIV, Mr. Maturin decided to include a study on the prevalence of hepatitis C virus (HCV), a virus that commonly affects IDUs, in this year's annual report. He was particularly concerned by the results of the HCV study which indicated that 87% of the IDU population PNEX serves tested positive for HCV antigens.

Background

HCV typically has a higher prevalence in IDU populations than does HIV. One explanation for this may be that HCV has the ability to survive outside of the body while HIV, typically, cannot. Because hypodermic syringes form a semi-vacuums environment, HIV can survive in a syringe long enough to potentially infect another person if the syringe is reused and not properly sterilized. Outside of syringes or the human body, there are few known places HIV can survive, limiting its spread to the exchange of fluids through sexual intercourse and blood-to-blood contact (which occurs with the reuse of infected syringes). Like HIV, HCV is a bloodborne pathogen but, unlike HIV, it can survive outside the body. Because of this, unlike HIV, HCV can be transmitted via a material medium. In the case of IDUs, this medium is often "cookers" (tools such as spoons, miniature metal cups, etc., used to prepare drugs through the process of heating), tourniquets, and pieces of cotton used in the injection process. Because HCV can survive outside of the body on inanimate objects, it can spread when these objects are shared. Such is the case when two or more people reusing their own syringes (not directly sharing) draw from the same "cooker." If one person has HCV in the group sharing the "cooker," everyone has been exposed to the virus, potentially becoming infected. This exposure happened despite taking some of the necessary precautions to avoid HIV exposure (not sharing used syringes).

Next Steps

The following week Stephen called a meeting with the outreach workers to discuss the findings of the study and their possible implications. Over the next 10 years, Stephen would like to reduce the prevalence of HCV by half. In the meeting, he plans to ask his team to suggest changes to the needle exchange program necessary to achieve this goal while maintaining the successful campaign against the spread of HIV.

Discussion Questions

1. With a grant from the Department of Health to address HCV, what strategies should the outreach workers recommend?

2. What are some of the possible challenges of addressing the HCV epidemic in an IDU population?

3. One can be infected with HCV for 20 or more years before symptoms begin to appear. What unique challenges may this present and how could they be overcome?

CASE 21: COMMUNITY COALITIONS AND THE BUILT ENVIRONMENT

Asal Mohamadi, Ph.D., M.P.H.

Situation

The Florida Department of Health (DOH) has created a new division entitled the Department of Development and Sustainability (DDS). One of the responsibilities of the new department is to address rising trends in poor health across the state as they relate to the built environment. DDS would like to approach this mission at the municipal level by building community coalitions that provide for the capacity to address these health issues by working together to effect change. A coalition is an agreement among individuals or groups, during which they cooperate in joint action, each in their own self-interest, joining forces together for a common cause. DDS suggests that addressing health at the community level will eventually reverse some of these undesirable trends and promote a sustainable health profile for the state. To realize this goal, DDS proposes a program called *Healthy Communities, Healthy Citizens.* This will consist of a conglomerate of smaller city-level programs that address the needs of that particular city through coalitions consisting of members and organizations from the community.

Elizabeth Ruth was recently named the director of *Healthy Communities, Healthy Citizens* and has been charged with engineering and implementing the program. In order to obtain budget approval for the fund of *Healthy Communities, Healthy Citizens*, the program must first implement a successful pilot program.

Background

Tallahassee is the capital of Florida and has an approximate population of 180,000. Along with a multitude of state and city government agencies, Tallahassee hosts two major universities: State University and A&M University; one public and one private hospital; and a county health department. Elizabeth plans to implement a pilot program in Tallahassee called *Citizens for a Healthy Tallahassee.* If the pilot program proves successful, it will be implemented in cities and communities across the state.

Next Steps

Elizabeth would like to work with the City of Tallahassee to, among other things, promote physical activity, reduce vehicular dependency, and reduce alcohol and tobacco use. Elizabeth recognizes that Tallahassee is a heterogonous population with its citizenship having multiple cultures and interests. Identifying a representative list of stakeholders (individuals or organizations that have a stake in the mission of the program) proves imperative for successful implementation and to achieve the desired health outcomes. She also recognizes that to effect greater change, policies are needed that promote healthy behavior and address socioeconomic issues such as neighborhood-concentrated poverty and neighborhood safety. It is important that the coalition be able to address the entire gambit of issues affecting health and the built environment.

Discussion Questions

1. Identify at least five health issues that may be related by the built environment. Explain how the built environment could possibly affect the identified health issue.

2. Identify at least 10 possible stakeholders (individuals or organizations that have a stake in the mission of the program) that could comprise a coalition.

3. Formulate a mission statement for the coalition that addresses identified health issues from Question 1 and accounts for stakeholders identified in Question 2.

CASE 22: NEGLECTED TROPICAL DISEASES—A LOCAL NGO'S CHALLENGES

Kevin Wiley, Jr. M.P.H.

Situation

Action on Disease, Development, and Sustainability (ADDS), a nongovernmental organization (NGO) operating in Southeast Asia, is committed to improving water systems in marginalized communities across Thailand, Cambodia, and Laos. ADDS is predominantly funded by the World Health Organization (WHO) and the University of South-East Asia. ADDS has been a major contributor in reducing the incidence of water-borne disease near the northeastern border of Thailand, specifically schistosomiasis. Schistosomiasis, caused by parasitic worms, is considered a neglected tropical disease (NTD) transmitted while bathing, swimming, or wading in contaminated water. The disease can persist in the brain or spinal cord causing seizures, paralysis, or spinal cord inflammation.

The WHO conducts biannual evaluations of ADDS programs, requiring that the NGO submit detailed incidence and financial reports. Dr. Daniel Inglehart, the director of ADDS Department of Neglected Disease, is instructed by the Thailand Ministry of Health (MOH) to withhold disease incidence reports because an exorbitant tourist season is expected. The WHO publishes information about the health status of Thailand provided by ADDS; furthermore, these reports are required for the continuation of funding from the WHO. The deadline to submit is in five days and Dr. Inglehart must receive approval from the MOH to release this information. Dr. Inglehart has yet to receive approval. Essential resources for ADDS's many ongoing programs are at stake if there is a failure to comply with WHO's guidelines. The MOH has also informed Dr. Inglehart that if the report is published, ADDS will no longer be able to conduct operations in Thailand.

Background

Most NTD-related infections can be reduced or eliminated by controlling vectors that transmit these diseases through improved sanitation, living conditions, and water systems. Many common NTDs are found in Asia, Africa, and Latin America, including Dengue Fever, Leishmaniasis, Leprosy, Guinea Worm Disease, and Rabies. These diseases disproportionately affect impoverished populations around the world in areas where access to clean water and proper human waste disposal remain nonexistent.

Next Steps

The request and threats by the MOH have put Dr. Inglehart in a financial and ethical dilemma. Dr. Inglehart has prepared the report but has yet to send it to the

WHO. He appealed to the MOH with no avail. Dr. Inglehart has two days before the WHO deadline lapses.

Discussion Questions

1. What concessions could Dr. Inglehart and WHO representatives make in future negotiations with the MOH to ensure timely report submission/publication without any disruption to the highly profitable tourist season?

2. How should Dr. Inglehart respond if the MOH requests that he withhold reports in the future?

3. If the WHO were to stop funding this program in Southeast Asia, what are some possible repercussions for WHO in the region? For ADDS?

4. Dr. Inglehart could seek funding from other institutions across the globe, but none as prestigious or reputable as the WHO. How could severing ties with the WHO affect ADDS's relationship with the international public health community?

Chapter 17

TERMS FOR PUBLIC HEALTH MANAGERS

James Allen Johnson III, M.P.H.
James E. Dotherow IV, M.P.A.

Learning Objectives

Upon completion of this chapter, you should be able to:

1. Define common terms used in public health management.
2. Better understand public health literature due to increased vocabulary.
3. Use this book more effectively.
4. Complete the discussion and action learning assignments.

Chapter Outline

Introduction
Terms and Definitions

INTRODUCTION

Students studying public health management must have a very wide grasp of terms and concepts since the field encompasses several domains: public health, public management, organization theory, and public policy. The glossary of terms and definitions provided here is comprehensive and seeks to serve as a resource for students and faculty. It can be used with this textbook, with other texts, and also in one's professional career and future management roles.

TERMS AND DEFINITIONS

A

access (physical) The ability to get doctors, facilities, and information. Hospitals, clinics, and other resources must be located where they can be reached and designed without barriers.

access (to health care) The ability to obtain health care. Access includes available physicians and facilities, transportation, acceptance by the facility, and a means of payment.

access control The ability and responsibility of a health care organization to control and account for access to medical records and other protected health information.

account An arrangement between a buyer and a seller in which goods or services are exchanged and payment is to be made later.

    closed account An account upon which full payment has been made.

    open account An account upon which not all payments have been made.

accountability The duty to provide, to all concerned, the evidence needed to establish confidence that the task or duty for which one is responsible is being or has been performed and describe the manner in which that task is being or has been carried out.

accountant An individual who specializes in examining, interpreting, or managing financial records.

    certified public accountant (CPA) A licensed individual who has met the requirements of the American Institute of Certified Public Accountants (AICPA).

    public accountant (PA) An individual who performs a variety of functions, such as the audit of a organization's financial statements and the design of financial systems.

accounting period The time, usually a month, quarter, or a year, covered by a financial statement.

accounts payable (AP) Amounts on an open account (*see account*) owed to creditors for goods and services.

accounts receivable (AR) Amount owed by others on an open account for goods or services.

accreditation A process of evaluation of an institution or education program to determine whether it meets the standards set up by an accrediting body and, if the institution or program meets the standards, granting recognition of the fact.

accredited Formally recognized by an accrediting body as meeting its standards for accreditation.

actuarial analysis A forecast developed by specialized actuarial methods, giving the probability of future events for a given population, such as life expectancy or frequency of hospitalization.

actuary A mathematician who specializes in estimating risks, rates, premiums, and other factors.

acute With respect to an illness, having a short course which often is relatively severe.

acute care Care for people with injuries or acute illness.

ad hoc committee A committee formed for a particular purpose, usually limited in duration until the purpose is completed. This is in contrast to a standing committee, which purportedly remains active over time.

adaptation Using information obtained during SWOT analysis and boundary spanning, the adaptation function helps organizations anticipate and adjust to change.

Adjusted Community Rate (ACR) A term used by CMS (see ***Centers for Medicare and Medicaid Services***) in its Medicare risk contracts with health care organizations to mean the premium the organization would charge for providing exactly the same Medicare-covered benefits to a community rated group, adjusted to allow for the greater intensity and frequency of utilization by Medicare recipients.

adjustment (bookkeeping) A bookkeeping entry made to correct errors, adjust balance-sheet balances to their true balance, and so forth.

   administrative adjustment A bookkeeping entry to account for services rendered but not billed.

adjustment (statistical) A statistical term referring to a procedure for correcting for differences in the composition of two or more populations so that valid comparisons can be made.

administration (government) A division of the federal government; a subdivision within a department. For example, the Food and Drug Administration is part of the Public Health Services, which in turn is within the Department of Health and Human Services (DHHS).

administration (management) The direction and management of an organization.

functional administration (FA) A type of administration of an organization in which the focus is on functional components the organization.

health care administration A type of administration that manages health care organizations.

market administration (MA) A type of administration of an organization in which the focus is on the institution's markets.

product administration (PA) A type of administration of an organization in which the focus is on products.

Administration for Children and Families (ACF) The agency within the Department of Health and Human Services (DHHS) responsible for federal programs that promote the economic and social well-being of families, children, individuals, and communities.

It includes the following programs:
Administration for Children and Families (ACF)
Administration on Developmental Disabilities (ADD)
Administration for Native Americans (ANA)
Child Care and Development Fund
Child Support Enforcement Program
Child Welfare
Community Services Programs
Domestic Violence
Head Start
Office of Refugee Resettlement (ORR)
President's Committee on Mental Retardation (PCMR)
Temporary Assistance for Needy Families
Youth Programs

Administration on Aging (AoA) The federal agency within the Department of Health and Human Services (DHHS) charged with serving the senior citizens of the United States.

It includes the following programs:
National Family Caregiver Support Program (NFCSP)
Elderly Nutrition Program (ENP)
Long-Term Care Ombudsman Program (LTCOP)
Alzheimer's Resource Room

administrative doctrine The rules, procedures, and ways of doing things that reflect the basic values of an organization.

administrative law The body of law which governs the powers of administrative agencies, the process of agency decision making, and the procedures by which a party can challenge an adverse decision of an agency.

administrative process The process by which an administrative agency makes a decision.

administrative systems The formal procedures designed to carry out routine coordinated work and programmable events.

administrator The individual responsible for carrying out policies established by the organization or agency which employs that person. An administrator is a line official, that is, an employee with authority over others.

admission (hospital) Formal acceptance of a patient by a hospital or other organization in order to provide care.

> **elective admission** An admission that can be scheduled in advance because the illness or injury is not life-threatening.
>
> **emergency admission** An admission that must take place immediately or else death or serious disability is likely to result.
>
> **inpatient admission** An admission to an institution which provides lodging and continuous care services.
>
> **outpatient admission** An admission to an institution which gives care but does not provide lodging.

advanced directive A statement executed by a person while of sound mind as to that person's wishes about the use of medical interventions for him or herself in case of the loss of his or her own decision-making capacity. A number of forms of advanced directives have been proposed and are used which are listed below.

> **durable power of attorney** A power of attorney which remains (or becomes) effective when the principal becomes incompetent to act for themselves.
>
> **health care proxy** A document which authorizes a designated person (who is also called a proxy) to make health care decisions in the event that the signer is incapable of making those decisions.
>
> **instructional advanced directive (IAD)** An advanced directive in which an attempt is made to allow the person executing the directive to record quite specifically those interventions which are not to be attempted in case of the loss of the person's own decision-making capacity.
>
> **living will** A will concerning the life of the individual executing the will in contrast to the usual last will and testament, in which the subject matter is the disposition of property and custody of minor children.
>
> **The Medical Directive** An instructional advance directive document which has been made available to the public. The person who completes the document checks off whether he would choose interventions in the case of each of the listed scenarios. The completed document is interpreted as an advance directive for the person who completes it.

advanced practice nurse (APN) A nurse with advanced skills, education, training, and certification in a nursing specialty. Each specialty has specific requirements for eligibility, education, training, certification and/or licensure of its practitioners.

advocate One that pleads the cause of another.

affirmative action A term that first meant the removal of "artificial barriers" to the employment of women and minority group members; now it refers to the compensatory opportunities for hitherto disadvantaged groups-specific efforts to recruit, hire, and promote qualified members of disadvantaged groups for the purpose of eliminating the present effects of past discrimination.

Agency for Healthcare Research and Quality (AHRQ) The lead federal agency for research to improve the quality of health care, reduce its cost, and broaden access to essential services. A component of the Department of Health and Human Services (DHHS).

Agency for Toxic Substances and Disease Registry (ATSDR) The ATSDR performs specific public health functions concerning hazardous substances in the environment. It works to prevent exposure and minimize adverse health effects associated with waste management emergencies and pollution by hazardous substances.

agency mission Responsibilities assigned to a specific agency for meeting national needs. Agency missions are expressed in terms of the purpose to be served by the programs authorized to carry out functions or subfunctions that, by law, are the responsibility of the agency and its component organizations. In contrast to national needs, generally described in context of major functions, agency missions are generally described in the context of subfunctions.

agenda A list or outline of things to be considered or done.

agenda setting The process by which ideas or issues bubble up through the various political channels to wind up for consideration by a political institution such as legislature or courts.

AIDS (acquired immunodeficiency syndrome) The disease caused by HIV (human immunodeficiency virus). The official definition of AIDS, a disease which was first described in 1981, has been changed repeatedly as the disease has become better understood. Currently AIDS is defined as any person with a blood count revealing fewer than 200 CD4-lymphocytes per cubic millimeter (mm^3) is considered to have AIDS. One should be aware that the labeling of an individual as having or not having AIDS has serious social, employment, and financial consequences, so the definition is of great importance.

Alcoholics Anonymous (AA) A worldwide organization formed in 1935 to provide support for people suffering from alcoholism.

Alderfer's ERG model Clayton Alderfer's idea of advanced needs that motivate people. Like Maslow, he believed that needs motivate people to take certain actions, and once lower-level needs are met, new needs can be sought. Alderfer stated three levels of needs: existence, relatedness, and growth.

allocate To apportion for a specific purpose or to particular persons or things.

all-payer system A system in which prices for health care services and payment methods are the same for all, regardless of payer. All those financing health care (government, individual, insurance company, health plan, self-insured employer) pay the same rates. Health care providers may not shift costs from one payer to another, as is often the case in the United States.

alternative dispute resolution (ADR) Methods of settling claims and disagreements other than by lawsuit.

alternative financing system (AFS) An alternative to the fee-for-service (FFS) payment system, such as a health maintenance organization (HMO) or competitive medical plan (CMP) in which some other mechanism, usually capitation, is the method of payment to the organization.

ambulatory care Care provided to a patient without hospitalization.

ambulatory care center A facility which provides health and allied services to patients who do not require overnight lodging in an inpatient facility. Ambulatory care centers can be either freestanding or hospital-based.

American Cancer Society (ACS) A national organization dedicated to eliminating cancer as a major health problem by preventing cancer, saving lives, and diminishing suffering from cancer through research, education, advocacy, and service. ACS is the largest source of private, nonprofit cancer research funds in the United States. **http://www.cancer.org**

American College of Healthcare Executives (ACHE) The leading professional association for health care executives. **http://www.ache.org**

American Hospital Association (AHA) The national association of hospitals in the United States. Non-hospital health care organizations may also hold membership. **http://www.aha.org**

American Management Association (AMA) A national organization of business management personnel. **http://www.amanet.org**

American Medical Association (AMA) The major national association of physicians, founded in 1847, in the United States.

American Nursing Association (ANA) The professional association for registered nurses in the United States.

American Osteopathic Association (AOA) The major national association of osteopathic physicians, founded in 1897, in the United States.

American Public Health Association (APHA) The national association which embraces all public health professions.

American Red Cross (ARC) A humanitarian organization committed to providing relief to victims of disasters and helping people prevent, prepare for, and respond to emergencies.

Americans with Disabilities Act (ADA) A federal law enacted in 1990 that extended rights of and services for persons with disabilities.

appropriation act A statute, under the jurisdiction of the House and Senate Committees on Appropriations, that generally provides authorization for federal agencies to incur obligations and to make payments out of the Treasury for specified purposes. An appropriation act, the most common means of providing budget authority, generally follows enactment of authorizing legislation unless the authoring legislation itself provides the budget authority. There are currently thirteen regular federal appropriation acts enacted annually. Congress occasionally enacts **supplemental appropriation acts** that provide additional budget authority beyond the original estimates for programs or activities in cases where the need for funds is too urgent to be postponed until the enactment of the next appropriation bill.

area wage adjustment A component of the payment formula under the prospective payment system (PPS) to allow for differences in wage scales in different parts of the country.

arm's length transaction A term meaning that a transaction conducted is beyond the reach of personal influence or control and that the parties involved in the transaction are independent.

assessment The delineation of health problems, their nature, and the means of dealing with them.

asset An object (property or money for example), a right (to royalties for example), or a claim (a title to a debt for example) which its owners consider to be of benefit to them.

> **capital asset** An asset with a life of more than one year that is not bought and sold in the ordinary course of business.
>
> **current asset** An asset with a life of less than one year.
>
> **fixed asset** Long-term assets that are not bought or sold in the normal course of business.
>
> **intangible asset** An asset which is not physical.
>
> **noncurrent asset** An asset with a life of more than one year.
>
> **tangible asset** An asset which is physical.

asset reduction Selling or giving away one's assets in order to be eligible for public assistance such as Medicaid.

assisted living The provision of services, including housing, health care, and support services to those who need help with the activities of daily living.

association health plan (AHP) A concept by which small businesses band together to gain an advantage in purchasing health insurance for their employees.

Association of American Medical Colleges (AAMC) An organization committed to improving the health of the public by enhancing the effectiveness of medical education.

assumption of risk A legal defense to a lawsuit when the lawsuit is based on negligence. If a person knowingly and voluntarily exposes himself to a risk of harm, he is said to "assume the risk" meaning that he has agreed to accept it.

assurance The implementation of policy, either by activities of others or direct public health activities.

audit A term which usually means a financial audit in which the organization's financial statement and the degree to which the statement reflects the actual affairs of the organization are examined. An audit also may include a review of financial and organizational procedures.

external audit An audit carried out by an independent organization.

fiscal audit An audit of the financial (fiscal) affairs of the institution.

internal audit An administrative process carried out in organizations, by the organization's own employees, in an effort to determine the extent to which the organization's internal operations conform with its own intended procedures and practices. When a similar review is done by an outside group, it is called an *external audit*.

performance audit An audit that compares the actions of an organization with the objectives that have been assigned to it.

quality management audit An audit of the quality of management of an institution.

average length of stay (ALOS) A standard hospital statistic. A length of stay (LOS) is the number of days between a patient's admission and discharge. To determine the average length of stay (ALOS) for a group of patients, their total lengths of stay are added together, and that total is divided by the number of patients in the group. The ALOS may be calculated not only for the entire hospital but also for specific groups.

B

base (measure) A reference quantity or reference time, often a given year. For example, the data used in calculating a consumer price index (CPI) include base prices, which are prices found in the year chosen as the base.

base (rate) A statistical term referring to the "per" number in a given rate. A ratio or proportion is often expressed as a percentage (per 100), but it may also be expressed per 1,000; per 10,000; per 100,000; or even per million. These "per" numbers are called the "base." Thus a percentage is said to have 100 as the base.

benchmarking Comparing the performance of an individual, department, institution, or organization with regard to a particular indicator against that of some other source of data.

beneficiary The person entitled to benefits from insurance or some other health care financing program, such as Medicare.

benefit package The array or set of benefits (services covered) included in or provided by a given insurance policy.

benefits The money, care, or other services to which an individual is entitled by virtue of insurance.

bias A factor or factors that systematically influence the judgments of individuals or the results of investigations so that the judgment is not impartial or so that one outcome of the investigation is unfairly preferred over another.

bioethics The field of ethics applied to medicine, public health, and the health sciences.

biostatistics The application of mathematics and statistics to the study of public health, medicine, and life sciences.

block grant A grant distributed in accordance with a statutory formula for use in a variety of activities within a broad functional area, largely at the recipient's discretion.

board (credentialing) A licensing or other qualifying or credential-awarding body.

board (governing) A common term for an organization's governing body, the body which is legally responsible for the organization's policies, organization, management, and quality of care. Board is usually short for board of trustees, board of directors, or board of governors.

bond A certificate sold by an organization or government entity to raise funds. It is basically a form of IOU upon which the organization or government entity will pay interest to the bondholder for a given period of time and pay the bondholder the amount borrowed (the principal amount) at the end of that time.

bond indenture The contract between a bondholder and the institution issuing the bond.

boundary spanning The interface between the organization and its external environment. Key concerns include technology, regulation, demographics, disease patterns, and community expectations.

break-even analysis An analytical technique for studying the relation among fixed costs and variable costs (*see cost*), volume or level of activity (sales), and profits.

break-even chart A chart graphically presenting the results of a break-even analysis.

break-even point The volume of activity (for example, sales) where revenues and expenses are exactly equal, that is, the level of activity where there is neither a gain nor a loss from operations. Activity above the break-even point produces profits; activity below it results in losses.

bribe Any money or equivalent of money which is offered to induce some action.

budget A financial plan serving as a pattern for and control over future operations—hence, any estimate of future costs or any systematic plan for the utilization of the workforce, material, or other resource.

budget cycle The timed steps of the budget process, which includes preparation, approval, execution, and audit.

budget process The total system a jurisdiction uses to make decisions on government spending needs and how to pay for them. The main difference between federal and state and local governments is that state and local jurisdictions must have balanced budgets each year.

budget reconciliation A part of the legislative budgeting process which defines federal programs in such a manner that program costs are consistent with Congress' decision as to how much money is to be spent for the program in question.

budget surplus The amount by which a government's budget receipts exceed its budget outlays for any given period.

building codes Regulations which owners must meet in the construction, use, and maintenance of buildings.

bureaucracy A termed coined by Max Weber to represent an ideal or completely rational form of organization. The organizational structure is based on the sociological concept of rationalization of collective activities. The key features Weber believed were necessary for an organization to achieve the maximum benefits of ideal bureaucracy include: 1) a clear division of labor to ensure that each task preformed is systematically established and legitimized by formal recognition as an official duty, 2) positions are arranged in a hierarchy so that each lower position is controlled and supervised by a higher one, leading to a chain of command, 3) formal rules and regulations uniformly guide the actions of employees, eliminating uncertainty in the performance of tasks resulting from differences among individuals, 4) managers should maintain impersonal relationships and should avoid involvement with employees personalities and personal preferences, and 5) employment should be based entirely on technical competence and protection against arbitrary dismissal. The term is now usually associated with large public-sector organizations to describe undesirable characteristics such as duplication, delay, waste, low morale, and general frustration.

bylaws A document adopted by an organization which governs its conduct and the rights and duties of its members. Bylaws may also authorize the separate issuance of rules and regulations to govern specific activities. The process for changing the rules and regulations is less cumbersome than that for changing the bylaws themselves.

C

cabinet The heads of executive departments of a jurisdiction who report to and advise its chief executive.

cap A limit on the amount of money which may be spent for a given purpose. A global budget for health care for a community would be such a cap.

capital The long-term assets of an organization which are not bought and sold in the course of its operation. These assets are primarily fixed assets such as land, equipment, and buildings.

  working capital The difference between current assets and current liabilities.

capital budgeting The process of planning expenditures on capital items.

capital expenditure An expenditure (chargeable to an asset account) made to acquire an asset which has an estimated life in excess of one year and is not intended for sale in the ordinary course of business.

capital financing Obtaining funds for building or renovation, that is, for additions to capital as opposed to the financing of operations. For the most part operations are financed by fees for services rendered.

capital rationing A situation where a constraint is placed on the total size of capital investment during a particular period.

capital structure The permanent long-term financing of an organization or institution represented by long-term debt, preferred stock, and net worth. Capital structure is distinguished from financial structure, which includes short-term debt plus all reserve accounts.

capitation Capitation is a flat periodic payment to a health care provider per person cared for per capita (per head). The provider assumes the risk that the payment will cover the costs for whatever the patient needs.

care The treatment, accommodations, and other services provided to a patient.

caregiver A term applied to any individual who provides care to another, from physician to friend.

carrier (disease) An individual who carries and can transmit a contagious disease without himself showing symptoms or signs of the disease.

carrier (genetics) An apparently unaffected individual who possesses a single copy of a recessive gene which is obscured by an alternative form of that gene.

carrier (insurance) An organization which handles the claims for beneficiaries on behalf of certain kinds of health insurance. A carrier may be an insurance company, a prepayment plan, or a government agency.

catastrophic illness An illness which requires very costly treatment; one which is catastrophic to the patient's or family's finances. The illness may be either acute or chronic.

categorical grant A grant that can be used only for specific, narrowly defined activities.

Centers for Disease Control and Prevention (CDC) An agency within the Department of Health and Human Services (DHHS), which is responsible for monitoring and studying diseases which are controllable by public health measures. The CDC is headquartered in Atlanta, Georgia.

Centers for Medicare and Medicaid Services (CMS) The agency within the Department of Health and Human Services (DHHS) which administers the Medicare, Medicaid, and the State Children's Health Insurance Program (SCHIP). CMS has three centers:

> **Center for Beneficiary Choices (CBC)** provides consumer education to help Medicare beneficiaries make health care decisions. The CBC will also manage the Medicare Advantage program, consumer research and demonstrations, and grievance and appeals.
>
> **Center for Medicaid and State Operations (CMSO)** manages programs administered by the states, including Medicaid, the State Children's Health Insurance Program, private insurance, survey and certification, and the Clinical Laboratory Improvement Amendments (CLIA).

Center for Medicare Management (CMM) manages the traditional fee-for-service Medicare program, including development and implementation of payment policy and management of the Medicare carriers and fiscal intermediaries.

centralized services Services which are carried out from a single location in an effort to improve efficiency, reduce cost, or both.

CEPH The Council on Education for Public Health is an independent agency recognized by the U.S. Department of Education to accredit schools of public health and public health programs. **http://www.ceph.org**

certificate A document verifying that someone or something has fulfilled specific requirements.

certificate of need (CON) A certificate, issued by a governmental or planning agency, which approves the organization's contention that it needs a given facility or service. A certificate of need is required under many regulatory situations in order to obtain approval to build, purchase, or institute the service in question.

certification The issuance of a certificate which gives evidence that its recipient (an individual, facility, or device) meets certain standards against which testing has been done by the certifying body.

change leadership The ability to energize stakeholders and sustain their commitment to changes, processes, and strategies.

charge The dollar amount asked for a service or product. It is contrasted with the cost, which is the dollar amount the provider incurs in furnishing the service or product.

charismatic leadership Leadership based on the compelling personality of a leader rather than upon position.

chief executive officer (CEO) The person appointed by the governing body to direct the overall management of a business, corporation, or organization. This person is sometimes called the executive director, especially within public organizations.

chief financial officer (CFO) The term is applied to the controller of the organization (the person in charge of the ongoing financial administration, including billing, accounting, budget management, and the like). This person is sometimes called the financial director.

chief information officer (CIO) The title often given to the person in charge of the organization's management information system (MIS).

chief medical officer (CMO) The person (usually a physician) responsible for the medical affairs of a corporation or organization. The actual duties will vary widely depending upon the context. This person is sometimes called the chief medical director.

chief operating officer (COO) The person in charge of the internal operation of the organization. The chief executive officer (CEO), while responsible for the internal operation of the organization, also has external responsibilities with the governing body, with the community, with other institutions, and so on.

chronic An illness which lasts for a long time and usually without prospect of immediate change either for the better or the worse. It is contrasted with acute, which refers to having a short course, which often is relatively severe.

civil service A collective term for all nonmilitary employees of a government.

civil service reform Efforts to improve the status, integrity, and productivity of the civil service at all levels of the governments by supplanting the spoils system with the merit system; efforts to improve the management and efficiency of the public service.

claim (finance) The usage in which the word is employed to describe one form of asset.

claim (insurance) A request for payment of insurance benefits to be paid to or on behalf of a beneficiary.

claim (legal) An allegation of legal liability and an accompanying demand for damages (money) or other rights due.

claims processing The procedure by which claims for payment for services are reviewed in order to determine whether they should be paid and for what amount.

clinical A term referring to direct contact with or information from patients and to the course of illness. Thus personal (bedside) contact with the patient is clinical contact; a laboratory which examines blood and other specimens from patients is a clinical laboratory; the patient's medical record is a clinical record; research involving patients is clinical research; a nurse taking care of patients is a clinical nurse.

clinician A person who uses a recognized scientific knowledge base and has the authority to direct the provision of personal health services to patients.

classical theory The original theory of organizational structure that closely resembles military structures.

code of ethics A statement of professional standards of conduct to which the practitioners of a profession say they subscribe to. Codes of ethics are usually not legally binding, so they may not be taken too seriously as constraints to behavior.

collective bargaining The process of negotiation regarding compensation, working conditions, benefits, and other matters between an employer and an organization representing the employees. In collective bargaining, the employees may be represented by a union or by some other form of association or organization.

committee A group of people set up for a specific purpose: to consider or investigate a matter, to report on a matter, or to carry out certain duties.

common law Law which has been created by the courts, through decisions of judges, rather than by the legislature (statutory law).

communication The exchange of information between individuals through a common system of signs, symbols, and behaviors. One simple way to see it is the public health manager as the sender and the employee as the receiver. Of course, this can and does go in the other direction. All effective communication has feedback that comes to the sender. This might be direct or indirect. Furthermore, all communication channels are subject to distortions that can interfere with the quality of the message received.

communication process A description or explanation of the chain of events involved in communication.

Community Health Center (CHC) A federal program to provide health care services to medically underserved areas and medically underserved populations.

community health network (CHN) A term sometimes employed as a label for a municipally operated system of providing health care for underserved populations.

community health services A term which encompasses preventive procedures, diagnosis, and treatment for residents of a community. It does not imply any organizational structure.

comorbidity *See morbidity.*

compliance Meeting the statutory or regulatory requirements set out for a particular activity or action.

conceptual skills Skills involving analytical ability, systems thinking, logic, creativity, problem solving, anticipation of change and recognition of opportunity, self awareness, and strategic thinking.

conflict of interest A situation where a person (or organization) has two separate and distinct duties owed concerning, or interests in, the same thing, and therefore cannot act completely impartially with respect to that thing.

congressional budget The budget as set forth by Congress in a concurrent resolution on the budget. By law, the resolution includes 1) the appropriate level of total budget outlays and of total new budget authority; 2) an estimate of budget outlays and new budget authority for each major functional category, for undistributed intergovernmental transactions, and other such matters relating to the budget as may be appropriate to carry out the purposes of the *1974 Congressional Budget and Impoundment Control Act*; 3) the amount, if any, of the surplus or deficit in the budget; 4) the recommended level of federal receipts; and 5) the appropriate level of public debt.

Congressional Budget Office (CBO) A federal agency that assists the House and the Senate Budget Committees and the Congress in the budget process by preparing objective reports and impartial analyses on proposed budgets.

congressional oversight The total means by which the United States Congress monitors the activities of executive branch agencies to determine if the laws are being faithfully executed.

Consolidated Omnibus Budget Reconciliation Act of 1985 (COBRA) A federal law which requires (among other things) that employers of 20 or more workers must continue former employees' health insurance coverage (at the former employee's expense) for up to three years for qualified beneficiaries. Qualified beneficiaries include widows and divorced and separated spouses of former employees, as well as their dependents (even dependents who lost their dependent status).

consortium An alliance between two or more parties to achieve a specific purpose.

constitutional architecture The administrative arrangements created by a government's constitution—from the separation of powers to the requirement that specific departments be created or services performed.

consultation (management) Advice from an expert given after a study of a situation or problem presented by the individual obtaining the consultation. In the public health field, such consultation often concerns organization, management, and strategic planning.

contingency theory An approach to leadership asserting that leadership styles will vary in their efforts in different situations. The situation (not traits or styles themselves) determines whether a leadership style or a particular leader will be effective.

continuing education (CE) Learning which takes place after formal education is completed. Most health professionals are required to acquire a specific number of hours or credits of CE each year in order to retain licensure or certification.

continuing medical education (CME) The education of practicing physicians through refresher courses, medical journals and texts, attendance at regularly scheduled teaching programs, and approved self-study courses.

continuing nursing education (CNE) The education of practicing nurses in order to update or advance their knowledge and skills. CNE is required in most areas of the profession to maintain licensure or certification.

continuing resolution Legislation enacted by Congress to provide budget authority for federal agencies and/or specific activities to continue in operation until the regular appropriations are enacted. Continuing resolutions are enacted when action on appropriations is not complete by the beginning of a fiscal year. The continuing resolution usually specifies a maximum rate at which the obligations may be incurred, based on the rate of the prior year, the President's budget request, or an appropriation bill passed by either or both houses of Congress.

contract An agreement between two or more parties which gives legally enforceable rights and duties to both. A contract need not be in writing to be enforceable unless it is a certain kind of agreement, such as one for the sale of real estate.

corporation A legal entity which exists separately, for all legal purposes, from the people or organizations which own it. To take advantage of legal advantages (limitation of liability and tax benefits, for example), a corporation must observe certain stipulations required by law such as meetings, minutes, and filing of annual reports and tax returns.

for-profit corporation A corporation whose profits (excess of income over expenses) are distributed, as dividends, to shareholders who own the corporation (in contrast to a nonprofit corporation, in which the profits go to corporate purposes rather than to individual shareholders).

nonprofit corporation A corporation whose profits (excess of income over expenses) are used for corporate purposes rather than returned to shareholders or investors (owners) as dividends. To qualify for tax exemption, no portion of the profits of the corporation may inure to the benefit of an individual.

corruption The unauthorized use of public office for private gain. The most common forms of corruption are bribery, extortion, and the misuse of inside information.

cost The expense incurred in providing a product or service.

capital cost The cost of developing or acquiring new equipment, facilities, or services; that is, the investment cost to the institution of such growth.

direct cost A cost which can be identified directly with any part of the organization. Direct costs are added on the basis of accounting formulae.

fixed cost A cost which is entirely independent of the volume of activity.

indirect cost Costs that are not directly accountable to a cost object, such as a particular function or product.

marginal cost The addition to total cost resulting from the production of an additional unit of service or product. This cost varies with the volume of the operation.

semi-variable cost A cost which is partly a variable cost and partly a fixed cost in its behavior in response to changes in volume.

variable cost A cost which is entirely dependent on the volume of activity, as opposed to a fixed cost, which is not affected by volume.

cost allocation An accounting procedure by which costs that cannot be clearly identified with any specific department are distributed among all or some departments.

cost-analysis A group of analyses from the discipline of economics which can be applied to a variety of public health interventions.

cost-benefit analysis (CBA) An economic analysis done to determine whether money was well spent or not. It is a comparison between the dollar value of the benefits realized and the dollar cost of the resources expended to obtain those benefits. The goal is to develop a cost-benefit ratio (CBR). In public administration/policy, CBA is an analytical technique that compares the social costs and benefits of proposed programs or policy actions. All losses and gains experienced by society are included and measured in dollar terms. The net benefits are calculated by subtracting the losses incurred by some sectors of society from the gains that accrue to others. Alternative actions are compared, so as to one or more that yield the greatest net benefits, or ratio of benefits to costs. The inclusion of all gains and losses to society in CBA distinguishes it from CEA, which is a more limited view of costs and benefits.

cost-benefit ratio (CBR) The mathematical result of dividing the benefits value by the cost value. If the ratio is greater than 1.0, the benefits more than outweigh the costs (good); if the ratio is less than 1.0, the costs are greater than the benefits (bad).

This analysis is difficult to use in public health where the benefits are frequently not assigned a dollar value.

cost containment Efforts to prevent increase in cost or to restrict its rate of increase. Cost containment is rarely addressed at reducing cost.

cost-effectiveness analysis (CEA) The comparison of the cost-benefit ratios, or net effectiveness, for the same benefits derived from different services or interventions. Effectiveness is defined as the degree to which the desired benefits are obtained from the particular service or intervention being analyzed.

council of government (COG) An organization of cooperating local governments seeking a regional approach to planning, development, transportation, environment, and other issues.

Council of Linkages A public health organization whose mission is to improve public health practices and education by fostering, coordinating, and monitoring links between academia and the public health community. They develop innovative strategies to build and strengthen public health infrastructure and create processes for continuing public health education throughout one's career.

cross-functional A term used in quality management teams to indicate that more than one department is involved.

cross-training Learning a new skill outside of one's primary area.

cultural competence Possession of the knowledge, skills, and attitudes needed to provide effective services for or working with diverse populations, taking into account the culture, language, values, and reality of the community.

D

data Material, facts, or figures on which discussion is held or from which inferences are drawn or decisions made.

database Any collection of data or information organized with some type of structure, such as rows and columns.

data set A specified set of items of data.

death rate The number of deaths divided by the number of persons at risk. The death rate is usually multiplied by 100, so as to be expressed as a percent. Note that the terms *death* and *mortality* are used interchangeably. For rare events, the death rate may use a different base, for example, per 10,000, and will be expressed not as a percent, but as "per 10,000."

debenture A bond or long-term loan (more than one year) that is not secured by a mortgage on specific property.

debt An obligation to pay, whether in cash, services, or goods.
   long-term debt Debt which does not have to be paid within one year.
   short-term debt Debt to be paid within one year.

debt limit/ceiling The maximum debt a government or government unit may incur under constitutional, statutory, or charter requirements either in total or as a percentage of assessed value. Limits typically encompass only full-faith and credit debt.

decentralized services Services which are carried out from several locations in an effort to improve efficiency, reduce cost, or both. A given type of service is usually under a single management division in an institution although, when decentralized, it may be under several managements.

deficit The amount by which expenditures exceed revenues during an accounting period.

deficit financing A situation in which a government's excess of outlays over receipts for a given period is financed primarily through borrowing from the public.

demographic data The class of data about a person or population which includes such items as age, sex, race, income, marital status, and education.

demographics Descriptions of populations in such terms as age, sex, race, educational level, income, family size, and ethnic background.

Department of Agriculture (USDA) The department of the executive branch of the federal government in charge of a variety of programs dealing with the environment, food production, and natural resource use and preservation.

Department of Commerce (DOC) The department of the executive branch of the federal government in charge of the business and economic sector. It also is responsible for such other issues as weather reports and the census, and includes the National Technical Information Service (NTIS).

Department of Defense (DOD) The department of the executive branch of the federal government in charge of the military and national defense.

Department of Education (DOE) The department of the executive branch of the federal government in charge of educational policy.

Department of Energy (DOE) The department of the executive branch of the federal government in charge of energy policy. Its stated mission is "to foster a secure and reliable energy system that is environmentally and economically sustainable, to be a responsible steward of the Nation's nuclear weapons; to clean up our own facilities and to support continued United States leadership in science and technology."

Department of Health and Human Services (DHHS) The department of the executive branch of the federal government responsible for the federal health programs in the civilian sector. The following agencies are under the direction of DHHS:

Office of the Secretary of Health and Human Services (OS)
Administration for Children and Families (ACF)
Administration on Aging (AoA)
Agency for Healthcare Research and Quality (AHRQ)
Agency for Toxic Substances and Disease Registry (ATSDR)
Centers for Disease Control and Prevention (CDC)
Centers for Medicare and Medicaid Services (CMS)

Food and Drug Administration (FDA)
Health Resources and Services Administration (HRSA)
Indian Health Service (IHS)
National Institutes of Health (NIH)
Substance Abuse and Mental Health Services Administration (SAMHSA)

Department of Justice (DOJ) The department of the executive branch of the federal government which enforces certain federal laws. The Department of Justice is headed by the U.S. Attorney General.

Department of Labor (DOL) The department of the executive branch of the federal government in charge of administering federal employer/employee policies and regulations.

Department of Transportation (DOT) The department in the executive branch of the federal government which is concerned with transportation. The DOT consists of seven units representing the different transportation modes.

depreciation A technique used in accounting to recognize the fact that certain kinds of property (assets), such as equipment, depreciate (lose their value) over time; assets may wear out or be made obsolete by new inventions or materials or techniques. Depreciated property must be replaced with the same or more modern equipment, or be abandoned as items no longer needed. Money must be spent on replacement, and a variety of accounting techniques have been developed to determine how much to allow for this purpose each year for each item.

Simply stated, the allowance is equal to the initial cost (or sometimes the future replacement cost) divided by the estimated life of the property. The total allowance for depreciation is shown on the balance sheet as a deduction from the initial value of the assets.

devolution The transfer of power from a central to a local authority.

diabetes A condition in which too much glucose (sugar) builds up in the blood. This can result in body cells not receiving enough energy and, over time, cause damage to the eyes, kidneys, nerves, and heart.

   type 1 diabetes A disease in which the beta cells in the pancreas are damaged and cannot produce insulin, the hormone which helps cells take in glucose. Insulin shots are necessary to provide the missing hormone.

   type 2 diabetes A disease in which the pancreas does not produce enough insulin (the hormone which helps cells take in glucose) or the cells are not taking in glucose despite the insulin. This is the most common form of diabetes and can usually be controlled with diet, exercise, and weight management.

diabetes educator A health professional with advanced education and training in the needs of people with diabetes who has acquired skills for passing on essential information to patients, their families, and the public.

   certified diabetes educator (CDE) A multidisciplinary credential for health professionals offered by the National Certification Board for Diabetes Education (NCBDE).

diabetic A person who has been diagnosed as having diabetes.

dietary risk factors Eating patterns which increase the likelihood for developing disease or other adverse health effects.

director (management) An operating officer. The title director is used by many institutions for their officers and executives.

disability The absence or loss of physical, mental, or emotional function and earning ability. Disability may be temporary or permanent.

disbursement Paying money to take care of an expense or a debt.

disease An illness or disorder of the function of the body or of certain tissues, organs, or systems. Diseases differ from injuries in that injuries are the result of external physical or chemical agents.

    acute disease A disease which normally is of short duration.

    chronic disease A disease which requires more than one episode of care or is of long duration.

Doctor of Health Administration degree (D.H.A.) An advanced practice degree in health administration and sometimes health policy for senior executives, clinician leaders, and policymakers in health care.

Doctor of Medicine degree (MD) An advanced practice degree in medicine that leads to approval for licensure. An equivalent degree offered by some medical schools is the D.O., Doctor of Osteopathy.

Doctor of Philosophy degree (Ph.D.) Often offered in the biomedical sciences such as microbiology, genetics, virology, biochemistry and the social sciences such as economics, public policy, psychology, sociology, and anthropology. Some Ph.D.'s, such as epidemiology and medical social science, have considerable overlap with other sciences.

Doctor of Public Health degree (Dr.P.H.) An advanced practice degree for public health leaders and professionals. This is sometimes offered with specializations such as epidemiology, community health, environmental health, outcomes research, and public health leadership.

Doctor of Science degree (Sc.D.) A research degree most often awarded in epidemiology, biostatistics, or health systems.

donated services The estimated monetary value of the services rendered by personnel who receive no monetary compensation or only partial monetary compensation for their services. The term is applied to services rendered by members of religious orders, societies, volunteers, and similar groups.

DSM-IV *Diagnostic and Statistical Manual of Mental Disorders*, Fourth Edition. The definitive authority in the United States on psychiatric terminology, published by the American Psychiatric Association.

E

ecological fallacy A statistical term for a logical fallacy in trying to take information from group studies and apply it to individuals.

economic system The way in which goods and services are produced, distributed, and consumed.

effectiveness The degree to which the effort expended, or the action taken, achieves the desired effect, result, or objective.

efficiency The relationship of the amount of work accomplished to the amount of effort required. Although efficiency is usually thought of in terms of cost, it can equally well be measured in other ways, such as time.

employee A person who works for and is paid by another (the employer), and who is under the control of the employer. An employee is to be distinguished from an independent contractor, who works for himself.

employee health benefit plan An organization's plan for health benefits for its employees and their dependents. The term generally refers to the benefits which are provided. Such plans are not part of the employee's salary. The employees may or may not contribute to paying the cost by deductions from their salaries.

empowerment Giving a person or organization the formal authority to do something.

endemic Constantly present in a specific population or geographic area. The adjective may be applied, for example, to a disease or an infectious agent.

end-of-life care Health care and other services provided to a person who is dying. The focus is to make the quality of life as high as possible during this time.

entropy prevention The set of management activities directed at maintaining quality and enthusiasm in the performance of established activities and duties which are not in need of change. Entropy is a term taken from physics for the tendency of any system (process) to lose energy, that is to run down, if no additional energy is provided. An appreciable amount of management energy is applied to change which, while resisted, is seen as "where the action is." However, an equal or even greater amount of management energy must be applied to keep ongoing activities (systems) interesting and exciting, and to prevent quality from declining and change from occurring.

environmental assessment A technique used in planning in which influences and events external to the organization which are felt likely to present either problems or opportunities are listed. An attempt is then made to predict the effects of these factors on the organization and to suggest the appropriate responses. It is to be contrasted with "environmental impact," in which the effects of actions of the organization on its environment are assessed.

Environmental Protection Agency (EPA) The agency of the federal government charged with administering the laws and regulations designed for the protection of our natural environment.

epidemic A group of cases of a specific disease or illness clearly in excess of what one would normally expect in a particular geographic area. There is no absolute criteria for using the term epidemic—as standards and expectations change, so might the definition of an epidemic (e.g., an epidemic of violence).

epidemiologist A public health practitioner, scientist, or physician who studies diseases or causes of disease in relationship to a population. An epidemiologist deals primarily with analysis of existing data rather than data collected prospectively in an experimental design.

epidemiology The study of diseases or causes of disease in relationship to a population.

equity (access) Fairness. This is one great impetus to health care reform; inequities among regions of the country—between rural and urban settings, among ethnic groups, and among socioeconomic groups—in access to and quality of both preventive and curative services, are widely reported.

equity (finance) Assets minus liabilities; also called *net worth.*

equity theory An extension of expectancy theory developed by Stacy Adams. In addition to preferences of outcomes or rewards associated with performance, individuals also assess the degree to which potential rewards will be equitably distributed. Equity theory states that people calculate the ratio of their efforts to the rewards they will receive and compare them to the ratios they believe exist for others in similar situations. People do this because they have a strong desire to be treated fairly.

ergonomics Commonly describes the study of ways to make a more comfortable and productive fit between humans and their machines and work environments.

ethics (moral) The study and theory of moral principles.

ethics (professional) The set of standards and rules promulgated by the various professions and enforced against their members. For example, physicians must follow the *Code of Ethics* of the American Medical Association (AMA).

evidenced-based decision making An approach to decision making that combines expertise, patient or client concerns, and information from scientific literature to derive a decision. The use of verifiable data and current information in the decision analysis.

evidence-based health care (EBHC) An evolutionary broadening of evidence-based medicine (EBM) which includes disciplines other than medicine in recognition of the many factors affecting a person's health.

exclusive dealing An agreement between a seller and buyer for the seller to sell only to the buyer (or the buyer to buy only from the seller). When such an arrangement unfavorably affects competition it may violate the federal antitrust laws.

executive An individual who is a high-level manager and who has authority to make significant decisions. Similar authority is implied by use of the terms employed for corporate officers, such as president and vice-president. The trend is to use these terms in public health organizations where formerly such persons might have been called administrators.

executive branch In a government with a separation of powers, the part that is responsible for the applying or administering the law.

executive budget The budget document for an executive branch of government that a jurisdiction's chief executive submits to legislature for review, modification, and enactment.

Executive Office of the President (EOP) The umbrella office consisting of the top presidential staff agencies that provide the President help and advice in carrying out his major responsibilities.

Expectancy theory Victor Vroom's formulation on how motivation occurs is based on the idea that people make decisions based on the expected outcomes. Individuals estimate how well the results of a given behavior will coincide with desired results and act accordingly. Three conditions affect their decisions: 1) people must believe that their through their own efforts they are more likely to achieve their desired levels of performance, 2) people must believe that by achieving a level of performance they receive an outcome or reward, and 3) people must value the outcome or reward.

expenditure 1) All amounts of money paid out by a government—net of recoveries and other correcting transactions—other than for retirement of national debt, investments in securities, extension of credit, or as agency transactions. Expenditures include only external transactions of a government and exclude noncash transactions such as the provision of prerequisites or other payment in kind. 2) The cost of goods received or services rendered whether cash payments have been made or not (accrual basis); payment of cost of goods received or services rendered (cash basis).

expenditure target A goal for attempting to hold down the rate of growth in expenditures.

expense The using up of an asset (as in depreciation), or the cost of providing services or making a product during an accounting period. The subtraction of expenses from revenue gives the net income.

F

FACHE Fellow of the American College of Healthcare Executives.

faith-based organization (FBO) A generic term covering all religious organizations, including nonprofit groups affiliated with a church or religion. Such organizations often address social issues by providing food, shelter, clothing, and health care to people in need. Began within a religion or group of religions that were established to meet the spiritual needs of a population.

Federal Emergency Management Agency (FEMA) An agency of the federal government, within the Department of Homeland Security (DHS), responsible for national preparedness for all kinds of emergencies, natural or otherwise.

federalism A system of governance in which a national, overarching government shares power with sub-national or state governments.

    cooperative federalism The notion that the national, state, and local governments are cooperating, interacting agents jointly working to solve common problems rather than conflicting, sometimes hostile competitors pursuing similar or conflicting ends.

    dual federalism Federalist theory in which the functions and responsibilities of the federal and state governments are distinguished and separate from each other.

    marble-cake federalism Concept that the cooperative relations among the varying levels of government result in an intermingling of activities; in contrast to the traditional layer-cake federalism, which holds that the three layers of government are almost totally separate.

    new federalism Republican efforts beginning in the Nixon era to decentralize governmental functions by returning power and responsibilities to the states. This trend continued into the 1990s and culminated in the "devolution movement."

    picket-fence federalism The concept that bureaucratic specialists at the various levels of government exercise considerable power over the nature of intergovernmental programs.

Federally Qualified Health Center (FQHC) A local, community-based organization that provides preventive, primary care and other services to those who might not otherwise have access to health care; sometimes called a community health center (CHC). To be considered a FQHC, the heath center must have the following features:

- Is tax-exempt nonprofit of the public

- Is located in or serves an underserved community

- Provides comprehensive primary health care services, referrals, and other services needed to facilitate access to care, such as case management, language translation, and transportation

- Serves everyone in the community regardless of ability to pay

- Is governed by a community board with the majority of members patients of the health center

fee-for-service (FFS) A method of paying physicians and other health care providers in which each service carries a fee.

Fiedler's contingency model Theory that effective leadership is contingent on whether the elements in a particular leadership situation fit the style of the leader.

Fieldler sought to identify leader styles that fit a particular situation and that could be used to increase leader effectiveness by: 1) changing leader styles to fit situations, 2) selecting leaders whose style fit a particular situation, 3) moving leaders to situations that fit their style, 4) changing situations to better fit leader styles. Fieldler viewed managers as being task-oriented or relations-oriented. The task-motivated leader is more concerned with task success and task-related problems. The relations-motivated manager prefers to have close interpersonal relations. Fieldler measured managers using the Least Preferred Co-worker (LPC) scale, in which managers answered questions about past and present co-workers with whom they liked least to work with.

financial administration Activities involving finance and taxation. It includes central agencies for accounting, auditing, and budgeting; the supervision of local government finance; tax administration; collection; custody, collection, and disbursement of funds; administration of employee-retirement systems and debt and investment administration.

financing (finance) A method of obtaining money. Types available include debt financing (borrowing money), equity financing (selling ownership—shares of stock—in the institution), tax-exempt bond financing (if available), and obtaining donations (of decreasing prominence at present).

fiscal federalism The financial relations between and among units of government in a federal system. The theory of fiscal federalism, or multi-unit government finance, is one part of applied economics known as "public finance." The pattern of taxation and grants provided by the federal government.

fiscal function The sum of the activities, wherever performed, through which the organization achieves fiscal soundness.

flexible spending account (FSA) An account managed by an employer that allows employees to set aside pretax funds for medical, dental, legal, and day-care services.

Flexner Report (The) The Flexner Report, authored by Adam Flexner, commissioned by the Carnegie Foundation and produced with help from the AMA in 1910, proposed that medical education follow the university-hospital model used by Johns Hopkins University. This report revolutionized medical education in the United States. The report suggested that the then used guild-apprenticeship model be abolished.

flowchart A type of diagram depicting the steps in a process and their sequence. Flowcharts are used, for example, in quality management to better view a process and find ways to simplify or otherwise improve it.

focus group A group of individuals convened to give their thoughts on a given subject.

Food and Drug Administration (FDA) An agency within the U.S. Department of Health and Human Services (DHHS) responsible for protecting the health of the nation against impure and unsafe foods, drugs, cosmetics, biological substances, and other potential hazards. A major part of the FDAs activity is controlling the sale, distribution, and use of pharmaceutical drugs and medical devices, including the licensing of new drugs for use by humans.

Food and Drug Administration Amendments Act of 2007 Legislation reauthorizing and expanding the *Prescription Drug User Fee Act* and the *Medical Device User Fee and Modernization Act*. This amendment allows the FDA to possess the resources needed to conduct the complex and comprehensive review of new drugs and medical devices.

Food and Safety Modernization Act of 2011 Sweeping reform to food safety legislation that shifts the focus from reacting to food contamination to preventing it.

for-profit An entity organized under any of various business forms (corporation, partnership, sole-proprietorship, etc.) whose profits (excess of income over expenses) are returned to its members (shareholders, investors, owners) as dividends.

Freedom of Information Act (FOIA) A federal law enacted in 1966 to establish an effective legal right of access to government information. The FOIA provides access to all federal agency records, except those that are specifically exempted.

full-time equivalent (FTE) A concept used in developing statistics on the size of a workforce. The idea is to express a workforce made up of both full-and part-time employees as the number of workers that would be employed if all were full time. It is computed by dividing the total hours worked by all employees in a given time period by the number of work hours in the time period.

fund (accounting) A device established to control receipt and disbursement of income from sources set aside to support specific activities or attain certain objectives. In the accounts of individual governments, each fund is treated as a distinct fiscal entity.

fund (noun) An asset set aside for a given purpose, e.g., a building fund, which is to be used only for that purpose.

fund (verb) To allocate or provide funds for (a program, project, etc.); for example, to fund depreciation means to set aside money at a rate determined by estimating the time before a given piece of equipment will have to be replaced so that, at the end of that time, there will be enough money to replace it.

fund balance A term often used by nonprofit organizations in their financial statements to indicate the difference between assets and liabilities. A positive fund balance is sometimes called a *gain*; in the profit sector, it would be called a profit. A negative fund balance is a loss in either sector. Nonprofit organizations may also refer to the fund balance as revenues over (under) expenses.

fund-raising Planned and coordinated activities by which the organization seeks gifts.

funds Available money resources.

G

gatekeeper The person responsible for determining the services to be provided to a patient and coordinating the provision of the appropriate care. The purposes of the gatekeeper's function are to improve the quality of care by considering all the patient's problems and other relevant factors, to ensure that all necessary care is obtained, and to reduce unnecessary care (and cost). When, as is often the case, the gatekeeper is a physician, she or he is a primary care physician and usually must, except in an emergency, give the first level of care to the patient before the patient is permitted to be seen by a secondary care physician.

gateway (organization) An organization or system which provides a single point of access to a given universe of products or services. A gateway organization usually provides service directly or, if it does not offer the desired service, makes sure that the consumer or client reaches the proper destination.

genomics The study of genomes on a large scale.

gerontology The multidisciplinary study of the biological, psychological, and social processes of aging and the elderly.

goal Broad statements of what needs to be accomplished.

goal setting theory Edwin Locke's theory that goal setting is a cognitive process through which conscious goals, as well as intentions about pursuing them, are developed and become primary determinants of behavior. The central premise in this perspective on the process of motivation is that people focus their attention on the concrete tasks related to attaining their goals, and they persist in the tasks until the goals are achieved.

global budget A limit on the total health care spending for a given unit of population, taking into account all sources of funds. In health care reform discussions and proposals, it usually means that caps will be placed on (1) employers' expenditures, based on payroll; (2) individuals' expenditures for insurance, based on income; (3) institutional budgets' core spending; and (4) personal out-of-pocket expenditures. Problem areas include how the information on total spending data is obtained or how the cap is enforced.

governance Organizational function that holds management and the organization itself accountable for its actions.

Government Accountability Office (GAO) A support agency of the United States Congress created by the *Budget and Accounting Act of 1921* to audit federal government expenditures and to assist Congress with its legislative oversight responsibilities.

grant 1) A sum of money given by the government, a foundation, or other organization to support a program, project, organization, or individual. 2) An assistance award in which substantial involvement is not anticipated between the federal government and the state or local government or other recipient during the performance of the contemplated activity.

gross domestic product (GDP) The market value of all goods and services produced by labor and property within the United States during a particular period of time. Income from overseas operations of a domestic corporation would not be included in the GDP, but activities carried on within United States borders by a foreign company would be.

gross national product (GNP) The market value of all goods and services produced by labor and property supplied by residents of the United States during a particular period of time. Income from overseas operations of a domestic corporation would be included in the GNP.

group A number of individuals assembled together or having common interest.

group cohesion The shared beliefs, values, and assumptions of a group that allow it to function as a team.

group dynamics The subfield of organizational behavior concerned with the nature of groups, how they develop, and how they interrelate with individuals and other groups.

group process Working in or with groups. Groups may be large or small, formal or informal, short-term or long-term, meet on a regular or infrequent basis, be static or ever-changing.

guidelines Directing principles which layout a suggested policy or procedure.
    administrative guidelines Suggestions promulgated by an administrative agency as to procedure or interpretations of law. Guidelines are not binding as are regulations, which have the force of law.
    clinical practice guidelines Statements by authoritative bodies as to the procedures appropriate for a physician to employ for certain diagnoses, conditions, or situations. They are intended to change providers' practice styles, reduce inappropriate and unnecessary care, and cut costs.

H

Hawthorne experiments The late 1920s and early 1930s management studies undertaken at the Hawthorne Works of the Western Electric Company near Chicago.

hazardous materials (HAZMAT) Substances, such as radioactive or chemical materials, that are dangerous to humans and other living organisms.

health The state of complete physical, mental, and social well-being and not merely the absence of disease. It is recognized, however, that health has many dimensions (anatomical, mental, and physiological) and is largely culturally defined. The relative importance of various disabilities will differ depending on the cultural milieu and the role of affected individuals in that culture. Most attempts at measurement have been in terms of morbidity and mortality.

health care or healthcare Services provided for health promotion, prevention of illness and injury, monitoring of health, maintenance of health, and treatment of diseases, disorders, and injuries in order to obtain cure or, failing that, optimum comfort and function (quality-of-life).

health care delivery A term that applies to providing any of the wide array of health care services.

health care delivery system A term without specific definition referring to all the facilities and services along with methods for financing them through which health care is provided.

health care executive An individual who works in administration and/or management within the health care field. Positions range from department head to chief executive officer (CEO) and may be within a hospital or other facility, health care association, home health agency, managed care organizations, or anywhere throughout the health care system.

   certified healthcare executive (CHE) A credential awarded by the American College of Healthcare Executives (ACHE) to members who meet certain requirements but who are not yet ready for Fellowship in the College. This credential may be used after the individual's name until such time as Fellowship status is achieved, after which FACHE replaces it.

health care institution As commonly used, any institution dealing with health. Some definitions state that an institution, to qualify for this term, must have an organized professional staff. However, there are no regulations such as standards for the licensure or registry of institutions which currently restrict the use of this term.

health care organization (HCO) An organizational form for health care delivery in which the financial risk (health care) is assumed by the organization rather than by individuals.

health care provider A term that can be generically used to mean any person or organization that provides health care.

health care reform A term without a clear definition which is applied to the efforts on the federal, state, and local levels to make changes in the health care delivery system so that costs are reduced or contained, the uninsured population is covered, all citizens have access to health care, financing is assured, and quality of care is controlled or improved.

health care system A system designed to take responsibility only for the care of those who seek it out. It responds to the needs of individual patients who present themselves with illness or injury.

health care worker (HCW) The definition depends upon the context, but will generally include physicians; residents; interns; supervising nurses, nurses, and nursing assistants; emergency medical technicians (EMTs); or anyone who comes into direct contact with patients.

health economics The branch of economics which deals with the provision of public health and health care services, their delivery and their use, with special attention to quantifying the demands for such services, the costs of such services and of their delivery, and the benefits obtained. More emphasis is given to the costs and benefits of health care to a population than to the individual.

health education Education which is directed at increasing the information of individuals and populations, especially communities, about health and its mainte-nance and the prevention of disease and injury; bringing about modifications in the behavior of individuals so as to achieve better health; and changing social policy in the direction of a more healthful environment and practices.

health fair A type of community health education activity in which exhibits are the main method used and in which free diagnostic services are sometimes offered.

health maintenance organization (HMO) A health care providing organization which ordinarily has a closed group of physicians (and sometimes other health professionals), along with either its own hospital or allocated beds in one or more hospitals. Individuals (usually families) join an HMO, which agrees to provide the medical and hospital care they need, for a fixed, predetermined fee. Each subscriber is under a contract stipulating the limits of the service.

health professional A comprehensive term covering people working in the field of public health or health care who have some special training and/or education. The degree of education, training, and other qualifications varies greatly with the nature of the profession, and with the state regulating its practice.

health promotion Efforts to change peoples' behavior in order to promote healthy lives and prevent illnesses and accidents and to minimize their effects. A health promotion program may include health risk appraisal of the individuals, and may give attention to fitness, stress management, smoking, cholesterol reduction, weight control, nutrition, cancer screening, and other matters on the basis of the risks detected.

Health Resources and Services Administration (HRSA) Improves access to health care for people who are uninsured or medically vulnerable by providing financial support to health care agencies in states and territories. The HRSA trains heath care professionals in rural communities and oversees organ donations and transplants, as well as maintains databases to protect against health care malprac-tice and health care waste, fraud, and abuse.

health services A term without specific definition which pertains to any services which are health-related.

health status The state of health of an individual or population.

health status index A statistic which attempts to quantify the health status of an individual or a population. Such indices are developed using health status indicators.

health status indicator A measurement of some attribute of individual or com-munity health which is considered to reflect health status. Each attribute is given a numerical value, and a score (a health status index) is calculated for the individual or community from the aggregate of these values. To the extent possible, the indicators are objective, that is, they are facts for which various observers or investigators would each find the same value. In the case of a community, such statistics as mortality and morbidity rates are sometimes used.

health system A system designed to take responsibility for the health of its defined community; it usually involves outreach rather than response or reaction. This is in contrast with a health care system.

Healthy People 2000 A report published by the U.S. Public Health Service in 1990 outlining health promotion and disease prevention goals for Americans for the year 2000. The report states that meeting the goals requires acceptance of shared responsibilities by citizens, health professionals, government at all levels, the media, and communities. The goals included such specifics as an increased life span accompanied by a high quality-of-life (QOL) factor, improve the health of populations now deemed to be particularly disadvantaged, and to provide all Americans with preventive health services.

Healthy People 2010 A national initiative setting forth goals of promoting health and preventing disease; an update of Healthy People 2000.

Herzberg Two-Factor theory Frederick Herzberg's theory of motivation in the workplace revolved around what satisfies and dissatisfies people at work. Herzberg added a new dimension to motivation theory by proposing a two-factor model of motivation whereby certain factors lead to satisfaction at work while others lead to dissatisfaction. Working from this two-factor model, Herzberg developed the *motivation-hygiene theory* to demonstrate that motivation factors are needed to motivate an employee to higher performance while hygiene factors are needed to ensure an employee is not dissatisfied.

HIPAA The *Health Insurance Portability and Accountability Act of 1996* (HIPAA) is federal legislation whose primary purpose is to provide continuity of health care coverage. It does this partly by providing limitations on preexisting condition exclusions, as well as prohibiting discrimination against individuals based on health status. The law also guarantees that insured workers will be eligible to keep their insurance if they leave their jobs. It created the medical savings account (MSA) to help individuals pay for their health care. HIPAA also made amendments to other legislation, including the *Employee Retirement Income Security Act* (ERISA), the Internal Revenue Code (IRC), and the *Public Health Service Act*. HIPAA also contains a section for requirements for the electronic transmission of health information.

HIV (human immunodeficiency virus) The virus which causes AIDS. HIV is usually passed from one person to another through blood-to-blood and sexual contact.

home health care Care at the levels of skilled nursing care and intermediate care provided in the patient's home through an agency or program that has the resources necessary to provide that care.

hospice A program that assists with the physical, emotional, spiritual, psychological, social, financial, and legal needs of the dying patient and their family.

The service may be provided in the patient's home or in an institution set up for that purpose.

Human Genome Project (HGP) A 13-year effort, begun in 1990, to discover all the estimated 20,000 to 25,000 human genes and make them accessible for further biological study. Another project goal was to determine the complete sequence of the 3 million DNA subunits (bases in the human genome). The project was completed in 2003.

human resource management The function of an organization where the focus is on job analysis, performance appraisal, recruitment, and selection. The human resources domain of public health management ultimately serves to promote healthy workplaces, thus keeping with the foundations and fundamentals of public health.

human resources The people who staff and operate an organization.

I

ICD *International Classification of Diseases.* A publication of the World Health Organization (WHO) revised periodically and now in the Tenth Revision, dated 1994. The full title is *International Statistical Classification of Diseases and Related Health Problems.* This classification, which originated for use in deaths, is used worldwide for that purpose. In addition, it has been used widely in the United States for hospital diagnosis classification since about 1955 through adaptations and modifications made in the United States of the Seventh, Eighth, and Ninth revisions. The current modification, *International Classification of Diseases Ninth Revision Clinical Modification* (ICD-9-CM), has been in official use in the United States since 1979.

immunity The condition of being immune or insusceptible to an agent. The term is most often used in regard to resistance to infectious disease. However, one may also speak, for example, of stress immunity, the ability to resist stress, or cold immunity, the ability to withstand cold.

> **acquired immunity** Immunity to infection which is the result of infection or the administration of an agent, such as a vaccine, either of which may stimulate the body to develop active immunity.
>
> **active immunity** A type of acquired immunity in which the body is stimulated to produce its own antibodies. This occurs either in response to an infection (which may or may not produce symptoms) or in response to the inoculation of a vaccine, either a strain of killed bacteria or other infectious agent or an attenuated (weakened) strain of the infectious agent (a strain which is able to stimulate the body to produce antibodies but not symptoms).
>
> **herd immunity** The relative immunity of a group of persons or animals as a result of the immunity of an adequate number (proportion) of the individuals in the group. The immunity may be active immunity or passive immunity. Herd immunity is actually immunity against an epidemic, rather than the immunity

of individuals against infection. For an epidemic to succeed, it must be possible for the disease to travel from one individual to another. When enough individuals are immune, the epidemic simply dies out.

passive immunity A type of acquired immunity that is conferred by giving to the person (or animal) immune substances developed in another animal or human. One example is tetanus antitoxin, an immune substance developed in a laboratory animal and transferred to the human by inoculation (injection). Such an antibody is prefabricated and immediately ready to repel the invasion of the infection (in this case, tetanus). Its protection is temporary because the body eliminates the antitoxin as fast as it can (it is a foreign substance) and thereafter the body is susceptible to tetanus again.

implementation Putting a government program into effect; the total process of translating a legal mandate, whether an executive order or an enacted statute, into appropriate program directives and structures that provide services or create goods.

incidence The number of specified new events taking place in a defined period of time in a given area or population. It usually refers to cases of disease or injury, and is the numerator in the calculation of an incidence rate for the event in question. The denominator is the population at risk within the given time period. Incidence is often confused with prevalence, which applies to the number of events or cases of disease present in a given population at a given time.

income Money earned during an accounting period, in contrast with revenue, which is the increase in assets or the decrease in liabilities during the accounting period.

income and expense statement A standard part of a financial statement in which are shown the revenues, costs, and expenses of the organization for the accounting period. The other part of the financial statement is the balance sheet.

incremental budgeting A method of budget review that focuses on the increments of increase or decrease in the budget of existing programs.

incremental funding The provision of budgetary resources for a program or project based on obligations estimated to be incurred within a fiscal year when such budgetary resources will cover only a portion of the obligations to be incurred while completing the program of project.

Indian Health Service (IHS) An agency within the Department of Health and Human Services (DHHS) whose goal is to assure that comprehensive, culturally acceptable personal and public health services are available and accessible to American Indian and Alaska Native people. The IHS manages a comprehensive health care delivery system for more than 561 federally recognized Indian tribes in 35 states. IHS provides services to approximately 1.8 million members in urban areas as well as on reservations.

informatics The science of gathering, storing, manipulating, managing, analyzing, visualizing, and utilizing information.

information systems Also known as *informatics*; system consisting of the network of all channels of communication within an organization.

information technology Technology involving the development, maintenance, and use of computer systems, software, and networking for the processing and distribution of data.

inpatient A patient who receives care while being lodged in an institution such as a hospital.

Institute of Medicine (IOM) A body formed by the National Academy of Sciences (NAS) in 1970 to secure the services of eminent members of appointed professions for the examination of policy matters pertaining to the health of the public. The Institute acts under the responsibility given to NAS in 1863 by its charter to be an advisor to the federal government and, upon its own initiative, to study problems of medical care, research, and education.

insurance A method of providing for money to pay for specific types of losses which may occur. Insurance is a contract between one party (the insured) and another (the insurer). The policy states what types of losses are covered, what amounts will be paid for each loss and for all losses, and under what conditions.

insurance coverage Generally refers to the amount of protection available and the kind of loss which would be paid for under an insurance contract.

intergovernmental relations The complex network of interrelationships among governments; the political, fiscal, programmatic, and administrative processes by which higher governments share resources and revenues with lower units of governments, generally accompanied by special conditions that the lower government units must satisfy as prerequisites to receiving assistance.

interpersonal skills Require an understanding of human behavior and interpersonal relationships; the ability to understand peoples' feelings, attitudes, and motivation; the ability to communicate in a clear and persuasive manner; the ability to foster cooperative relationships; and well-developed emotional intelligence.

J

The Joint Commission An independent, nonprofit, voluntary organization which develops standards and provides accreditation surveys and certification to hospitals and to other health organizations. **http://jointcommission.org**

joint resolution A joint resolution requires the approval of both houses of Congress and the signature of the President, just as a bill does, and has the force of law when approved. There is no real difference between a bill and a joint resolution. Joint resolutions are generally used in dealing with limited matters, such as a single appropriation for a specific purpose.

K

Kaiser Family Foundation One of the nation's largest private foundations devoted exclusively to health. Created in 1948 by industrialist Henry J. Kaiser, it focuses on four main areas: health policy, reproductive health, HIV policy, and health and development in sub-Sahara Africa. **http://www.kff.org**

Kaiser-Permanente Medical Care Program America's largest nonprofit health maintenance organization (HMO). Considered to be a pioneer in comprehensive prepayment systems, Kaiser-Permanente includes the following three components:

Kaiser Foundation Health Plan The health maintenance organization (HMO) under which the members are organized.

Kaiser Foundation Hospitals A nonprofit corporation that provides the hospital services to the HMO members.

Permanente Medical Groups The physician partnerships and professional corporations which provide the medical services to the HMO.

knowledge-based management Management practices and decisions supported by valid data.

L

leadership The exercise of authority, whether formal or informal, in directing or coordinating the work of others.

adaptive leadership The practice of mobilizing people to tackle tough challenges. It is specifically about change, building on the past, and being both conservative and progressive. Adaptation occurs best when there is experimentation and relies heavily upon diversity. It is important to remember that organizational adaption takes time and culture changes slowly.

autocratic leaders Make decisions and then hand them down to participants. The role of participants is to carry out tasks with no opportunities to alter decisions.

consultative leaders Convince other participants of the correctness of the decision by carefully explaining the rationale of the decision and its effect upon other participants and on the program or project itself. A second style of consultative leadership occurs when a leader permits slightly more involvement from participants—the manager presents the decision to the participants and invites questions to enhance the understanding and acceptance.

democratic leaders Define the limits of the situation and problem to be solved and permit other participants to make the decision.

laissez-faire leaders Permit participants to have great discretion in decision making. The manager bears no more influence than other participants in decision making. The leader's and other participants' roles in decision making are indistinguishable in this style.

participative leaders Present tentative decisions that will be changed if other participants can make a convincing case. A second style of participative leadership is when a manager presents a problem to participants, seeks their advice and suggestions, but then makes the decisions. This style of leadership makes greater use of participation and less use of authority than autocratic and consultative styles.

servant-leader Stresses the importance of the role a leader plays as a steward of the resources of an organization and teaches leaders to serve others, such as fellow employees, the public, or a cause, while still achieving the goals of the organization. In theory, this type of leadership is found in the public sector, where managers and officials serve the people of their state or community.

transactional leaders Permit some of the needs of followers to be met if they perform to the leader's expectations; leaders and followers undertake transactions in which each receives something of value.

transformational leaders Managers are more focused on creating change than on transactions. They focus on creating changes that are organization- or system-wide in scope.

learning organization Peter Senge's term for organizations in which new patterns of thinking are nurtured and where people are continually learning together to improve both the organization and their personal lives.

level of care The amount (intensity) and kind of professional care required for an individual in order to achieve the desired outcomes.

leverage Financing by borrowing.

capital leverage See *financial leverage*.

financial leverage The ratio of total debt to total assets. Financial leverage is also called capital leverage. An institution uses financial leverage when it believes it has *positive* leverage, that is, that it can use the money obtained by debt financing (see *financing*) to earn more money than it costs to borrow the money (interest and taxes). Should the cost of borrowing exceed the added revenue, the situation is one of *negative* leverage.

negative leverage See *financial leverage*.

operating leverage The ratio of fixed costs to variable costs (see *cost*). When it takes very little added labor or materials to provide added units of service or products, the operating leverage is high (and the marginal cost of added units is low); a greater volume brings accelerated profits, once the break-even point is reached. The higher the proportion of the costs that are variable (that is, the lower the operating leverage) the greater an increase in units of service or products will be required to increase profits.

positive leverage See *financial leverage*.

leveraged Financed largely by borrowed funds.

liability (financial) In finance, a liability is an obligation to pay.

current liability A liability due within one year.

liability (legal) An actual or potential responsibility to do something, pay something, or refrain from doing something. Liability is used to refer to a legal duty or other obligation, often one which must be enforced by a lawsuit.

corporate liability Legal responsibility of a corporation rather than of an individual.

joint liability The responsibility of more than one defendant to share in legal liability to a plaintiff.

product liability An area of law which imposes legal responsibility on manufacturers (and in some cases distributors and retailers) of goods which leave the factory in an unreasonably dangerous condition, and which in fact cause harm to someone because of that condition.

professional liability A legal duty which is the result of performing (or failing to perform) something which one does (or should have done) as a professional.

license A legal term that represents a specific right to do or use something or to refrain from it.

licensure A method used to ensure that persons who provide services are adequately qualified. The licensure law will often define the scope of practice for that profession and anyone performing services within that scope must first have a license to do so.

life expectancy A statistically-derived estimate as to how long a given individual or population may be expected to live.

lifetime reserve A Medicare term referring to the pool of 60 days of hospital care upon which a patient may draw after they have used up the maximum Medicare benefit for a single event.

limited liability company (LLC) A form of organization which allows all owners and managers to have limited liability for the debts of the company or organization but also favorable tax treatment which avoids traditional corporate taxation.

line-item budget The classification of budgetary accounts according to narrow, detailed objects of expenditure used within each particular agency of government, generally without reference to the ultimate purpose or objective served by the expenditure.

lobbying Attempts to influence the passage or defeat of legislation.

local health department A unit of local government which implements local, national, and state public health policy. It typically carries out some clinical services, environmental services, and support services. Clinical services may include, for example, dental health, occupational health, nursing, maternal and child health, family planning, communicable disease, and Women, Infants, and Children's Programs (WIC). Environmental services may include general environment, vector control, animal control, and pollution control. Support services may include, in addition to administration, vital statistics, laboratory, and health education.

long-term care (LTC) Care for patients, regardless of age, who have chronic diseases or disabilities and who require preventive, diagnostic, therapeutic, and supportive services over long periods of time.

long-term care facility (LTCF) A facility which provides lodging and health care services to patients with chronic health care needs who require long-term care.

loss (financial) Excess of expense over income resulting in a decrease in assets.

M

MacArthur Foundation The John D. and Catherine T. MacArthur Foundation is a private, independent grant awarding institution dedicated to helping groups and individuals foster lasting improvement in the human condition. **http://www. macfound.org**

macroeconomics The economic theory which pertains to forces which determine the decisions and actions of populations rather than of individuals; the latter theory concerning individuals is called *microeconomics.*

maintenance Organizational function responsible for the fiscal, physical, and human resource infrastructure of the organization.

malpractice A failure of care or skill by a professional which causes loss or injury and results in legal liability.

managed care Any arrangement for health care in which someone is interposed between the patient and physician and has authority to place restraints on how and from whom the patient may obtain medical and health services, and what services are to be provided in a given situation. Managed care was originally designed to control costs, encourage efficient use of resources, and ensure that care given is appropriate.

management A word that refers both to the people responsible for running an organization and to the running process itself; the use of numerous resources (such as employees and machines) to accomplish an organizational goal. Permeates all other functions and subsystems of the organization. It involves those in charge of all the other functions.

management by objectives (MBO) A method of goal setting to enhance the contributions of everyone in an organization. The process involves participation in developing specific, attainable, and measurable personal objectives or goals. These personal goals and objectives are aligned with organizational objectives.

management control The aspect of management concerned with the comparison of actual versus planned performance as well as the development and implementation of procedures to correct substandard performance.

management revolution James Burham's concept that control of large businesses moved from the original owners to professional managers. Society's new governing class would not be the traditional possessors of wealth, but those who have the professional expertise to manage and lead large organizations.

manager Any individual who is responsible for directing the activities of an organization or one of its components.

managerialism An entrepreneurial approach to public management that emphasizes management rights and a reinvigorated scientific management.

mandate To require or a requirement; one level of government requiring another to offer—and/or pay for—a program as a matter of law or as a prerequisite to partial or full funding for either the program in question or other programs.

market forces The economic forces of supply and demand.

marketing Activity to publicize an organization or service and to increase its use.

Maslow's hierarchy of needs Abraham Maslow's five sets of basic human needs arranged in a hierarchy of prepotency: physiological needs (food, water, shelter, etc.), safety needs, affiliation needs, esteem needs, and self-actualization.

Master of Business Administration degree (M.B.A.) This may have a concentration in health administration or multi-sector health management. An advanced college degree, earned by those who successfully graduate from their college or university's MBA program. A typical MBA program deals with multiple aspects of business, including finance and management skills.

Master of Health Administration (M.H.A.) A management and administration degree for health care that is prevalent in hospitals and health delivery settings. It sometimes requires a postgraduate residency in health administration.

Master of Public Administration degree or sometimes Master of Public Affairs degree (M.P.A.) Many offer concentrations in health administration and health policy. This is a commonly held degree for public-sector and non-profit managers and administrators, including many in federal public health organizations and state and county health departments.

Master of Public Health degree (M.P.H.) Students can specialize in health administration and health policy or other areas of focus such as environmental health, community health, epidemiology, etc. The Council on Education in Public Health is a strident advocate.

Master of Science in Administration degree (M.S.A.) A management and administration degree for health care that is used in hospitals, government agencies, the military, and health delivery settings.

Master of Science in Nursing degree (M.S.N.) Often offers a concentration in administration and can also include specialization in community health nursing or public health nursing

Maternal and Child Health Bureau (MCHB) One of the key program areas of the Health Resources and Services Administration (HRSA), an agency in the Department of Health and Human Services (DHHS). It is charged with the primary responsibility for promoting and improving the health of mothers and children. **http://mchb.hrsa.gov**

maternal and child health (MCH) program A program providing preventive and treatment services for pregnant women, mothers, and children. The services may include health education and family planning. Funding may be from federal, state, or local sources.

McCelland's Acquired Needs model David McCelland's theory that needs are learned through life experiences. These needs develop throughout a person's life. He stated three levels of needs: achievement, power, and affiliation.

Medicaid The federal program that provides health care to indigent and medically indigent persons. Although partially federally funded (and managed by CMS), the Medicaid program is administered by the states, in accordance with an approved plan for that state. Each state has considerable flexibility in designing its plan and operating its Medicaid program but must comply with federal requirements. This is in contrast with Medicare, which is federally funded and administered at the federal level by CMS. The Medicaid program was established in 1965 by amendment to the *Social Security Act*.

medical director (organization) A physician retained to coordinate the medical care in the organization, to ensure adequacy and appropriateness of the medical services provided to each patient, and to maintain surveillance of the health status of employees. Most county health departments are required to have a medical director.

medically underserved area A rural or urban area that does not have enough health care resources to meet the needs of its population or whose population has relatively low health status. The term is defined in the *Public Health Service Act* and used to determine which areas have priority for assistance.

medically underserved population A population group which does not have enough health care resources to meet its needs. The group may reside in a medically underserved area or may be a population group with certain attributes; for example, migrant workers, Native Americans, or prison inmates may constitute a medically underserved population. The term is defined in the *Public Health Service Act* and used to determine which areas have priority for assistance.

Medicare The federal program that provides payment for health care for persons sixty-five years of age and older and other qualifying individuals. The program is administered at the federal level by the Centers for Medicare and Medicaid Services (CMS). Medicare was established in 1965 by amendment to the *Social Security Act*. **http://www.medicare.gov**

Medicare Advantage A program that permits those with Medicare Part A and Part B to choose among several types of health plans including health maintenance organizations (HMO), preferred-provider organizations (PPO), provider-sponsored organizations (PSO), and private fee-for-service plans (FFS). This program covers more than original Medicare.

Medicare Part A The Medicare program that pays for hospital services, as well as for nursing facility care, home health care, and hospice care following a covered hospital stay.

Medicare Part B The Medicare program through which persons entitled to Medicare Part A may obtain assistance with payment for physician services, diagnostic tests, and other professional and outpatient services. Individuals participate voluntarily through enrollment and payment of a monthly fee and annual deductible.

Medicare Part D The Medicare program that pays for prescription drugs. The program is voluntary for Medicare beneficiaries who may enroll in a choice of plans and pay an extra premium each month for the coverage. There is also a deductible.

merit system A public-sector concept of staffing that implies that no test of party membership is involved in the selection, promotion, or retention of government employees and that a constant effort is made to select the best-qualified individuals available for appointment and advancement.

moral leadership Leading people in specific directions of action and thought based on morals and decency.

motivation An amalgam of all of the factors in one's working environment that foster or inhibit productive efforts. Defined as the set of processes that drive, direct, and maintain human behavior toward attaining some goal or meeting a need.

N

National Academy of Sciences (NAS) A private, nonprofit, self-perpetuating society of distinguished scholars engaged in scientific and engineering research, dedicated to the furtherance of science and technology and to their use for the general welfare. Upon the authority of the charter granted to it by the Congress when it was formed in 1863, the NAS has a mandate that requires it to advise the federal government on scientific and technical matters. Under the NAS charter, the National Research Council (NRC) was established in 1916, the National Academy of Engineering (NAE) in 1964, and the Institute of Medicine (IOM) in 1970. **http://www.nasonline.org**

national health insurance A federally established and operated system of health care financing encompassing all (or nearly all) citizens. Such a system, not in effect in the United States, would provide uniform benefits to all and be paid for via taxes. Distinguish this from national health service, in which the government is not only the payer, but also the provider.

National Health Service (NHS) An organization created by the United Kingdom in 1948 to provide health care for all of its citizens. Its core principles include providing quality health care that meets the needs of everyone, is free at the point of service, and is based on the patient's clinical need, not their ability to pay. The NHS is funded by taxes and is accountable to Parliament. **http://www.nhs.uk**

National Institutes of Health (NIH) The nation's premier biomedical research organization. The NIH is an agency within the Department of Health and Human Services (DHHS). Based in Bethesda, Maryland, the NIH is comprised of 28 separate institutes and centers. The institutes carry out research and programs related to certain specific types of diseases, such as mental and neurological disease, arthritis, cancer, and heart disease. There is an institute for each of the categories of disease for which NIH has programs, and a number of other components not specific to any disease categories.

neoclassical theory Theoretical perspectives that revise, expand, and/or are critical of classical organization theory.

net worth Assets minus liabilities.

new public administration An academic advocacy movement for social equity in the performance and delivery of public services; it called for a proactive administrator with a desire for social equity to replace the traditional impersonal and neutral bureaucrat.

new public management A disparate group of structural reforms and informal management initiatives that reflect the doctrine of managerialism in the public sector.

nongovernmental organization (NGO) A legal entity created by private individuals, private organizations, publicly traded organizations, or in some combination where government influence, supervision, and management are removed, or at least greatly minimized, from the NGO's strategic and operational mission.

nonprofit An entity whose profits (excess of income over expenses) are used for its own purposes rather than returned to its members (shareholders, investors, owners) as dividends. To qualify for tax exemption, no portion of the profits of the entity may inure to the benefit of an individual.

nurse practitioner (NP) A registered nurse who has completed a nurse practitioner program at the master's degree or certificate level. NPs have qualifications which permit them to carry out expanded health care evaluation and decision making regarding patient care with focus on primary care and patient education. In most states, NPs may prescribe medication.

O

objective A short-term goal; something that must be achieved on the way to a larger achievement. More specific than goals and have defined outcomes that can be measured.

obesity The condition of being obese, or significantly overweight. Determining a person's ideal body weight is now typically done by calculating the body mass index (BMI), a number that takes into account an individual's height and weight. People with a BMI of 25 to 29.9 are considered overweight. Those with a BMI of 30 and above are considered obese.

occupational health An area of specialization in public health which concerns the factors (such as working conditions and exposure to hazardous materials) in an occupation that influence the health of workers in that occupation, and which is concerned generally with the prevention of disease and injury and the maintenance of fitness.

Occupational Safety and Health Administration (OSHA) A federal agency responsible for developing and enforcing regulations regarding safety and health among workers in the United States. **http://www.osha.gov**

Office of Disease Prevention and Health Promotion (ODPHP) An agency within the Department of Health and Human Services (DHHS) charged with developing and coordinating national disease prevention and health promotion strategies. **http://odphp.osophs.dhhs.gov**

Office of Public Health and Science (OPHS) An agency within the Department of Health and Human Services (DHHS) under the direction of the Assistant Secretary for Health (ASH), which includes a number of divisions:

Office of Disease Prevention and Health Promotion
Office of Global Health Affairs
Office of HIV/AIDS Policy
Office for Human Research Protection
Office of Minority Health
Office of Population Affairs
Office of Research Integrity
Office of the Surgeon General
Office on Women's Health
President's Council on Physical Fitness and Sports
Regional Health Administrators

officer A person in an organization holding a position of authority either by election or appointment.

Omnibus Budget Reconciliation Act (OBRA) A series of federal legislations that made several significant changes in the provisions to Medicaid. The first OBRA was passed in 1980. Multiple OBRAs were passed in subsequent years ending with the *Omnibus Budget Reconciliation Act of 1993*. Collectively the OBRAs expanded Medicaid eligibility, provided for ambulatory surgery benefits, established the *Nursing Home Reform Act*, and called for significant physician payment reform by establishing payment schedule and increased funding for effectiveness research. *The Omnibus Budget Reconciliation Acts of 1980 and 1981* collectively are referred to as the Boren Amendment.

organization A structured social system consisting of groups and individuals working together to meet agreed-upon objectives.

organizational awareness The ability to understand and learn the formal and informal decision-making structures and power relationships in an organization or industry. This includes the ability to identify who the real decision makers are and the individuals who can influence them, and to predict how new events will affect individuals and groups within the organization.

organizational behavior The study of individual and group behaviors in organizations, analyzing motivation, work satisfaction, leadership, work-group dynamics, and the attitudes and behaviors of the members of organizations.

organizational culture The pattern of shared values, beliefs, and norms—along with associated behaviors, symbols, and rituals—that are acquired over time by members of an organization. It is the historically developed sense of the institution's "legacy"—what it is and what it stands for—that permeates throughout the organization and is known to all who work for it.

organizational development An approach or strategy for increasing organizational effectiveness. As a process it has no value biases, but is usually associated with the idea that effectiveness is found by integrating the individual's desire for growth with organizational goals.

organizational theory A sociological approach to the study of organizations focusing on topics that affect the organization as a whole, such as organizational environments, goals and effectiveness, strategy and decision making, change and innovation, and structure and design.

outcome Refers to the "outcome" (finding) of a given diagnostic procedure. It may also refer to cure of a patient, restoration of function, or extension of life. When used for populations or the health care system, it typically refers to changes in birth or death rates or some similar global measure.

P

panel A group of individuals who are given a specific task.

paradigm An intellectual model for a situation or condition.

path-goal theory The path-goal model attempts to predict leader behaviors that will be most effective in particular situations. The focus of this model is how leaders influence participants' perceptions of their work goals and the paths they follow toward attaining these goals. The leader's functions are to increase personal payoffs to followers for attaining their work-related goals and to make the path to these payoffs smoother. Leaders influence the follower's perceptions of their work goals, personal goals, and the paths to goal attainment.

Patient's Bill of Rights This phrase was first widely used in a statement by the American Hospital Association (AHA) in 1973, giving 12 rights to which it felt that hospital patients were entitled. These include the right of the patient to be included in making treatment decisions, to be treated with dignity, to have privacy, and so forth. In several states, legislation has been passed codifying and augmenting these rights with some states extending these rights to non-hospitalized patients. Over the years, the idea of patient's rights has grown to include legal rights concerning treatment decisions, insurance, and payment for care.

patronage The power of elected and appointed officials to make partisan appointments to office or to confer contracts, honors, or other benefits on behalf of their political supporters. Patronage has always been one of the major tools by which political executives consolidate their power and attempt to control bureaucracy.

pay-as-you-go (PAYGO) The financial policy of a government unit that finances capital outlays from current revenues rather than from borrowing. Under BEA90, the requirement is that revenue changes and entitlement changes carry a means of financing any change that would otherwise increase the federal deficit.

peer review Review by individuals from the same discipline and with essentially equal qualifications (peers).

performance The actual carrying out of an activity. To be able to evaluate performance accurately requires considerable sophistication in the collection and analysis of data about the performance demonstrated.

performance appraisal The formal methods by which an organization documents the work performance of its employees. Performance appraisals are typically designed to change dysfunctional work behavior, communicate perceptions of work quality, assess the future potential of an employee, and to provide a documented record for disciplinary and separation actions.

performance data Data which are developed from the activities of an individual or institution. More sophisticated performance data can be developed from ongoing information systems which can describe patterns.

performance management The systematic integration of an organization's efforts to achieve its objectives.

performance measure Something used to gather data on and evaluate activities and outcomes.

per member per month (PMPM) Refers to the cost (or charge) for a health care premium for an individual for one month.

philanthropic organizations Organizations and foundations that raise funds for research, disease control and treatment, health promotion, and service delivery.

physician A person qualified by a doctoral degree in medicine (allopathy, homeopathy, or osteopathy). To practice, a physician must also be licensed by the state in which she or he practices.

physician assistant (PA) A health worker with advanced training who is licensed to practice medicine under the supervision of a physician. PAs take patient histories, perform examinations, order tests and x-rays, suture wounds, set casts, do other minor procedures, and make preliminary diagnoses. Most states permit PAs to prescribe drugs.

Planned Approach to Community Health (PATCH) A model for planning, conducting, and evaluating community health promotion and disease prevention programs developed by the Centers for Disease Control and Prevention (CDC).

planning The analysis of needs, demands, and resources, followed by the proposal of steps to meet the demands and needs by use of the current resources and obtaining other resources as necessary.

community-based planning Planning where the attempt is made to have the planning initiative within the local community rather than external to the community.

comprehensive health planning Planning that attempts to coordinate environmental measures, health education, health care, and occupational and other health efforts to achieve the greatest results in a community.

pluralism A theory of government that attempts to reaffirm the democratic character of society by asserting that open, multiple competing, and responsive groups preserve traditional democratic values in a mass industrial state. Pluralism assumes that the power will move from group to group as elements in the mass transfer allegiance in response to their perceptions of their individual interest.

policy A stable, purposeful course of action dealing with a problem or matter of concern. Policy comes in many forms, including: legislative statutes, executive orders, court opinions, and agencies (FDA, EPA, FEMA, and so forth). Additionally, policy is the absence of making a decision or taking action. The three main types of policy are distributive, regulatory, and redistributive.

policy development The formulation and advocacy of what should be done.

policy formulation The development of a course of action.

political culture The part of the overall societal culture that determines a community's attitudes toward the quality, style, and vigor of its political processes and government operations.

politics 1) The art or science concerned with guiding or influencing governmental policy. 2) The total complex of relations between people living in a society. 3) Relations or conduct in a particular area of experience, especially as seen or dealt with from a political point of view. 4) In public policymaking, "who gets what, when, and how."

population A group of individuals occupying a specified area at the same time.

position classification The use of formal job descriptions to organize all jobs in a civil service merit system into classes on the basis of duties and responsibilities for the purpose of delegating authority, establishing chains of command, and providing equitable salary scales.

postbureaucratic organization Constantly changing temporary organizational systems; task forces composed of groups of relative strangers with diverse skills created in response to a special problem, as opposed to a continuing need.

power The potential to exert influence.

coercive power Power based on the ability to punish people or prevent them from receiving rewards.

ecological power Power derived from the leader's control over the physical environment in the workplace, as well as some control over technology and organization designs used in the workplace.

expert power Power derived from having knowledge valued by the organization or system.

information power Access to vital information and control over the distribution of it.

legitimate power Power derived from a person's position in an organization.

referent power Referent power results when individuals engender admiration, loyalty, and emulation to the extent that they gain the power to influence others.

practitioner An individual entitled by training and experience to practice a profession. Often such practice requires licensure, and the boundaries of the practice are prescribed by law.

precautions Actions taken to prevent an undesired effect or outcome.

universal precautions (UP) A set of policies and procedures recommended by the Centers for Disease Control and Prevention (CDC) and required by the Occupational Safety and Health Administration (OSHA) for protecting patients, health workers, and physicians from the risk of contracting diseases. Universal means that the precautions are to be taken with respect to every patient, not just those who are known to be particularly vulnerable or contagious. Recommended precautions include the use of gloves and special disposal of hypodermic needles to reduce accidental needle sticks.

preferred provider option (PPO) A form of health plan in which certain physicians with whom the payer has contracted are designated as preferred providers. When a beneficiary elects to receive care from these physicians, the physicians' charges are paid in full and there is no additional charge to the beneficiary. The beneficiary may elect to obtain care from other physicians, but if so, there is a financial penalty to the beneficiary and they must pay part of the charges.

preferred provider organization (PPO) An alternative delivery system designed to compete with health maintenance organizations (HMOs) and other delivery systems. A PPO is stated to be an arrangement involving a contract between health care providers (both professional and institutional) and organizations such as employers and third-party administrators (TPAs), under which the PPO agrees to provide health care services to a defined population for predetermined fixed fees. There is little uniformity among the organization of various PPOs.

prevalence The number of events or cases of disease present in a given population at a given time. Prevalence is distinguished from incidence, which is the number of new events taking place in a defined period of time in a specified area or population. Usually both incidence and prevalence refer to cases of disease or injury.

preventive health services Services designed to prevent disease or injury from occurring, detect it early, minimize its progression, and control resulting disability.

primary care The Institute of Medicine (IOM) defines primary care as "the provision of integrated, accessible health care services by clinicians who are accountable for addressing a large majority of personal health care needs, developing a sustained partnership with patients, and practicing in the context of family and community." It may be provided by physicians or by other health professionals such as physician assistants (PAs) and nurse practitioners.

problem An issue that needs to be addressed.

process measure Process measures examine all steps and activities taken in implementing a program and the outputs they generate.

productivity A measured relationship between the quantity (and quality) of results produced and the quantity of resources required for production. Productivity is, in essence, a measure of the work efficiency of an individual, a work unit, a system, or an organization.

program Generally defined as an organized set of activities directed toward a common purpose, or goal, undertaken by an agency in order to carry out its responsibilities. In practice, the term has many uses and does not have a well-defined and standard meaning in the legislative process. Program is used to describe an agency's mission, programs, activities, functions, services, projects, and processes.

program evaluation The process of assessing program alternatives, including research and results, and the options for meeting program objectives and future expectations. Program evaluation is the process of appraising the manner to which programs 1) achieve their stated objectives, 2) meet the performance perceptions and expectations of responsible federal officials and other interested groups, and 3) produce other significant effects of either a desirable or undesirable character.

projection In statistics, a projection is a calculated estimate for a whole calculated from data for a part of the whole, or an estimate of a future situation based on information currently available.

public administration Public administration can be broadly described as the development, implementation, and study of branches of government policy. The pursuit of the public good by enhancing civil society, ensuring a well-run, fair, and effective public service are some of the goals of the field. Today public administration is often regarded as including also some responsibility for determining the policies and programs of governments. Specifically, it is the planning, organizing, directing, coordinating, and controlling of government operations. Public administration is carried out by public servants who work in public departments and agencies, at all levels of government, and perform a wide range of tasks.

public health The science and art of preventing disease, prolonging life, and promoting physical health and efficiency through organized community efforts for the sanitation of the environment, the control of community infections, the education of the individual in principles of personal hygiene, the organization of medical and nursing services for the early diagnosis and preventive treatment of disease, and the development of the social machinery which will ensure to every individual in the community a standard of living adequate for the maintenance of health.

public health informatics The systematic application of information, computer science, and technology to public health practice, research, and technology.

public health policy An attempt by the government at all levels to address a public health issue, problem, or concern.

Public Health Service (PHS) The division of the federal government charged with protecting and advancing the health of the American people. The PHS is a part of the Department of Health and Human Services and consists of the Office of Public Health and Science, ten Regional Health Administrators, and eight operating divisions including the Agency for Healthcare Research and Quality (AHRQ), Agency for Toxic Substances and Disease Registry (ATSDR), Centers for Disease Control and Prevention (CDC), Food and Drug Administration (FDA), Health Resource Service Administration (HRSA), Indian Health Service (IHS), National Institutes of Health (NIH), and Substance Abuse and Mental Health Services Administration (SAMHSA).

Public Health Service Act Legislation passed in 1944 that authorizes a number of federal health-related activities. There have been numerous amendments to the act since that time. Among other things, the act provides grants for community health services and the development of community health centers. The act established the National Health Service Corps and provided for a Loan Repayment Program and scholarship opportunities. The act also authorizes federally regulated public health programs, biomedical research, family planning, emergency medical service systems, regulation of drinking water supplies, and health planning and resource development. Authority to enforce the act is delegated to the Secretary of the Department of Health and Human Services (DHHS).

public policy Decision making by government. Governments are concerned with what they should and should not do. What they do or do not do is policy.

public program All activities designed to implement public policy.

Pure Food and Drug Act of 1906 Legislation passed by Congress to provide federal inspection of meat products and to prohibit the manufacture, sale, and distribution of adulterated food products and poisonous medicines.

Q

quality control (QC) The sum of all the activities which prevent unwanted change in quality. This usually involves the identification of any problems or opportunities for improvement, and prompt corrective action so that the quality is maintained.

quality improvement (QI) The sum of all the activities which create desired change in quality. This often involves an analysis of patterns in order to identify opportunities for improvement.

quality management (QM) Efforts to determine the quality of the service being rendered to develop and maintain programs to keep it at an acceptable level, to institute improvements when the opportunity arises or the quality does not meet standards, and to provide the evidence required to establish confidence that quality is being managed and maintained at the desired level.

quality of care The degree of conformity with accepted principles and practices (standards), the degree of fitness for the patient's needs, and the degree of attainment of achievable outcomes (results), consonant with the appropriate allocation or use of resources.

R

random A statistical term used in sampling which means that every element or event in the whole universe being sampled has an equal chance of being drawn.

rate (charge) A financial term referring to a hospital or other institution's charges.

rate (ratio) A ratio or proportion, often expressed as a percentage (per 100); but may also be expressed per 1,000; per 10,000; per 100,000; or per million. These per numbers are called the base. Thus a rate expressed per 100,000 is said to have 100,000 as the base. The base chosen is usually large enough to ensure that the rate will be expressed in whole numbers; the more rare the event, the larger the base chosen. A death rate of 7 per 10,000 is easier to understand than a rate of 0.07 percent (although both actually give the same information).

  infant mortality rate The number of deaths of children less than 1 year old per 1,000 live births.

  morbidity rate The number of occurrences of a particular disease per year within a certain population.

  mortality rate The number of deaths per year within a certain population as a proportion of that population.

ratio A value obtained by dividing one number (the numerator) by another (the denominator).

  current ratio A financial term used to express liquidity. It is the ratio of current assets to current liabilities.

  debt ratio Total debt divided by total assets.

  quick ratio The ratio of cash plus accounts receivable to current liabilities. This differs from the *current* ratio in that inventories are not included in the quick ratio (since they may not easily be convertible into cash in order to meet short term obligations). A good ratio would be 1:1.

rational decision-making model A view of the public policy-making process that assumes complete information and a systematic, logical, and comprehensive approach to change.

reciprocity An agreement among specific states under which one state will grant a license to a physician or other health professional if that person produces evidence that she is licensed in any other state which is a party to the agreement. Usually the initial license must have been granted on the basis of an examination, either that of the National Board of Medical Examiners (NBME) or of the state of origin.

red tape The symbol of excessive official formality and over-attention to prescribed routines.

reengineering The fundamental rethinking and redesign of organizational processes to achieve significant improvements in critical measures of performance, such as cost and quality of services.

regression A statistical method used to measure and express the effect one variable, the independent variable, has on another variable, the dependent variable. A common form of regression is a linear regression, in which the model chosen for the analysis is a linear equation.

regulation The totality of government controls on the social and economic activities of its citizens; the rule-making process of those administrative agencies charged with the official interpretation of laws.

regulatory commission An independent agency created by the government to regulate some aspect of economic life.

reinforcement 1) To give added emphasis to, stress, or support. 2) To reward or punish an action or response so that it becomes more or less likely to occur.

reinventing government The latest manifestation of the progressive tradition of continuously improving government.

revenue Increase in an organization's assets or a decrease in its liabilities during an accounting period. This is in contrast with *income* which refers to money earned during an accounting period.

> **marginal revenue** The addition to or subtraction from total revenue resulting from the sale of one more or one less unit of service or product.

review The processes of examination and evaluation.

risk (financial) A chance of monetary loss.

risk (health) The likelihood of disease, injury, or death among various groups of individuals and from different causes. Individuals are said to be at risk if they are in a group in which a given causal factor is present.

risk factors Factors in the individual's genetic and physical makeup, lifestyle and behavior, and environment which are known (or thought) to increase the likelihood of physical or mental problems.

risk management The process of minimizing risk to an organization at a minimal cost in keeping with the organization's objectives.

Robert Wood Johnson Foundation (RWJF) The nation's largest philanthropic organization devoted exclusively to health issues. It concentrates its grant allocations in four areas: access to health care, delivery of care to the chronically ill, substance abuse, and healthy communities and lifestyles.

S

sample A part of a population intended to be in some way representative of the entire population.

sampling A technique used in statistics in which a part of a whole is examined with the intent that the results of the examination can be taken as representing the condition of the whole.

satisficing Aiming to achieve only satisfactory results because the satisfactory process is familiar, whereas aiming for the best-achievable results would call for costs, effort, and the incurring of risks. Due to time pressures, emotional issues, or limited information, the manager will not arrive at an optimal decision but will instead make a satisfactory decision.

scientific management A systematic approach to managing that seeks the "one best way" of accomplishing a task by discovering the fastest, most efficient, and least-fatiguing methods.

scoring A term used in connection with legislative budgeting in estimating the effects on revenue of tax policy changes, depending on their influence on behavior. *Static scoring* is used when no effect on behavior is expected from the change in tax policy; *dynamic scoring* is used when behavior is expected to change. The Congressional Budget Office (CBO) tends to use static scoring in its budget predictions.

self-directed work team A work group that will accept responsibility for their processes and products, as well as the behavior of other group members.

self-pay patient A patient who pays either all or part of the hospital bill from their own resources as opposed to a third-party payer.

separation of powers The allocation of powers among the different branches of government so that they are a check upon each other.

sexually transmitted disease (STD) A disease which may be transmitted by sexual contact.

single-payer plan A method of health care financing in which there is only one source of money for paying health care providers.

situational leadership model Model of leadership that attempts to explain effective leadership as interplay among 1) the leader's relationship behavior, defined as the extent to which a leader engages in two-way or multi-way communication, listening, facilitating behaviors, and supportive behaviors with followers through open communication and actions toward them; 2) the leader's task behavior, which is the extent to which the leader organizes, defines roles, and guides and directs followers; and 3) the followers' readiness level, which is defined as the readiness to perform a task or function or pursue an objective. The central premise of this model is that the most effective leadership style is determined by the readiness of the people whom the leader is trying to influence.

SMART rule A method used to write clear objectives. S = short; M = measurable; A = action oriented; R = realistic; T = time-bound.

social consciousness The awareness by an individual of the needs of society and of the impact of events on society.

social organizations Like faith-based organizations, social organizations are formed to meet a social need.

Social Security Act A major piece of legislation originally signed into law on August 14, 1935. It created an insurance program to pay retired workers age 65 or older a continuing income after retirement, as well as several other provisions related to the general welfare.

social services Assistance to patients and their families in handling social, environmental, and emotional problems.

spoils system The practice of awarding government jobs to one's political supporters, as opposed to awarding them on the basis of merit.

stakeholder 1) Any individual or group that might be affected by the outcome of something. All decisions have their stakeholders. 2) The affected individuals or communities along with those who are influential in forming a plan to address the problem in question.

standard (threshold) A measure of quality or quantity, established by an authority, by a profession, or by custom, which serves as a criterion for evaluation. It is in the nature of a threshold, below which one should not fall. This type of standard is distinguished from a standard which is simply a "norm."

State Children's Health Insurance Program (SCHIP) A federal program that uses a block grant mechanism to help states set up health care programs for needy children and families not otherwise covered by health insurance (including Medicaid). Typical children in this target group have parents who earn too much to qualify for Medicaid, but not enough to afford private health insurance.

statistic A number calculated from data.

steering committee A generic term for a committee set up to provide broad guidance for a program, project, or activity.

strategic management A philosophy of management that links strategic planning with day-to-day decision making.

strategic planning Planning which is long-range and that is intended to lay out the nature and sequence of the steps to be taken to achieve the large goals of the organization. Strategic planning is based on the principle that, with goals and objectives specified, strategies can be developed for achieving them, resources can be generated to implement the strategies, and progress can be continually monitored.

strategy The overall conduct of a major enterprise to achieve long-term goals; the pattern to be used in a series of organizational decisions.

Substance Abuse and Mental Health Services Administration (SAMHSA)
Provides grants and data collection activities to promote quality behavioral
health services. Major activities include the improvement of the quality and
availability of prevention, treatment, and recovery support services in order to
help reduce illness, death, disability, and cost to society caused by substance
abuse and mental illness.

Surgeon General of the United States The head of the Office of the Surgeon
General, a division within the Department of Health and Human Services
(DHHS). The Surgeon General is responsible for administering the Public Health
Service Commissioned Corps (PHSCC) and being a spokesperson for national
health concerns.

sustainability Creating and maintaining the conditions under which humans
and nature can exist in productive harmony that permits fulfilling the social,
economic, and other requirements of present and future generations. Focuses
on the organization's environmental practices in balance with fiscal and social
responsibility to assure the long-term success of the organization and its
programs.

SWOT analysis A review of an organization's Strengths, Weaknesses, Opportunities, and Threats. The review of strengths and weaknesses provides an internal
assessment for organization while the review of opportunities and threats provides
the organization with an analysis of the external environment. SWOT analyses are
generally used in the strategic planning process.

systems analysis An analysis of the resources (personnel, facilities, equipment,
materials, funds, and other elements), organization, administration, procedures,
and policies needed to carry out a given task. The analysis typically addresses alternatives in each category and their relative efficiency and effectiveness.

systems theory A view of an organization as a complex set of dynamically intertwined and interconnected elements, including all its inputs, processes, outputs,
feedback loops, and the environment in which it operates and with which it continuously interacts.

T

target A desired performance, outcome, or result.

tax-exempt A nonprofit organization which is not required to pay certain federal
and/or state taxes. A tax-exempt organization may also qualify to receive tax-deductible
donations.

tax incentive A method of encouraging behavior by providing favorable tax treatment such as exemptions, deductions, or credits.

team A number of persons associated together in work or activity. Often used in
the field of public health to examine problems or issues, provide recommendations

on matters facing an organization or community, or analyze and investigate the efficacy of a process.

technical skills Require knowledge about the procedures, regulations, policies, technology, tools, and techniques for conducting the activities of the manager's unit, division, or department.

theory x The assumption that the average human has an inherent dislike of work; that most people must be threatened to get them to produce adequate work effort; and that people prefer to be directed and avoid responsibility.

theory y The assumption that work is as natural as play; that workers can exercise self-direction and self-control; and that imagination, ingenuity, and creativity are widespread among workers.

total quality management (TQM) A phrase for quality control in its most expanded sense of a total and continuing concern for quality in the production of goods and services.

trait theory An approach to leadership that assumes leaders possess traits that make them fundamentally different from followers. Advocates of trait theory believe that some people possess unique leadership qualities and characteristics (such as attractiveness, charisma, family status) that enable them to assume responsibilities not everyone can execute. Therefore, they are " born" leaders.

transformational leadership Leadership that strives to change organizational culture and directions. It reflects the ability of a leader to develop a values-based vision for the organization, to convert the vision into reality, and to maintain it over time.

TRICARE The program which provides supplemental benefits to the Uniformed Services direct medical care system. It pays for health care for eligible persons, who include retired members of the uniformed services of the United States and their dependents, dependents of deceased members of the military services, and dependents of North Atlantic Treaty Organization (NATO) members if the NATO member is stationed in or passing through the United States on official business.

triple bottom line A new trend worldwide with a focus on sustainability, the triple bottom line focuses not only on the financial/economic bottom line, but includes social responsibility and the environment.

trust fund Accounts, designed by law, for receipts earmarked for specific purposes and the associated expenditure of those receipts.

Tuckman's Stages of Team Development Five stages covering the lifespan of a team, from formation to adjournment. 1) Forming—the first stage of team development as the members are selected, brought together, and identify objectives to be completed. 2) Storming—members begin to develop personal relationships, put aside past conflicts, and often select a group leader. 3) Norming—members develop group rules, procedures, etc. 4) Performing—team begins to reach consensus on implementing ideas and suggestions. 5) Adjourning—as most teams are short-term in nature, members return to their individual assignments.

U

uncompensated care Care for which no payment is expected or no charge is made.

unified budget The present form of the federal budget, in which receipts and outlays from federal funds and trust funds (such as Social Security) are consolidated.

United States Public Health Service Commissioned Corps (USPHS) One of seven uniformed services of the United States. The USPHS is under the direction of the Surgeon General within the Public Health Service. Its mission is to protect, promote, and advance the health and safety of the American people. The USPHS has approximately 6,000 officers.

V

vaccine A preparation which, when introduced into a human or other animal, stimulates the development of immunity against specific infections. Most vaccines are either killed bacteria or viruses of strains which, when alive, are able to cause the disease in question, or live bacteria or viruses of attenuated (weakened) strains of the disease-causing organism (closely related bacteria or viruses which are not able to cause the disease but are able to stimulate the production of the specific immunity required).

Vaccines for Children (VFC) A federal program that provides free vaccines to physicians who serve eligible children, those without health insurance or whose insurance does not cover vaccinations. It is administered by the Centers for Disease Control and Prevention (CDC) through the National Immunization Program (NIP).

value-added Reflecting the position that something done to a given product or service has increased its value.

vision A view of an organization's future. The purpose of strategic management is to transform the vision into a reality.

vision statement The identification of objectives to be achieved in the future.

volunteer A person who performs services without pay.

volunteer services Services provided by volunteers.

W

World Health Organization (WHO) The division of the United Nations (UN) that is concerned with health. Headquartered in Geneva, Switzerland, the WHO came into being in April of 1948 when the United Nations ratified the WHO's

Constitution. Its objective is the attainment by all peoples of the highest possible level of health. It is governed by the World Health Assembly which meets annually. **http://www.who.ch**

Z

zero-based budgeting A process emphasizing management's responsibility to plan, budget, and evaluate. Zero-based budgeting provides for analysis of alternative methods of operation and various levels of effort. It places new programs on equal footing with existing programs by requiring that program priorities be ranked, thereby providing a systematic basis for allocating resources.

References

Alderfer, C. P. (1972). *Existence, relatedness, and growth: Human needs in organizational settings.* New York, NY: Free Press.

Barsukiewicz, C., Raffel, M., & Raffel, N. (2010). *The U.S. health system: Origins and functions* (6th ed.). Clifton Park, NY: Delmar, Cengage Learning.

Beauchamp, D. (1976). Public health as social justice. *Inquiry, 13*(1), 1–14.

Beauchamp, T., & Childress, J. (2008). *Principles of biomedical ethics* (6th ed.). New York, NY: Oxford University Press.

Begun, J., Zimmerman, B. & Dooley, K. (2003). Health care organizations as complex adaptive systems. In Mick, S. & Wyttenbach, M. (Eds.), *Advances in health care organization theory* (pp. 253–288). San Francisco, CA: Jossey-Bass.

Breslow, L. (2002). *Encyclopedia of public health.* Farmington Hills, MI: MacMillian Reference USA. Gale Cengage Learning.

Burns, L., Bradley, E., & Weiner, B. (2012). *Shortell and Kaluzny's Health care management: Organization Design & Behavior* (6th ed.). Clifton Park, NY: Delmar, Cengage Learning.

Carney, J. (2006). *Public health in action: Practicing in the real world.* Sudbury, MA: Jones and Bartlett.

Committee on Public Health Strategies to Improve Health, & Institute of Medicine. (2011). *For the public's health: The role of measurement in action and accountability.* Washington, DC: National Academies Press.

Committee on Quality of Health Care in America, & Institute of Medicine, Corrigan, J., Donaldson, M., & Kohn, L. (Eds.). (2000). *To err is human: Building a safer health system.* Washington, DC: National Academies Press.

Committee on Quality of Health Care in America, & Institute of Medicine. (2001). *Crossing the quality chasm: A new health system for the 21st century.* Washington, DC: National Academies Press.

Covey, S. (1992). *Principle centered leadership.* New York, NY: Free Press.

Denhardt, R., Denhardt, J., & Aristigueta, A. (2012). *Managing human behavior in public and non-profit organizations* (3rd ed.). Thousand Oaks, CA: Sage.

Fallon, L. F., Jr., & Zgodzinski, E. (2011). *Essentials of public health management* (3rd ed.). Sudbury, MA: Jones and Bartlett.

Fee, E. (1993). Public health, past and present: A shared social vision. In Rosen, G. (Ed.), *A history of public health* (expanded edition) (pp. ix–lxiv). Baltimore, MD: Johns Hopkins University Press.

Fee, E. (1994). Public health and the state: The United States. In Porter, D. (Ed.), *The history of public health and the modern state* (pp. 224–275). Atlanta, GA: Editions Rodopi.

Fee, E. (2009). History and development of public health. In Scutchfield, F. D. & Keck, C. W. (Eds.), *Principles of public health practice* (3rd ed., pp. 12–35). Clifton Park, NY: Delmar, Cengage Learning.

Ferlie, E., Lynne, L., Jr., & Pollitt, C. (2007). *The Oxford handbook of public management.* New York, NY: Oxford University Press.

Friesen, M., & Johnson, J. (1995). *The success paradigm: Creating organizational effectiveness through quality and strategy.* Westport, CT: Quorum Books.

Fugate, M., & Kiniki, A. (2011). *Organization behavior: Key concepts, skills, and best practices* (5th ed.). New York, NY: McGraw Hill.

Garrett. L. (2001). *Betrayal of trust: The collapse of global public health.* New York, NY: Hyperion.

Graber, D., & Johnson, J. (2001). Spirituality and healthcare organizations. *Journal of Healthcare Management, 46*(1), 39–50.

Greenberg, J. (2011). *Behavior in organizations* (10th ed.). Upper Saddle River, NJ: Prentice Hall.

Hackman, M., & Johnson, C. (2008). *Leadership: A communication perspective* (5th ed.). Long Grove, IL: Waveland Press.

Hammaker, D. (2011). *Health care management and the law: Principles and applications.* Clifton Park, NY: Delmar, Cengage Learning.

Hays, S., Kearney, R., & Coggburn, J. (2009). *Public human resources management: Problems and prospects* (5th ed.). Upper Saddle River, NJ. Prentice Hall.

Heifetz, R., Grashow, A., & Linsky, M. (2009). *The practice of adaptive leadership:Tools and tactics for changing your organization and the world.* Boston, MA: Harvard Business Press.

Institute for the Future (2003). *Health and health care 2010: The forecast, the challenge* (2nd ed.). San Francisco, CA: Jossey-Bass.

Institute of Medicine. (1996). *The future of public health.* Washington, DC: National Academies Press.

Issel, M. (2008). *Health program planning and evaluation: A practical, systematic approach for community health* (2nd ed.). Sudbury, MA: Jones and Bartlett.

Ivanov, L., & Blue, C. (Eds.) (2008). *Public health nursing: Leadership, policy, and practice.* Clifton Park, NY: Delmar, Cengage Learning.

Johnson, C. (2011). *Meeting the ethical challenges of leadership: casting light or shadow* (4th ed.). Thousand Oaks, CA: Sage.

Johnson, D., & Johnson, F. (2012). *Joining together: Group theory and skills* (11th ed.). Upper Saddle River, NJ: Prentice-Hall.

Johnson, J. (2005). Training and development (pp 161–170). In Fried, B., Fottler, M., & Johnson, J., *Human resources in healthcare: Managing for success* (2nd ed.). Chicago, IL: Health Administration Press.

Johnson, J. (2009). *Health organizations: Theory, behavior, and development.* Sudbury, MA: Jones and Bartlett.

Johnson, J. (2009). International health education and promotion. In Minelli, M. & Brackon, D., *Community health education* (5th ed., pp. 325–334). Sudbury, MA: Jones and Bartlett.

Johnson, J., & Breckon, D. (2007). *Managing health education and promotion programs: Leadership for the 21st century* (2nd ed.). Sudbury, MA: Jones and Bartlett.

Johnson, J., Kennedy, M., & Delener, N. (2005). *Community preparedness: The role of community organizations and business.* Westport, Connecticut: Praeger.

Johnson, J., & Omachonu, V. (1999). Total quality management as health care strategy. In Johnson, J. & Jones, W., *The AMA and organized medicine.* New York, NY: Garland Publishing.

Johnson, J., & Stoskopf, C. (2010). *Comparative health systems: Global perspectives.* Sudbury, MA: Jones and Bartlett.

Kass, N. (2001). An ethics framework for public health. *American Journal of Public Health, 91*(11), 1776–1782.

Katz, D., & Kahn, R. (1978). *The social psychology of organizations.* Hoboken, NJ: John Wiley & Sons.

Keck, W. (2000). Lessons learned from an academic health department. *Journal of Public Health Management Practice, 6*(1), 47–52.

Keck, C. W., & Scutchfield, F. D. (Eds.) (2009). The future of public health. In Scutchfield, F. D. & Keck, C. W., *Principles of public health practice* (3rd ed., pp. 736–756). Clifton Park, NY: Delmar, Cengage Learning.

Kelly, P. (2012). *Nursing leadership and management* (3rd ed.). Clifton Park, NY: Delmar, Cengage Learning.

Kettl, D. (2011). *Politics of the administrative process* (5th ed.). Washington, DC: CQ Press.

Kilpatrick, A., & Johnson, J. (1999). *Handbook of health administration and policy.* New York, NY: Marcel-Dekker.

Kilpatrick, A., & Johnson, J. (2007). *Human resources and organizational behavior: Cases in health services management.* Chicago, IL: Health Administration Press.

Kirch, W. (Ed.) (2008). *Encyclopedia of public health* (4 vol.). New York, NY: Springer.

Koh, H. (2010). A 2020 vision for healthy people. *New England Journal of Medicine, 362,* 1653–1656.

Ledlow, G., Johnson, J., & Hakoyama, M. (2008). Social marketing and organizational communication efficacy. In Wright, K. & Moore, S., *Applied health communications.* New York, NY: Hampton Press.

Lewis, C., & Elnitsky, C. (2008). Program development and evaluation. In Ivanov, L. & Blue, C. (Eds.), *Public health nursing: Leadership, policy, & practice* (pp. 303–324). Clifton Park, NY: Delmar, Cengage Learning.

Lloyd, P. (1994). Management competencies in health for all/new public health settings. *Journal of Health Administration Education, 12*(2), 187–207.

Marmot, M. (2001). Inequalities in health. *New England Journal of Medicine, 345*(2), 134–136.

Mattingly, R. (1997). *Management of health information: Functions & Applications.* Clifton Park, NY: Delmar, Cengage Learning.

Mays, G., Halverson, P., Lenaway, D., McHugh, M., Moonshinge, R., Perry, N., & Shim, K. (2004). Identifying dimensions of performance in local public health systems: Results from the national public health performance standards programs. *Journal of Public Health Management Practice, 10*(3), 193–203.

McClelland, D. (1961). *The achieving society.* New York, NY: Free Press.

McIlwain, T., & Johnson, J. (1999). Strategy: Planning, management, and critical success factors. In Kilpatrick, A. & Johnson, J., *Handbook of health administration and policy* (pp. 637–644). New York, NY: Marcel-Dekker.

Meadows, D. (2008). *Thinking in systems: A Primer.* White River Junction, VT: Chelsea Green Publishing.

Mick, S., & Wyttenback, M. (Eds.) (2003). *Advances in health care organization theory.* San Francisco, CA: Jossey-Bass.

Minelli, M., & Breckon, D. (2009). *Community health education: Settings, roles, and skills,* (5th ed.). Sudbury, MA: Jones and Bartlett.

Miringgoff, M. (1999). *Social health of the nation.* New York, NY: Oxford University Press.

Mor Barak, M. (2011). *Managing diversity: Toward a globally inclusive workplace.* Thousands Oaks, CA: Sage.

Neighbors, M., & Tannehill-Jones, R. (2010). *Human diseases* (3rd ed.). Clifton Park, NY: Delmar, Cengage Learning.

Northouse, P. (2013). *Leadership: Theory and practice* (6th ed.). Thousand Oaks, CA: Sage.

Nutt, P. (1984). *Planning methods: For health and related organizations.* New York, NY: John Wiley & Sons.

Owens, R., & Valesky, T. (2010). *Organization behavior in education: Leadership and school reform* (10th ed.). Upper Saddle River, NJ: Prentice-Hall.

Pecora, P., & Austin, M. (1997). *Managing human services personnel.* Thousands Oaks, CA: Sage.

Pollitt, C. (2003). *The essential public manager.* New York, NY: Open University Press.

Porter, D. (Ed.) (1994). *The history of public health and the modern state.* Atlanta, GA: Editions Rodopi B.V.

Rabin, J., Hildreth, W. B., & Miller, G. (Eds.) (2007). *Handbook of public administration* (3rd ed.). Boca Raton, FL: CRC Press.

Rainey, H. (2009). *Understanding and managing public organizations* (4th ed.). San Francisco, CA: Jossey-Bass.

Ramsey, M. (1994). Public health in France. In Porter, D. (Ed.), *The history of public health and the modern state* (pp. 45–118). Atlanta, GA: Editions Rodopi B.V.

Ricketts, T. (2009). Public health policy and the policy making process. In Scutchfield, F. D. & Keck, C. W. (Eds.) (2009), *Principles of public health practice* (3rd ed.) (pp. 86–115). Clifton Park, NY: Delmar, Cengage Learning.

Rovner, J. (2009). *Health care policy and politics A-Z* (3rd ed.). Washington, DC: CQ Press.

Rowitz, L. (2008). *Public health leadership: Putting Principles into Practice* (2nd ed.). Sudbury, MA: Jones and Bartlett.

Ructman, L., & Mowbray, G. (1983). *Understanding program evaluation.* Thousand Oaks, CA: Sage.

Schulz, R., & Johnson, A. (1990). *Management of hospitals and health services* (3rd ed.). Frederick, MD: Beard Books.

Scutchfield, F. D., & Keck, C. W. (Eds.) (2009). *Principles of public health practice* (3rd ed.). Clifton Park, NY: Delmar, Cengage Learning.

Shortell, S., & Kaluzny, A. (1997). *Essentials of health care management.* Clifton Park, NY: Delmar, Cengage Learning.

Shortliffe, E. (2006). *Biomedical informatics: Computer applications in health care and biomedicine* (3rd ed.). New York, NY: Springer.

Slee, D., Slee, V., & Schmidt, J. (2008). *Slee's health care terms* (5th ed.). Sudbury, MA: Jones and Bartlett.

Turshen, M. (1989). *The politics of public health.* New Brunswick, NJ: Rutgers University Press.

U.S. Department of Health and Human Services (2004). *Public health in America.* Washington, DC.

Walshe K., & Rundell, T. (2001). Evidence-based management: From theory to practice in health care. *Millbank Quarterly, 79,* 429–457.

Wheatley, M. (1999). *Leadership and the new science: Discovering order in a chaotic world* (3rd ed.). San Francisco, CA: Berrett-Koehler.

Witkin, B., & Altschuld, J. (1995). *Planning and conducting needs assessments.* Thousand Oaks, CA: Sage.

World Health Organization (2006). *Working together for health.* Geneva, Switzerland: WHO Press.

Glossary

A

adaptation   An organization's capacity to change in response to external or internal factors.

adaptive leadership   The practice of mobilizing people to tackle tough challenges and thrive. Adaptive leadership has three characteristics: 1) it preserves the DNA essential for continued survival; 2) it repels, reregulates, or rearranges the DNA that no longer serves current needs; and 3) it creates new DNA arrangements enhancing the ability to flourish in new ways and in new challenging environments. Successful adaptations enable a living system to take the best of its past into the future.

Administration for Children and Families (ACF)   The agency within the Department of Health and Human Services (DHHS) responsible for federal programs that promote the economic and social well-being of families, children, individuals, and communities.

Administration on Aging (AoA)   The federal agency within the Department of Health and Human Services (DHHS) charged with serving the senior citizens of the United States.

advocacy bond   When an agency, a legislative body, and a professional group reach consensus on a public health issue and what needs to be done to address it.

Agency for Healthcare Research and Quality (AHRQ)   The lead federal agency for research to improve the quality of health care, reduce its cost, and broaden access to essential services. A component of the Department of Health and Human Services (DHHS).

Agency for Toxic Substances and Disease Registry (ATSDR)   The ATSDR performs specific public health functions concerning hazardous substances in the environment. It works to prevent exposure and minimize adverse health effects associated with waste management emergencies and pollution by hazardous substances.

agenda   A list or outline of things to be considered or done.

Alderfer's ERG model   Clayton Alderfer's idea of advanced needs that motivate people. Like Maslow, he believed that needs motivate people to take certain actions, and once lower-level needs are met, new needs can be sought. Alderfer stated three levels of needs: existence, relatedness, and growth.

allocate   To apportion for a specific purpose or to particular persons or things.

assessment   The delineation of health problems, their nature, and the means of dealing with them.

assurance   The implementation of policy, either by activities of others or by direct public health activities.

B

block grants   A grant distributed in accordance with a statutory formula for use in a variety of activities within a broad functional area, largely at the recipient's discretion; grants that are allocated more broadly, with activities determined more by the grant recipient.

boundary spanning   An organization's relationship to its external environment.

bureaucracy A termed coined by Max Weber to represent an ideal or completely rational form of organization. The organizational structure is based on the sociological concept of rationalization of collective activities. The key features Weber believed were necessary for an organization to achieve the maximum benefits of ideal bureaucracy include: 1) a clear division of labor to ensure that each task preformed is systematically established and legitimized by formal recognition as an official duty; 2) positions are arranged in a hierarchy so that each lower position is controlled and supervised by a higher one, leading to a chain of command; 3) formal rules and regulations uniformly guide the actions of employees, eliminating uncertainty in the performance of tasks resulting from differences among individuals; 4) managers should maintain impersonal relationships and should avoid involvement with employees' personalities and personal preferences; 5) an employment should be based entirely on technical competence and protection against arbitrary dismissal. The term is now usually associated with large public-sector organizations to describe undesirable characteristics such as duplication, delay, waste, low morale, and general frustration.

C

categorical grants A grant that can be used only for specific, narrowly defined activities; grants that are very specific and targeted at selected public health programs and population groups.

Centers for Disease Control and Prevention (CDC) An agency within the Department of Health and Human Services (DHHS), which is responsible for monitoring and studying diseases which are controllable by public health measures. The CDC is headquartered in Atlanta, Georgia.

Centers for Medicare and Medicaid Services (CMS) The agency within the Department of Health and Human Services (DHHS) which administers the Medicare, Medicaid, and the State Children's Health Insurance Program (SCHIP). CMS has three centers: Center for Medicare Management (CMM); Center for Beneficiary Choices (CBC); Center for Medicaid and State Operations (CMSO).

code of ethics A statement of professional standards of conduct to which the practitioners of a profession say they subscribe. Codes of ethics are usually not legally binding, so they may not be taken too seriously as constraints to behavior.

communication The exchange of information between individuals through a common system of signs, symbols, and behaviors.

communication process A description or explanation of the chain of events involved in communication.

conceptual skills Skills involving analytical ability, systems thinking, logic, creativity, problem solving, anticipation of change and recognition of opportunity, self-awareness, and strategic thinking.

Council on Linkages A public health organization whose mission is to improve public health practices and education by fostering, coordinating, and monitoring links between academia and the public health community.

D

discrimination Occurs when individuals, organizations, or governments (a) treat people differently because of personal characteristics like race, gender, age, religion, disability, national origin, or sexual orientation rather than their ability to perform their jobs and (b) these actions have a negative impact on access to employment, promotions, or compensation.

Doctor of Health Administration (D.H.A.) An advanced practice degree in health administration and sometimes health policy for senior executives, clinician leaders, and policymakers in health care.

Doctor of Medicine (MD) An advanced practice degree in medicine that leads to approval for licensure. An equivalent degree offered by some medical schools is the D.O., Doctor of Osteopathy.

Doctor of Public Health (Dr.P.H.) An advanced practice degree for public health leaders and professionals. This is sometimes offered with specializations such as epidemiology, community health, environmental health, outcomes research, and public health leadership.

Doctor of Science (Sc.D.) A research degree most often awarded in epidemiology, biostatistics, or health systems.

E

effectiveness The degree to which the effort expended, or the action taken, achieves the desired effect, result, or objective.

efficiency The relationship of the amount of work accomplished to the amount of effort required.

endemic Constantly present in a specific population or geographic area. The adjective may be applied, for example, to a disease or an infectious agent.

epidemic A group of cases of a specific disease or illness clearly in excess of what one would normally expect in a particular geographic area. There is no absolute criteria for using the term epidemic—as standards and expectations change, so might the definition of an epidemic (e.g., an epidemic of violence).

equity theory An extension of expectancy theory developed by Stacy Adams. In addition to preferences of outcomes or rewards associated with performance, individuals also assess the degree to which potential rewards will be equitably distributed. Equity theory states that people calculate the ratio of their efforts to the rewards they will receive and compare them to the ratios they believe exist for others in similar situations. People do this because they have a strong desire to be treated fairly.

ethical issue An issue either implicitly or explicitly involved in any decision made in the public health arena.

ethical theory A system of rules or principles that serve as guides to making decisions in a particular situation.

ethics The kinds of values, morals, and behaviors an individual, profession, or society finds desirable or appropriate.

evidence-based decision making An approach to decision making that combines expertise, patient or client concerns, and information from scientific literature to derive a decision. The use of verifiable data and current information in the decision analysis.

expectancy theory Individuals estimate how well the results of a given behavior will coincide with desired results and act accordingly. Three conditions affect their decisions: 1) people must believe that their through their own efforts they are more likely to achieve their desired levels of performance; 2) people must believe that by achieving a level of performance they receive an outcome or reward; and 3) people must value the outcome or reward.

F

faith-based organizations (FBO) A generic term covering all religious organizations, including nonprofit groups affiliated with a church or religion. Such organizations often address social issues by providing food, shelter, clothing, and health care to people in need. Began within a religion or group of religions that were established to meet the spiritual needs of a population.

federalism A system of governance in which a national, overarching government shares power with sub-national or state governments.

federal system A political and philosophical concept that describes how power is given to governments.

fiscal federalism The financial relations between and among units of government in a federal system. The theory of fiscal federalism, or multi-unit government finance, is one part of applied economics known as "public finance." The pattern of taxation and grants provided by the federal government.

Food and Drug Administration (FDA) An agency within the U.S. Department of Health and Human Services (DHHS) responsible for protecting the health of the nation against impure and unsafe foods, drugs, cosmetics, biological substances, and other potential hazards. A major part of the FDA's activity is controlling the sale, distribution, and use of pharmaceutical drugs and medical devices, including the licensing of new drugs for use by humans.

Food and Drug Administration Amendments Act of 2007 Legislation reauthorizing and expanding the *Prescription Drug User Fee Act* and the *Medical Device User Fee and Modernization Act*. This amendment allows the FDA to possess the resources needed to conduct the complex and comprehensive review of new drugs and medical devices.

Food Safety Modernization Act of 2011 Sweeping reform to food safety legislation that shifts the focus from reacting to food contamination to preventing it.

G

goals Broad statements of what needs to be accomplished.

goal setting Cognitive process through which conscious goals, as well as intentions about pursuing them, are developed and become primary determinants of behavior.

governance Holds those within the organization, especially management, accountable. It also governs the organization's direction and guides its actions.

group A number of individuals assembled together or having common interests.

group decision making An important component of the group process. Reaching consensus can be done through voting or general consensus, depending on whether the group is formal or informal.

group process Working in or with groups. Groups may be large or small, formal or informal, short-term or long-term, meet on a regular or infrequent basis, be static or ever-changing.

H

health   A state of complete physical, mental, and social well-being and not merely the absence of disease and infirmity.

health professionals   A comprehensive term covering people working in the field of public health or health care who have some special training and/or education. The degree of education, training, and other qualifications varies greatly with the nature of the profession, and with the state regulating its practice.

Health Resources and Services Administration (HRSA)   Improves access to health care for people who are uninsured or medically vulnerable by providing financial support to health care agencies in states and territories. The HRSA trains health care professionals in rural communities and oversees organ donations and transplants, as well as maintains databases to protect against health care malpractice and health care waste, fraud, and abuse.

Healthy People 2010   A national initiative setting forth goals of promoting health and preventing disease; an update of *Healthy People 2000*.

Healthy People 2020   Prepares for the next decade; the initiative aims to unify national dialogue about health, motivate action, and encourage new directions in health promotion, providing a public health roadmap and compass for the country.

human resources department   Sometimes labeled the *personnel department*, has several core functions and numerous management and development responsibilities. The primary functions include planning, recruitment, selection, training, legal compliance, compensation and benefits, career development, performance appraisal, and employee discipline and termination.

human resources management   The function of an organization where the focus is on job analysis, performance appraisal, recruitment, and selection. The human resources domain of public health management ultimately serves to promote healthy workplaces, thus keeping with the foundations and fundamentals of public health.

I

Indian Health Service (IHS)   An agency within the Department of Health and Human Services (DHHS) whose goal is to assure that comprehensive, culturally acceptable personal and public health services are available and accessible to American Indian and Alaska Native people. The IHS manages a comprehensive health care delivery system for more than 561 federally recognized Indian tribes in 35 states. IHS provides services to approximately 1.8 million members in urban areas as well as on reservations.

information systems   Also known as *informatics*; system consisting of the network of all channels of communication within an organization.

information technology   Technology involving the development, maintenance, and use of computer systems, software, and networking for the processing and distribution of data.

interpersonal skills   Require an understanding of human behavior and interpersonal relationships; the ability to understand peoples' feelings, attitudes, and motivation; the ability to communicate in a clear and persuasive manner; the ability to foster cooperative relationships; and well-developed emotional intelligence.

K

knowledge, skills, and abilities (KSAs)   Performance-related inputs. KSAs are more likely to lead to desired performance when motivational factors or needs have been addressed effectively.

L

laissez faire   Non-interference.

M

maintenance   Deals with the aspects (fiscal, physical, human) that need maintenance in some form or another.

management   A word that refers both to the people responsible for running an organization and to the running process itself; the use of numerous resources (such as employees and machines) to accomplish an organizational goal. Permeates all other functions and subsystems of the organization. It involves those in charge of all the other functions.

Maslow's hierarchy of needs   Abraham Maslow's five sets of basic human needs arranged in a hierarchy of prepotency: physiological needs (food, water, shelter, etc.), safety needs, affiliation needs, esteem needs, and self-actualization.

Master of Business Administration (M.B.A.)
This may have a concentration in health administration or multi-sector health management. An advanced college degree, earned by those who successfully graduate from their college or university's MBA program. A typical MBA program deals with multiple aspects of business, including finance and management skills.

Master of Health Administration (M.H.A.)
A management and administration degree for health care that is prevalent in hospitals and health delivery settings. It sometimes requires a postgraduate residency in health administration.

Master of Public Administration (M.P.A.)   Master of Public Administration degree or sometimes Master of Public Affairs degree. Many offer concentrations in health administration and health policy. This is a commonly held degree for public-sector managers and administrators, including many in federal public health organizations and state and county health departments.

Master of Public Health (M.P.H.)   Students can specialize in health administration and health policy or other areas of focus such as environmental health, community health, epidemiology, etc. The Council on Education in Public Health is a strident advocate.

Master of Science in Administration (M.S.A.)   A management and administration degree for health care that is used in hospitals, government agencies, the military, and health delivery settings.

McClelland's Acquired Needs model   David McClelland's theory that needs are learned through life experiences. These needs develop throughout a person's life. He stated three levels of needs: achievement, power, and affiliation.

Millennium Declaration   The Declaration asserts that every individual has the right to dignity, freedom, equality, a basic standard of living that includes freedom from hunger and violence, and encourages tolerance and solidarity. The Declaration also emphasizes the role of developed countries in aiding developing countries to achieve a "global partnership for development." These goals, referred to as the Millennium Development Goals (MDG), have served to guide global policy and many public health initiatives by foundations, governments, and nongovernmental organizations. There are eight goals with 21 targets, and a series of measurable indicators for each target.

motivation   An amalgam of all of the factors in one's working environment that foster or inhibit productive efforts. Defined as the set of processes that drive, direct, and maintain human behavior toward attaining some goal or meeting a need.

National Institutes of Health (NIH)   The nation's premier biomedical research organization. The NIH is an agency within the Department of Health and Human Services (DHHS). Based in Bethesda, Maryland, the NIH is comprised of nearly 30 separate institutes and centers. The institutes carry out research and programs related to certain specific types of diseases, such as mental and neurological disease, arthritis, cancer, and heart disease. There is an institute for each of the categories of disease for which NIH has programs, and a number of other components not specific to any disease categories.

nongovernmental organizations   Legal entities created by private individuals, private organizations, publicly traded organizations, or in some combination where government influence, supervision, and management are removed, or at least greatly minimized, from the NGO's strategic and operational mission.

objectives   A short-term goal; something that must be achieved on the way to a larger achievement. More specific than goals and have defined outcomes that can be measured.

Occupational Safety and Health Act of 1970   The federal law that sets certain safety standards to eliminate threats to workplace safety.

organization   A structured social system consisting of groups and individuals working together to meet agreed-upon objectives.

organizational behavior   The study of individual and group behaviors in organizations, analyzing motivation, work satisfaction, leadership, work-group dynamics, and the attitudes and behaviors of the members of organizations.

organizational culture   The pattern of shared values, beliefs, and norms—along with associated behaviors, symbols, and rituals—that are acquired over time by members of an organization.

organization theory   A sociological approach to the study of organizations focusing on topics that affect the organization as a whole, such as organizational environments, goals and effectiveness, strategy and decision making, change and innovation, and structure and design.

outcomes   Events or conditions that indicate program effectiveness.

P

performance appraisal   The formal methods by which an organization documents the work performance of its employees. Performance appraisals are typically designed to change dysfunctional work behavior, communicate perceptions of work quality, assess the future potential of an employee, and to provide a documented record for disciplinary and separation actions.

philanthropic organizations   Organizations and foundations that raise funds for research, disease control and treatment, health promotion, and service delivery.

policy   A stable, purposeful course of action dealing with a problem or matter of concern. Policy comes in many forms, including: legislative statues, executive orders, court opinions, and agencies (FDA, EPA, FEMA, and so forth). Additionally, policy is the absence of making a decision or taking action. The three main types of policy are distributive, regulatory, and redistributive.

policy development   The formulation and advocacy of what should be done.

politics   1) The art or science concerned with guiding or influencing governmental policy. 2) The total complex of relations between people living in a society. 3) Relations or conduct in a particular area of experience, especially as seen or dealt with from a political point of view. 4) In public policymaking, "who gets what, when, and how."

problem   An issue that needs to be addressed.

process measures   Examine all the steps and activities taken in implementing a program and the outputs they generate.

production   An organization's essential product or service.

public health   The science and art of preventing disease, prolonging life, and promoting physical health and efficiency through organized community efforts for the sanitation of the environment, the control of community infections, the education of the individual in principles of personal hygiene, the organization of medical and nursing services for the early diagnosis and preventive treatment of disease, and the development of the social machinery which will ensure to every individual in the community a standard of living adequate for the maintenance of health.

public health informatics   The systematic application of information, computer science, and technology to public health practice, research, and technology.

public health policy   An attempt by the government at all levels to address a public issue, problem, or concern.

Pure Food and Drugs Act of 1906   Passed by the United States Congress to provide federal inspection of meat products and prohibit the manufacture, sale, or transportation of adulterated food products and poisonous medicines.

R

recruitment   Positions are created based on organizational needs and policies, and individuals are recruited accordingly.

regulation   A law, rule, or other order prescribed by authority.

reinforcement   1) To give added emphasis to, stress, or support. 2) To reward or punish an action or response so that it becomes more or less likely to occur.

S

satisficing   Aiming to achieve only satisfactory results because the satisfactory process is familiar, whereas aiming for the best-achievable results would call for costs, effort, and the incurring of risks. Due to time pressures, emotional issues, or limited information, the manager will not arrive at an optimal decision but will instead make a satisfactory decision.

scientific management   A systematic approach to managing that seeks the "one best way" of accomplishing a task by discovering the fastest, most efficient, and least-fatiguing methods.

selection   Positions are created based on organizational needs and policies, and individuals are selected accordingly. Employees must often be developed through training and other support to be effective in a given position and within the agency they have been hired by.

servant-leader   The leadership approach public health managers and professionals should embrace; consists of five foundational principles: 1) a concern for people, 2) stewardship, 3) equity or justice, 4) indebtedness, and 5) self-understanding.

situational leadership Based substantially on aspects of a given situation, which in turn determines the style of leadership that is most likely to be effective.

the SMART rule A method used to write clear objectives. S = short, M = measurable, A = action oriented, R = realistic, and T = time-bound.

social organizations Like faith-based organizations, social organizations are formed to meet a social need.

stages of team development Consists of five steps or stages: forming, storming, norming, performing, and adjourning.

stakeholders 1) Any individual or group that might be affected by the outcome of something. All decisions have their stakeholders. 2) The affected individuals or communities along with those who are influential in forming a plan to address the problem in question.

Substance Abuse and Mental Health Services Administration (SAMHSA) Provides grants and data collection activities to promote quality behavioral health services. Major activities include the improvement of the quality and availability of prevention, treatment, and recovery support services in order to help reduce illness, death, disability, and cost to society caused by substance abuse and mental illness.

sustainability Creating and maintaining the conditions under which humans and nature can exist in productive harmony that permits fulfilling the social, economic, and other requirements of present and future generations; focuses on the organization's environmental practices in balance with fiscal and social responsibility to assure the long-term success of the organization and its programs.

systems theory A view of an organization as a complex set of dynamically intertwined and interconnected elements, including all its inputs, processes, outputs, feedback loops, and the environment in which it operates and with which it continuously interacts.

systems thinking Generally has four stages: situational analysis, strategy formulation, strategy implementation, and strategy control.

T

teams Often used in the field of public health to examine problems or issues, provide recommendations on matters facing an organization or community, or analyze and investigate the efficacy of a process.

technical skills Require knowledge about the procedures, regulations, policies, technology, tools, and techniques for conducting the activities of the manager's unit, division, or department.

transformational leadership Leadership that strives to change organizational culture and directions. It reflects the ability of a leader to develop a values-based vision for the organization, to convert the vision into reality, and to maintain it over time.

triple bottom line A new trend worldwide with a focus on sustainability, the triple bottom line focuses not only on the financial/economic bottom line, but includes social responsibility and the environment.

U

United Nations Organization (UN) Formed in 1945; multiple-nation body to promote health and humanitarian goals worldwide; headquartered in New York, NY.

V

voluntary health organizations When a citizen or group of citizens identify a need that has not been met to their satisfaction.

W

World Health Organization (WHO) The division of the United Nations (UN) that is concerned with health. Headquartered in Geneva, Switzerland, the WHO came into being in April of 1948 when the United Nations ratified the WHO's Constitution. Its objective is the attainment by all peoples of the highest possible level of health. It is governed by the World Health Assembly which meets annually.

Index

Note: Page numbers with f indicate figures; those with t indicate tables; those with e indicate exhibits.

A

AA. *See* Alcoholics Anonymous (AA)

AAA. *See* Area Agencies on Aging (AAA)

AAMC. *See* Association of American Medical Colleges (AAMC)

Acceptance, conveying as communication skill, *257t*

Access (physical), 387

Access (to health care), 387

Access control, 387

Account, 387

Accountability, 387

Accountant, 387

Accounting period, 387

Accounts payable (AP), 387

Accounts receivable (AR), 388

Accreditation, 315, 388

Accredited, 388

ACF. *See* Administration for Children and Families (ACF)

ACHE. *See* American College of Healthcare Executives (ACHE)

Acquired immunity, 418

Acquired immunodeficiency syndrome (AIDS). *See* AIDS (acquired immunodeficiency syndrome)

ACR. *See* Adjusted Community Rate (ACR)

ACS. *See* American Cancer Society (ACS)

Action on Disease, Development, and Sustainability (ADDS), 384–385

Active immunity, 418

Actuarial analysis, 388

Actuary, 388

Acute, 388

Acute care, 388

Acute disease, 406

ADA. *See* Americans with Disabilities Act (ADA)

Adaptation, 90, 388

Adaptive leadership, 192, 193, 421

ADD. *See* Administration on Developmental Disabilities (ADD)

ADDS. *See* Action on Disease, Development, and Sustainability (ADDS)

Ad hoc committee, 388

Adjourning, *275t,* 441

Adjusted Community Rate (ACR), 388

Adjustment (bookkeeping), 388

Adjustment (statistical), 388

Administration (government), 388

Administration (management), 388–389

Administration for Children and Families (ACF), 111, 389, 404

mission and goals of, 111, *111e*

Administration for Native Americans (ANA), 389

Administration on Aging (AoA), 111, 389, 404

mission and goals of, *112e*

Administration on Developmental Disabilities (ADD), 389

Administrative adjustment, 388

Administrative doctrine, 389

Administrative guidelines, 414

Administrative law, 389

Administrative process, 389

Administrative systems, 389

Administrator, 390

Admission (hospital), 390

ADR. *See* Alternative dispute resolution (ADR)

Advanced directive, 390

Advanced practice nurse (APN), 390

Advocacy, 73–774, *74f*

Advocacy bond, 74

Advocate, 390

Affiliation needs, 425

Affirmative action, 390

Affordable Care Act, *75e*

AFS. *See* Alternative financing system (AFS)

Agency for Healthcare Research and Quality (AHRQ), 111, 391, 404, 435

mission and goals of, *112e*

Agency for Toxic Substances and Disease Registry (ATSDR), 112, 391, 404, 435

mission and goals of, *113e*